ZERO TO FINALS

Medicine

First Edition 2019
ISBN: 9781091859890

Dr Thomas Watchman
MbChB (hons), BSc (Psychology), MSc (Medical Education), FHEA
General Practice Specialty Trainee Year 2
Manchester, United Kingdom

Copyright Zero to Finals 2019. All rights reserved.

No part of this book can be reproduced or transmitted in any way without prior permission from Dr Thomas Watchman at Zero to Finals. Email: tom@zerotofinals.com.

About Zero to Finals

My name is Tom. I started Zero to Finals in 2016 to build the resource I wish I had during medical school. As you can imagine for someone that created an educational platform, I love learning and teaching medicine. I spend my time split between training to become a GP, working on Zero to Finals, studying for exams and hanging out with family and friends. You can find out more about me on the Zero to Finals website at zerotofinals.com/about-tom.

I always dreamed of setting up a resource that focuses on helping medical students achieve more in medical school and eases the burden of facing complicated and overwhelming textbooks, lectures and journals. I took a year out of training after the UK foundation program with the objective of making this dream a reality. I have been working on it non-stop ever since.

Zero to Finals is designed to provide you with learning resources to help you break through those sticking points, finally get your head around a topic you have struggled with and prepare efficiently and effectively for your exams.

The Zero to Finals books are designed to be studied from cover to cover in preparation for your exams. I have removed the waffle and focused on the key information you need for your exams. I have added helpful "Tom Tips" I have picked up during a decade of sitting medical exams, that will help you score those extra marks. The focus is on learning the concepts, vocabulary and latest guidelines so you take the fastest route to exam success and proficiency as a new doctor.

The Zero to Finals books are supplemented by the resources on the website (zerotofinals.com). If you struggle to follow the notes in this book or to get your head around a topic, head over to the website. There is a webpage on each topic with illustrations, diagrams, podcasts and videos that tackle the problem from every angle. You can also find carefully crafted practice questions, with feedback to help you develop your exam technique. All the resources on the webpage are free to use without having to sign up or give away your information.

If you still can't get your head around a topic, find an error or want to provide feedback email me at tom@zerotofinals.com.

Disclaimer

It is important that you use Zero to Finals for its intended purpose: as a resource to help students and health professionals prepare for exams. It is not intended to be used as a resource, guideline or reference for clinical practice or decision making or by patients looking for medical information or advice. There are plenty of very good resources for this, not least your senior colleagues or personal doctor. By using these resources you agree that Zero to Finals and those involved in creating the resources are not responsible for any actions you take or don't take based on the information provided.

The skills needed for medicine and other healthcare professions are board and complex. There is a limit to what you can learn from one resource. You need to develop clinical judgment, experience and context specific decision making skills that cannot be learned in one place. Attend clinical placements, listen to your tutors and supervisors, ask for help and use a variety of up to date guidelines, protocols, research and other resources when preparing for exams and treating patients.

I employ extensive effort to ensure the information is accurate and up to date, however I am not perfect, and research, guidelines and best practice are always changing. There will be errors despite my best efforts. I'd be very grateful if you point them out when you find them so I can correct them. Don't accept anything as fact without questioning it.

For Merili

This would not be possible without your ongoing love, humour and support.

CONTENTS

1	Cardiology	5
2	Endocrinology	39
3	Gastroenterology	70
4	Respiratory	105
5	Infectious Diseases	135
6	Haematology	170
7	Rheumatology	206
8	Renal	246
9	Neurology	267
10	Ophthalmology	307

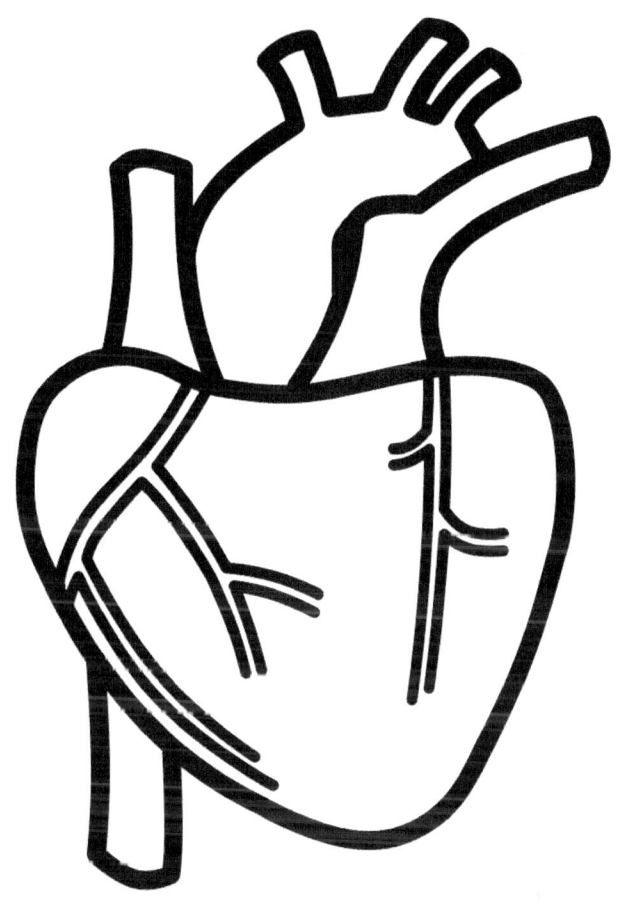

CARDIOLOGY

1.1	Cardiovascular Disease	6
1.2	Stable Angina	8
1.3	Acute Coronary Syndrome	10
1.4	Acute LVF and Pulmonary Oedema	14
1.5	Chronic Heart Failure	17
1.6	Cor Pulmonale	19
1.7	Hypertension	19
1.8	Murmurs	22
1.9	Prosthetic Valves	25
1.10	Atrial Fibrillation	26
1.11	Arrhythmias	31
1.12	Pacemakers	37

Cardiovascular Disease

Atherosclerosis

Athero- refers to soft or porridge like and **-sclerosis** refers to hardening. **Atherosclerosis** is a combination of **atheromas** (fatty deposits in the artery walls) and **sclerosis** (the process of hardening or stiffening of the blood vessel walls). **Atherosclerosis** affects the medium and large arteries. It is caused by **chronic inflammation** and **activation of the immune system** in the artery wall. This causes deposition of **lipids** in the artery wall, followed by the development of fibrous **atheromatous plaques**.

These plaques cause:
- **Stiffening** of the artery walls leading to **hypertension** (raised blood pressure) and strain on the heart trying to pump blood against resistance
- **Stenosis** leading to reduced blood flow (e.g. in angina)
- **Plaque rupture** results in a **thrombus** that can block a distal vessel and cause **ischaemia**. An example of this is in **acute coronary syndrome** where a **coronary artery** becomes blocked.

Atherosclerosis Risk Factors

It is important to break these down into **modifiable** and **non-modifiable** risk factors. There is nothing we can do about non-modifiable risk factors, but we can do something about the modifiable ones.

Non-Modifiable Risk Factors

- Older age
- Family history
- Male

Modifiable Risk Factors

- Smoking
- Alcohol consumption
- Poor diet (high sugar and trans-fat and reduced fruit and vegetables and omega 3 consumption)
- Low exercise
- Obesity
- Poor sleep
- Stress

Medical Co-Morbidities

Medical co-morbidities increase the risk of atherosclerosis and should be carefully managed to minimise the risk:
- Diabetes
- Hypertension
- Chronic kidney disease
- Inflammatory conditions such as rheumatoid arthritis
- Atypical antipsychotic medications

TOM TIP: Think about risk factors when taking a history from someone with suspected atherosclerotic disease (such as someone presenting with chest pain) and ask about their exercise, diet, past medical history, family history, occupation, smoking, alcohol intake and medications. This will help you perform well in exams and when presenting to seniors.

End Results of Atherosclerosis

- Angina
- Myocardial infarction
- Transient ischaemic attacks
- Strokes
- Peripheral vascular disease
- Chronic mesenteric ischaemia

Prevention of Cardiovascular Disease

Prevention of cardiovascular disease falls in to two main categories:

Primary Prevention - for patients that have never had cardiovascular disease in the past.

Secondary Prevention - for patients that have developed angina, myocardial infarction, TIA, stroke or peripheral vascular disease already.

Optimise Modifiable Risk Factors:

For primary and secondary prevention of cardiovascular disease it is essential to optimise the modifiable risk factors:
- Advise on diet, exercise and weight loss
- Stop smoking
- Stop drinking alcohol
- Optimise treatment of co-morbidities (such as diabetes)

Primary Prevention of Cardiovascular Disease

Perform a **QRISK 3 score**. This will calculate the percentage risk that a patient will have a stroke or myocardial infarction **in the next 10 years**. If they have **more than a 10% risk** of having a stroke or heart attack **over the next 10 years** (i.e. their QRISK 3 score is above 10%) **they you should start a statin**. The current NICE guidelines are for **atorvastatin** 20mg at night.

All patients with **chronic kidney disease** (CKD) or **type 1 diabetes** for more than 10 years should be offered **atorvastatin 20mg**.

NICE recommend checking lipids at 3 months and increasing the dose to aim for a greater than 40% reduction in non-HDL cholesterol. Always check adherence before increasing the dose.

NICE also recommend checking LFTs within 3 months of starting a statin and again at 12 months. They don't need to be checked after that. Statins can cause a transient and mild rise in ALT and AST in the first few weeks of use. They usually don't need to be stopped if the rise is less than 3 times the upper limit of normal.

Secondary Prevention of Cardiovascular Disease

Secondary prevention after developing cardiovascular disease can be remembered as the **4 As**:
- **A** - **A**spirin (plus a second antiplatelet such as clopidogrel for 12 months)
- **A** - **A**torvastatin 80mg
- **A** - **A**tenolol (or other beta blocker - commonly ***bisoprolol***) titrated to maximum tolerated dose
- **A** - **A**CE inhibitor (commonly ***ramipril***) titrated to maximum tolerated dose

Notable Side Effects of Statins

- Myopathy (check ***creatine kinase*** in patients with muscle pain or weakness)
- Type 2 Diabetes
- Haemorrhagic strokes (very rarely)

Usually the benefits of statins far outweigh the risks and newer statins (such as atorvastatin) are very well tolerated.

Stable Angina

Angina

A narrowing of the **coronary arteries** reduces blood flow to the **myocardium** (heart muscle). During times of high demand, such as exercise, there is insufficient supply of blood to meet the demand. This causes the symptoms of angina, typically constricting chest pain with or without radiation to jaw or arms. Angina is "**stable**" when symptoms are always relieved by rest or **glyceryl trinitrate** (GTN). It is "**unstable**" when the symptoms come on randomly whilst at rest. **Unstable angina** is a type of **acute coronary syndrome**.

Investigations

CT coronary angiography is the **gold standard** diagnostic investigation. This involves injecting contrast and taking CT images timed with the heart beat to give a detailed view of the coronary arteries, highlighting any narrowing.

All patients with angina should have to following as baseline investigations:
- Physical examination (heart sounds, signs of heart failure, BMI)
- ECG
- FBC (check for anaemia)
- U&Es (prior to starting an ACE inhibitor and other medications)
- LFTs (prior to starting a statins)
- Lipid profile
- Thyroid function tests (check for hypo- or hyperthyroid)
- HbA1C and fasting glucose (for diabetes)

Management

The management described here is based on 2018 NICE CKS on Angina and 2018 SIGN guidelines. There are four principles to management. You can remember this with the mnemonic "***RAMP***":

- **R** - **R**efer to cardiology (urgently if unstable)
- **A** - **A**dvise them about the diagnosis, management and when to call an ambulance
- **M** - **M**edical treatment
- **P** - **P**rocedural or surgical interventions

Medical Management

There are three aims to medical management:
- Immediate symptomatic relief
- Long term symptomatic relief
- Secondary prevention of cardiovascular disease

Immediate Symptomatic Relief
- GTN spray is used as required. It causes vasodilation and helps relieves the symptoms.
- Instruct them to take GTN when symptoms start, then repeat after 5 minutes if required. If there is still pain 5 minutes after the repeat dose - call an ambulance.

Long Term Symptomatic Relief is with either (or used in combination if symptoms are not controlled on one):
- Beta blocker (e.g. bisoprolol 5mg once daily)
- Calcium channel blocker (e.g. amlodipine 5mg once daily)

Other options for long term symptomatic relief may be considered by a specialist. These are long acting nitrates (e.g. *isosorbide mononitrate*), *ivabradine*, *nicorandil* and *ranolazine*.

Secondary Prevention (4 As)
- **A** - **A**spirin (i.e. 75mg once daily)
- **A** - **A**torvastatin 80mg once daily
- **A** - **A**CE inhibitor
- **A** - **A**lready on a beta-blocker for symptomatic relief.

Procedural / Surgical Interventions

Percutaneous Coronary Intervention (PCI) with **coronary angioplasty** (dilating the blood vessel with a balloon and/or inserting a stent) is offered to patients with "proximal or extensive disease" on **CT coronary angiography**. This involves putting a catheter into the patient's **brachial** or **femoral** artery, feeding that up to the **coronary arteries** under **xray guidance** and injecting **contrast** so that the coronary arteries and any areas of stenosis are highlighted on the xray images. This can then be treated with **balloon dilatation** followed by insertion of a **stent**.

Coronary Artery Bypass Graft (CABG) surgery may be offered to patients with severe stenosis. This involves opening the chest along the sternum (causing a **midline sternotomy scar**), taking a graft vein from the patient's leg (usually the **great saphenous vein**) and sewing it on to the affected coronary artery to bypass the stenosis. The recovery is slower and the complication rate is higher than PCI.

TOM TIP: When examining a patient that you think may have coronary artery disease, check for a midline sternotomy scar (previous CABG), scars around the brachial and femoral arteries (previous PCI) and along the inner calves (saphenous vein harvesting scar) to see what procedures they may have had done and to impress your examiners.

Acute Coronary Syndrome

Pathophysiology

Acute coronary syndrome is usually the result of a **thrombus** from an **atherosclerotic plaque** blocking a **coronary artery**. When a thrombus forms in a fast flowing artery it is made up mostly of **platelets**. This is why **anti-platelet medications** such as **aspirin**, **clopidogrel** and **ticagrelor** are the mainstay of treatment.

The Coronary Arteries

The **left coronary artery** becomes the **circumflex** and **left anterior descending (LAD)**.

Right coronary artery (RCA) curves around the right side and under the heart and supplies the:
- Right atrium
- Right ventricle
- Inferior aspect of the left ventricle
- Posterior septal area

Circumflex artery curves around the top, left and back of the heart and supplies the:
- Left atrium
- Posterior aspect of left ventricle

Left Anterior Descending (LAD) travels down the middle of the heart and supplies the:
- Anterior aspect of the left ventricle
- Anterior aspect of the septum

Three Types of Acute Coronary Syndrome

- **Unstable angina**
- **ST elevation myocardial infarction (STEMI)**
- **Non-ST elevation myocardial infarction (NSTEMI)**

Making a Diagnosis

When a patient presents with possible ACS symptoms (i.e. chest pain) perform an ECG:

If there is **ST elevation** or **new left bundle branch block** the diagnosis is **STEMI**.

If there is **no ST elevation** then perform **troponin** blood tests:
- If there are raised **troponin** levels and/or other ECG changes (**ST depression** or **T wave inversion** or **pathological Q waves**) the diagnosis is **NSTEMI**
- If **troponin levels are normal** and the **ECG does not show pathological changes** the diagnosis is either **unstable angina** or another cause such as **musculoskeletal** chest pain

Cardiology

Symptoms

Central, constricting chest pain associated with:
- Nausea and vomiting
- Sweating and clamminess
- Feelings of impending doom
- Shortness of breath
- Palpitations
- Pain radiating to the jaw or arms

Symptoms should continue at rest for more than 20 minutes. If they settle with rest consider angina. Diabetic patients may not experience typical chest pain during an acute coronary syndrome. This is often referred to as a "*silent MI*".

ECG Changes in Acute Coronary Syndrome

STEMI:
- *ST segment elevation* in leads consistent with an area of ischaemia
- New *Left Bundle Branch Block* also diagnoses a *STEMI*

NSTEMI:
- *ST segment depression* in a specific region
- *Deep T wave inversion*
- *Pathological Q waves*. This suggests a deep infarct and is a late sign.

Artery	Heart Area	ECG Leads
Left Coronary Artery	Anterolateral	I, aVL, V3-6
LAD	Anterior	V1-4
Circumflex	Lateral	I, aVL, V5-6
Right Coronary Artery	Inferior	II, III, aVF

Troponins

Troponins are proteins found in cardiac muscle. The specific type of troponin, the normal range and diagnostic criteria vary based on different laboratories (so check the local policy). A diagnosis of ACS typically requires **serial troponins** (e.g. at baseline and 6 or 12 hours after the onset of symptoms). A rise in troponin is consistent with **myocardial ischaemia** as the proteins are released from the ischaemic muscle. They are **non-specific**, meaning that a raised troponin does not automatically mean ACS.

There are alternative causes of raised troponins:
- Chronic renal failure
- Sepsis
- Myocarditis
- Aortic dissection
- Pulmonary embolism

Other Investigations

Perform all the investigations you would normally arrange for stable angina (see stable angina section) plus:
- **Chest xray** to investigate for pulmonary oedema and other causes of chest pain
- **Echocardiogram** after the event to assess the functional damage to the heart
- **CT coronary angiogram** to assess for coronary artery disease

Acute STEMI Treatment (always check local protocol)

Patients with **STEMI** presenting within 12 hours of onset should be discussed urgently with local cardiac centre for either:
- **Primary PCI** (if available within 2 hours of presentation)
- **Thrombolysis** (if PCI is not available within 2 hours)

The local cardiac centre will advise about further management such as further loading with aspirin and ticagrelor.

Percutaneous coronary intervention (PCI) involves putting a catheter into the patient's brachial or femoral artery, feeding that up to the coronary arteries under xray guidance and injecting contrast to identify the area of blockage. This can then be treated using balloons to widen the gap or devices to remove or aspirate the blockage. Usually a stent is put in to keep the artery open.

Thrombolysis involves injecting a **fibrinolytic** medication (they break down **fibrin**) that rapidly dissolves clots. There is a significant risk of bleeding which can make it dangerous. Some examples of thrombolytic agents are **streptokinase**, **alteplase** and **tenecteplase**.

Acute NSTEMI Treatment: BATMAN

B – **B**eta blockers unless contraindicated
A – **A**spirin 300mg stat dose
T – **T**icagrelor 180mg stat dose (clopidogrel 300mg is an alternative)
M – **M**orphine titrated to control pain
A – **A**nticoagulant: **low molecular weight heparin** (**LMWH**) at treatment dose (e.g. **enoxaparin** 1mg/kg twice daily for 2-8 days)
N – **N**itrates (e.g. GTN) to relieve coronary artery spasm

Give oxygen only if their oxygen saturations are dropping (i.e. <95%).

GRACE Score to assess for PCI in NSTEMI:

This scoring system gives a 6-month risk of **death** or **repeat MI** after having an NSTEMI:
- <5% Low Risk
- 5-10% Medium Risk
- >10% High Risk

If they are medium or high risk they are considered for early PCI (within 4 days of admission) to treat underlying coronary artery disease.

Complications of MI (DREAD)

D - **D**eath
R - **R**upture of the heart septum or papillary muscles
E - "o**E**dema" (*heart failure*)
A - **A**rrhythmia and **A**neurysm
D - **D**ressler's Syndrome

Dressler's Syndrome

This is also called *post-myocardial infarction syndrome*. It usually occurs around **2 - 3 weeks after an MI**. It is caused by a **localised immune response** and causes *pericarditis* (inflammation of the *pericardium* around the heart). It is less common as the management of ACS becomes more advanced.

It presents with *pleuritic* chest pain, low grade fever and a *pericardial rub* on auscultation. It can cause a *pericardial effusion* and rarely a *pericardial tamponade* (where the fluid constricts the heart and prevents function).

A diagnosis can be made with an **ECG** (*global ST elevation* and *T wave inversion*), echocardiogram (*pericardial effusion*) and raised **inflammatory markers** (*CRP* and *ESR*).

Management is with **NSAIDs** (*aspirin / ibuprofen*) and in more severe cases **steroids** (*prednisolone*). They may need *pericardiocentesis* to remove fluid from around the heart.

Secondary Prevention Medical Management (6 As)

- **A**spirin 75mg once daily
- **A**nother antiplatelet: e.g. *clopidogrel* or *ticagrelor* for up to 12 months
- **A**torvastatin 80mg once daily
- **A**CE inhibitors (e.g. *ramipril* titrated as tolerated to 10mg once daily)
- **A**tenolol (or other beta blocker titrated as high as tolerated)
- **A**ldosterone antagonist for those with **clinical heart failure** (i.e *eplerenone* titrated to 50mg once daily)

Dual antiplatelet duration will vary following **PCI procedures** depending on the type of stent that was inserted. This is due to a higher risk of thrombus formation with different types of stent.

Secondary Prevention Lifestyle Advice

- Stop smoking
- Reduce alcohol consumption
- Mediterranean diet
- Cardiac rehabilitation (a specific exercise regime for patients post MI)
- Optimise treatment of other medical conditions (e.g. diabetes and hypertension)

Types of MI

This is slightly unnecessary knowledge for everyday practice but worth being aware of. It is worth avoiding as it could confuse people unless they are a medical registrar or cardiologist.

- **Type 1**: Traditional MI due to an acute coronary event
- **Type 2**: Ischaemia secondary to increased demand or reduced supply of oxygen (e.g. secondary to severe anaemia, tachycardia or hypotension)
- **Type 3**: Sudden cardiac death or cardiac arrest suggestive of an ischaemic event
- **Type 4**: MI associated with procedures such as PCI, coronary stenting and CABG

Acute LVF and Pulmonary Oedema

Acute Left Ventricular Failure (LVF)

You will come across **acute left ventricular failure** often during your medical jobs. This occurs when the **left ventricle** is unable to adequately move blood through the left side of the heart and out into the body. This causes a **backlog** of blood (like too many buses waiting to pick up people at a bus stop) that increases the amount of blood stuck in the **left atrium**, **pulmonary veins** and **lungs**. As the vessels in these areas are engorged with blood due to the increased volume and pressure they leak fluid and are unable to reabsorb fluid from the surrounding tissues. This causes **pulmonary oedema**, which is where the lung tissue and alveoli become full of **interstitial fluid**. This interferes with the normal **gas exchange** in the lungs causing shortness of breath, reduced oxygen saturation and the other signs and symptoms.

Triggers

- Iatrogenic (e.g. aggressive IV fluids in frail elderly patient with impaired left ventricular function)
- Sepsis
- Myocardial Infarction
- Arrhythmias

Presentation

Acute LVF typical presents as a **rapid onset breathlessness**. This is exacerbated by lying flat and improves on sitting up. Acute LVF causes a **type 1 respiratory failure** (low oxygen without an increase in carbon dioxide in the blood).

Symptoms:
- Shortness of breath
- Looking and feeling unwell
- Cough with frothy white or pink sputum

On examination:
- Increase respiratory rate
- Reduced oxygen saturations
- Tachycardia
- 3rd Heart Sound
- Bilateral basal crackles (sounding "wet") on auscultation
- Hypotension in severe cases (**cardiogenic shock**)

There may also be signs and symptoms related to **underlying cause**, for example:
- Chest pain in ACS
- Fever in sepsis
- Palpitations with arrhythmias

If they also have **right sided heart failure** you could find:
- Raised **Jugular Venous Pressure (JVP)** caused by a backlog on the right side of the heart leading to an engorged internal jugular vein in the neck.
- Peripheral oedema in the ankles, legs and sacrum)

TOM TIP: When you are on the wards and a nurse asks you to review a patient that has just started desaturating ask yourself how much fluid that patient has been given and whether they will be able to cope with that amount. For example, an 85 year old lady with chronic kidney disease and aortic stenosis is prescribed 2 litres of fluid over 4 hours and then starts to drop her oxygen saturations. This is a common scenario and a dose of IV furosemide can often work like magic to clear some fluid and ease their breathing.

Work Up

- History
- Clinical examination
- ECG to look for ischaemia and arrhythmias
- Arterial blood gas (ABG)
- Chest xray
- Routine bloods for infection, kidney function, **BNP** and consider **troponin** if suspecting myocardial infarction
- Echocardiogram

Investigations

If the clinical presentation is acute LVF then initiate treatment before having the diagnosis confirmed by BNP or echo. Without treatment they can deteriorate before getting the investigations.

B-type Natriuretic Peptide (BNP) Blood Test

B-type natriuretic peptide (BNP) is a hormone that is released from the heart **ventricles** when the cardiac muscle (***myocardium***) is stretched beyond the normal range. Finding a high result indicates the heart is overloaded (with blood) beyond its normal capacity to pump effectively.

The action of BNP is to relax the smooth muscle in blood vessels. This reduces the **systemic vascular resistance** making it easier for the heart to pump blood through the system. BNP also acts on the kidneys as a diuretic to promote the excretion of more water in the urine. This reduces the circulating volume helping to improve the function of the heart.

Testing for BNP is ***sensitive*** but not ***specific***. This means that when the result is negative it is useful in **ruling out** heart failure, but it can be positive due to other causes. Other causes of a raised BNP include:
- Tachycardia
- Sepsis
- Pulmonary embolism
- Renal impairment
- COPD

Echocardiography (Echo)

Echocardiography (echo) is useful in assessing the function of the left ventricle and any structural abnormalities in the heart. The main measure of the left ventricular function is the **ejection fraction**. This is the percentage of blood in the left ventricle that is squeezed out with each **ventricular contraction**. An ejection fraction **above 50%** is considered normal.

Chest Xray Findings

Cardiomegaly on a chest xray is defined as a **cardiothoracic ratio** of **more than 0.5**. This is when the diameter of the widest part of the heart (the widest part of the **cardiac silhouette**) is more than half the diameter of the widest part of the **lung fields**.

Upper lobe **venous diversion** may also be seen. Usually when standing erect the lower lobe veins contain more blood and the upper lobe veins remain relatively small. In LVF there is such a back-pressure that the upper lobe veins also fill with blood and become engorged. This is referred to as **upper lobe diversion**. This is visible as increased prominence and diameter of the upper lobe vessels on a chest xray.

Fluid leaking from oedematous lung tissue causes additional xray findings of:
- Bilateral **pleural effusions**
- Fluid in **interlobar fissures**
- Fluid in the septal lines (**Kerley lines**)

Management

You can use the simple mnemonic **Pour SOD** for remembering the management of acute LVF:
- **Pour** away (stop) their IV fluids
- **S**it up
- **O**xygen
- **D**iuretics

Sit the patient upright. When lying flat the fluid in the lungs spreads to a larger area. When upright gravity takes it to the bases leaving the upper lungs clear for better gas exchange.

Oxygen if their oxygen saturations are falling (<95%). As always be cautious in patients with COPD.

Diuretics (e.g. IV **furosemide** 40mg stat). This reduces the circulating volume and means the heart is less overloaded allowing it to pump more effectively.

Monitor fluid balance. Measuring fluid intake, urine output, U&E bloods and daily body weight is essential to balance their fluid input and output.

Other options to consider in **severe** acute pulmonary oedema or **cardiogenic shock** (not routinely used) include:
- **Intravenous opiates**. Opiates such as morphine act as **vasodilators** but are not routinely recommended.
- **Non-invasive ventilation (NIV). Continuous positive airway pressure (CPAP)** involves using a tight fitting mask to forcefully blow air into their lungs. This helps to open the airways and alveoli to improve gas exchange. If NIV does not work they may need full **intubation and ventilation**.
- "**Inotropes**", for example an infusion of **noradrenalin**. **Inotropes** strengthen the force of heart contractions and improve heart failure, however they need close titration and monitoring, so by this point you would need to send the patient to the **local coronary care unit**, **high dependency unit** or **intensive care unit**.

Chronic Heart Failure

Chronic heart failure is essentially the chronic version of acute heart failure. It is caused by either impaired left ventricular contraction (**systolic heart failure**) or left ventricular relaxation (**diastolic heart failure**). This impaired left ventricular function results in a chronic back-pressure of blood trying to flow into and through the left side of the heart.

Presentation

There are some key features that patients with chronic heart failure present with:
- Breathlessness worsened by exertion
- Cough. They may produce frothy white/pink sputum.
- **Orthopnoea**. This is the sensation of shortness of breathing when lying flat, relieves by sitting or standing. Ask them how many pillows they use at night.
- **Paroxysmal Nocturnal Dyspnoea** (see below)
- Peripheral oedema (swollen ankles)

Paroxysmal Nocturnal Dyspnoea (PND)

Paroxysmal nocturnal dyspnoea is a term used to describe the experience that patients have of suddenly waking at night with a severe attack of shortness of breath and cough.

Patients will describe waking up and feeling acutely short of breath, with a cough and wheeze. They have to sit on the side of the bed or walk around the room and gasp for breath. They feel like they are suffocating and may want to open a window in an attempt to get air. Symptoms improve over several minutes.

PND is caused by a few proposed mechanisms:

Firstly, fluid settling across a large surface area of their lungs as they sleep lying flat. As they stand up the fluid sinks to the lung bases and their upper lungs clear and can be used more effectively.

Secondly, during sleep the respiratory centre in the brain becomes less responsive so their respiratory rate and effort does not increase in response to reduced oxygen saturation like it normally would when awake. This allows the person to develop more significant **pulmonary congestion** and **hypoxia** before waking up and feeling very unwell.

Thirdly, there is less **adrenalin** circulating during sleep. Less adrenalin means the **myocardium** is more relaxed and this reduces the cardiac output.

Diagnosis

- Clinical presentation
- BNP blood test, specifically the **N-terminal pro-B-type natriuretic peptide** (NT-proBNP)
- Echocardiogram
- ECG

Causes

- Ischaemic heart disease
- Valvular heart disease (commonly *aortic stenosis*)
- Hypertension
- Arrhythmias (commonly *atrial fibrillation*)

Management

This is based on NICE guidelines 2018. See the full guidelines before implementing treatment.

- Refer to specialist (NT-proBNP > 2,000 ng/litre warrants an urgent referral)
- Careful discussion and explanation of the condition
- Medical management (see below)
- Surgical treatment in severe *aortic stenosis* or *mitral regurgitation*
- Heart failure specialist nurse input for advice and support

Additional management:
- Yearly flu and pneumococcal vaccine
- Stop smoking
- Optimise treatment of co-morbidities
- Exercise as tolerated

First Line Medical Treatment (ABAL)

- **A** - **A**CE inhibitor (e.g. *ramipril* titrated as tolerated up to 10mg once daily)
- **B** - **B**eta Blocker (e.g. *bisoprolol* titrated as tolerated up to 10mg once daily)
- **A** - **A**ldosterone antagonist when symptoms not controlled with A and B (*spironolactone* or *eplerenone*)
- **L** - **L**oop diuretics improves **symptoms** (e.g. *furosemide* 40mg once daily)

Extra details on medical treatment:

An *angiotensin receptor blocker (ARB)* can be used instead of an ACE inhibitor if ACE inhibitors are not tolerated (for example *candesartan* titrated up to 32mg once daily).

Avoid ACE inhibitors in patients with valvular heart disease until initiated by a specialist.

Aldosterone antagonists are used when there is a reduced ejection fraction and symptoms are **not** controlled with an ACEi and beta blocker.

Patients should have their **U&Es** monitored closely whilst on **diuretics**, **ACE inhibitors** and **aldosterone antagonists** as all three medications can cause **electrolyte disturbances**.

Cor Pulmonale

Cor pulmonale is **right sided heart failure** caused by **respiratory disease**. The increased pressure and resistance in the **pulmonary arteries** (**pulmonary hypertension**) results in the **right ventricle** being unable to effectively pump blood out of the ventricle and into the pulmonary arteries. This leads to back pressure of blood in the right atrium, the **vena cava** and the **systemic venous system**.

Respiratory Causes

- COPD is the **most common** cause
- Pulmonary embolism
- Interstitial lung disease
- Cystic fibrosis
- Primary pulmonary hypertension

Presentation

Often patients with early cor pulmonale are **asymptomatic**. The main presenting complaint is **shortness of breath**. Unfortunately shortness of breath is also caused by the the chronic lung diseases that lead to cor pulmonale. Patients may also present with **peripheral oedema**, increased breathlessness of exertion, **syncope** (dizziness and fainting) or chest pain.

Examine the patient for the **signs of cor pulmonale**:
- Hypoxia
- Cyanosis
- Raised JVP (due to a back-log of blood in the *jugular veins*)
- Peripheral oedema
- Third heart sound
- Murmurs (e.g. **pan-systolic** in *tricuspid regurgitation*)
- **Hepatomegaly** due to back pressure in the hepatic vein (pulsatile in *tricuspid regurgitation*)

Management

Management involves treating the symptoms and the underlying cause. Long term oxygen therapy is often used. The prognosis is poor unless there is a reversible underlying cause.

Hypertension

Hypertension is the term used to describe **high blood pressure**. The **American College of Cardiology** (ACC) and **American Heart Association** (AHA) joint guidelines from 2017 define normal blood pressure as **less than** 120/80. The UK **NICE guideline** on the diagnosis and management of hypertension is from 2011, therefore is quite outdated. It is likely to be replaced with more aggressive treatment guidelines but for now the treatment described below is still based on the older guideline.

Causes of Hypertension

Essential hypertension accounts for **95% of hypertension**. This is also known as **primary hypertension** and essentially means that the hypertension has developed on its own and does not have a secondary cause.

There are **secondary causes of hypertension** that you can remember with the mnemonic **ROPE**:
- **R** - **R**enal disease is the most common cause of secondary hypertension. If the blood pressure is very high or does not respond to treatment consider **renal artery stenosis**.
- **O** - **O**besity
- **P** - **Pregnancy induced hypertension / pre-eclampsia**
- **E** - **E**ndocrine. Most endocrine conditions can cause hypertension but primarily consider **hyperaldosteronism** ("**Conns syndrome**") as this may represent 2.5% of new hypertension. A simple test for this is a **renin:aldosterone ratio** blood test.

Complications

- Ischaemic Heart Disease
- Cerebrovascular accident (i.e. stroke or haemorrhage)
- Hypertensive retinopathy
- Hypertensive nephropathy
- Heart failure

Hypertension diagnosis

The diagnosis of **hypertension** can be made based on several readings in the clinic, 24 hour **ambulatory** blood pressure or home readings.

Having your blood pressure taken by a doctor or nurse often results in a higher reading. This is commonly called "**white coat syndrome**". The latest thinking is that **home readings** taken by the patient at different times throughout the day are the **gold standard** investigation and are most likely to represent the true blood pressure.

Stage	Clinic Reading	Ambulatory / Home Readings
Stage 1 Hypertension	>140/90	>135/85
Stage 2 Hypertension	>160/100	>150/95

These are based on NICE guidelines from 2011 and are likely to be lowered in the next set of guidelines. The ACC / AHA guidelines from 2017 define **stage 1 hypertension** as >130/80 and **stage 2 hypertension** as >140/90.

Medications

- **A** = **A**CE inhibitor (e.g. **ramipril** 1.25mg up to 10mg once daily)
- **B** = **B**eta blocker (e.g. **bisoprolol** 5mg up to 20mg once daily)
- **C** = **C**alcium channel blocker (e.g. **amlodipine** 5mg up to 10mg once daily)
- **D** = Thiazide-Like **D**iuretic (e.g. **indapamide** 2.5mg once daily)
- **ARB** = **A**ngiotensin II **R**eceptor **B**locker (e.g. **candesartan** 8mg to up 32mg once daily)

Angiotensin Receptor Blockers are used if the person does not tolerate an ACE inhibitor (commonly due to a dry cough) or the patient is black of African or Caribbean descent.

Initial Management

Investigate for possible causes and end organ damage.

Advise on lifestyle. This includes recommending a healthy diet, reducing salt intake to under 6g per day, stopping smoking and taking regular exercise.

Medical Management

There are slightly different guidelines for younger patients and those aged over 55 or black. These are based on the 2011 NICE guidelines:
- **Step 1**: Aged less than 55 and non-black use **A**. Aged over 55 or black use **C**.
- **Step 2**: Non-black use **A + C**. If black then use **ARB** instead of **A**.
- **Step 3**: **A + C + D**
- **Step 4**: **A + C + D + D**

For step 4, if the serum potassium is **more than 4.5 mmol/l** then the added diuretic is a **higher dose thiazide-like diuretic** such as *indapamide*. If the serum potassium is **less than or equal to 4.5 mmol/l** then the added diuretic is a **potassium sparing diuretic** such as *spironolactone*.

Potassium Balance

Spironolactone is a "*potassium-sparing diuretic*" that works by blocking the action of **aldosterone** in the kidneys resulting in **sodium excretion** and **potassium reabsorption**. This can be helpful when **thiazide diuretics** are causing **hypokalaemia**.

Using *spironolactone* increases the risk of **hyperkalaemia**. **ACE inhibitors** can also cause **hyperkalaemia**. For this reason it is important to monitor U+Es regularly when using ACE inhibitors and all diuretics.

Treatment Targets

Age	Systolic Target	Diastolic Target
< 80 years	< 140	< 90
> 80 years	< 150	< 90

These are based on NICE guidelines from 2011 and are likely to be lowered in the next set of guidelines. The SPRINT Study and a Lancet 2016 review shows that more aggressive targets (i.e. < 120 systolic) further reduces cardiovascular events.

Hypertension in Diabetes

SIGN guidelines aim for a systolic of less than 130 and a diastolic of less than 80 in diabetic patients. **ACE inhibitors** have been consistently found to significantly reduce complications in hypertensive patients with diabetes, particularly renal complications.

First line treatment for hypertension in diabetic patients is an ACE inhibitor in everyone except:
- Women with child bearing potential: calcium channel blocker
- Black patients: ACE inhibitor + calcium channel blocker

Murmurs

S1 and S2

The *first heart sound* (*S1*) is caused by the closing of the **atrioventricular valves** (the **tricuspid** and **mitral valves**) at the start of the **systolic contraction** of the **ventricles**.

The *second heart sounds* (*S2*) is caused by the closing of the **semilunar valves** (the **pulmonary** and **aortic valves**) once the systolic contraction is complete.

3rd Heart Sound (S3)

A *third heart sound* (*S3*) is heard roughly 0.1 seconds after the second heart sound. I think of it as rapid ventricular filling causing the **chordae tendineae** to pull to their full length and twang like a guitar string. This can be normal in young (15-40 years) healthy people because the heart functions so well that the ventricles easily allow rapid filling. In older patients it can indicated heart failure, as the **ventricles** and **chordae** are stiff and weak so they reach their limit much faster than normal. Picture this like tight hamstrings in an old de-conditioned patient sharply tightening as they start to bend over.

4th Heart Sound (S4)

A *fourth heart sound* (*S4*) is heard directly before *S1*. This is always abnormal and relatively rare to hear. It indicates a stiff or hypertrophic ventricle and is caused by turbulent flow from an atria contracting against a non-compliant ventricle.

Listening to Murmurs

Auscultate with the **bell** of your stethoscope to better hear **low pitched** sounds and the **diaphragm** to listen to **high pitched** sounds. To remember this think of a child's **high-pitched** screaming from their **diaphragm** and a church **bell** giving a **deep** "bong".

Listen over the **4 valve areas** in turn for murmurs:
- *Pulmonary*: 2nd I.C.S left sternal boarder
- *Aortic*: 2nd I.C.S right sternal boarder
- *Tricuspid*: 5th I.C.S left sternal boarder
- *Mitral*: 5th I.C.S mid clavicular line (apex area)

Listen to "*Erb's point*". This is in the **third intercostal space** on the **left sternal boarder** and is the best area for listening to heart sounds (*S1* and *S2*).

Special manoeuvres can be used to emphasise certain murmurs:
- Patient on their left hand side (*mitral stenosis*)
- Patient sat up, learning forward and holding exhalation (*aortic regurgitation*)

Cardiology

Assessing a Murmur (SCRIPT)

- **S** - **S**ite: where is the murmur loudest?
- **C** - **C**haracter: soft / blowing / crescendo (getting louder) / decrescendo (getting quieter) / crescendo-decrescendo (louder then quieter)
- **R** - **R**adiation: can you hear the murmur over the carotids (AS) or left axilla (MR)?
- **I** - **I**ntensity: what grade is the murmur?
- **P** - **P**itch: is it high pitched or low and grumbling? Pitch indicates velocity.
- **T** - **T**iming: is it systolic or diastolic?

Murmur Grade

Grading a murmur is quite subjective but is helpful is assessing the severity of the defect and will make you sound clever. If in doubt it is probably grade 2 or 3.

1. Difficult to hear
2. Quiet
3. Easy to hear
4. Easy to hear with a palpable thrill
5. Can hear with stethoscope barely touching chest
6. Can hear with stethoscope off the chest

Describing a Murmur

You can use this script for describing a murmur in your exams. If you practice it during your OSCE practice sessions it will become second nature and you will sound very slick when presenting to your examiner.

"This patient has a **harsh / soft / blowing**, **Grade ...**, **systolic / diastolic** murmur, heard loudest in the **aortic / mitral / tricuspid / pulmonary** area, that **does not / radiates to the carotids / left axilla**. It is **high / low pitched** and has a **crescendo / decrescendo / crescendo-decrescendo** shape. This is suggestive of a diagnosis of **mitral stenosis / aortic stenosis**"

Hypertrophy vs Dilatation

Valvular heart disease can cause **hypertrophy** (thickening both outwards and into the chamber) or **dilatation** (thinning and expanding, like blowing up a balloon) of the **myocardium** in different heart areas. This affects the chamber immediately before the pathological valve (i.e. the left ventricle in aortic pathology and the left atrium in mitral pathology).

When pushing against a stenotic valve the muscle has to try harder resulting in hypertrophy:
- *Mitral stenosis* causes **left atrial hypertrophy**.
- *Aortic stenosis* causes **left ventricular hypertrophy**.

When a leaky valve allows blood to flow back into a chamber it stretches the muscle resulting in dilatation:
- *Mitral regurgitation* causes **left atrial dilatation**.
- *Aortic regurgitation* causes **left ventricular dilatation**.

Mitral Stenosis

This is a narrow *mitral valve* making it difficult for the left atrium to push blood through to the ventricle. It is caused by:
- **Rheumatic heart disease**
- **Infective endocarditis**

It causes a *mid-diastolic*, **low pitched** "rumbling" murmur due to a low velocity of blood flow. There will be a loud S1 due to thick valves requiring a large systolic force to shut, then shutting suddenly. You can palpate a **tapping apex beat**, which is due to the loud S1.

It is associated with:
- **Malar flush**. This is due to back-pressure of blood into the pulmonary system causing a rise in CO_2 and vasodilation.
- **Atrial fibrillation**. This is caused by the left atrium struggling to push blood through the stenotic valve causing strain, electrical disruption and resulting fibrillation.

Mitral Regurgitation

Mitral regurgitation is when an incompetent mitral valve allows blood to lead back through during systolic contraction of the left ventricle. It causes a **pan-systolic**, **high pitched** "whistling" murmur due to high velocity blood flow through the leaky valve. The murmur radiates to left axilla.

It results in **congestive cardiac failure** because the leaking valve causes a reduced ejection fraction and a backlog of blood that is waiting to be pumped through the left side of the heart. Therefore you may hear a **third heart sound**.

Causes:
- Idiopathic weakening of the valve with age
- Ischaemic heart disease
- Infective endocarditis
- Rheumatic heart disease
- Connective tissue disorders such as **Ehlers Danlos syndrome** or **Marfan syndrome**

Aortic Stenosis

Aortic stenosis is the **most common** valve disease you will encounter. It causes an **ejection-systolic**, **high pitched** murmur due to the high velocity blood flow during systole. This has a **crescendo-decrescendo** character due to the speed of blood flow across the value during the different periods of **systole**. Flow during systole is slowest at the very start and end and fastest in the middle.

Other signs:
- The murmur radiates to the **carotids** as the turbulence continues up into the neck
- **Slow rising pulse** and **narrow pulse pressure**
- Patients may complain of **exertional syncope** (light headedness and fainting when exercising) due to difficulty maintaining good flow of blood to the brain

Causes:
- Idiopathic age related calcification
- Rheumatic heart disease

Aortic Regurgitation

Aortic regurgitation typically causes an **early diastolic**, **soft murmur**. It is also associated with a **Corrigan's pulse** (AKA **collapsing pulse**). A Corrigan's pulse is a rapidly appearing and disappearing pulse at carotid as the blood is pumped out by the ventricles and then immediately flows back through the aortic valve back into the ventricles. Aortic regurgitation results in heart failure due to a back pressure of blood waiting to get through the left side of the heart.

It can also cause an "**Austin-Flint**" murmur. This is heard at the **apex** and is an early diastolic "**rumbling**" murmur. This is caused by blood flowing back through the aortic valve and over the mitral valve causing it to vibrate.

Causes:
- Idiopathic age related weakness
- Connective tissue disorders such as **Ehlers Danlos syndrome** or **Marfan syndrome**

Prosthetic Valves

Patients that have had a valve replacement will have a scar. Usually this will be a **midline sternotomy scar** straight down the middle of the sternum indicating a **mitral** or **aortic** valve replacement or a **coronary artery bypass graft** (**CABG**). Less commonly a **lateral thoracotomy** incision can be used for **mitral valve** replacement surgery.

Bioprosthetic versus mechanical

Valves can be either replaced by a **bioprosthetic** or a metallic **mechanical** valve. "**Porcine**" bioprosthetic valves come from a pig.

Bioprosthetic valves have a limited lifespan of around 10 years.

Mechanical valves have a good lifespan (well over 20 years) but require **lifelong** anticoagulation with **warfarin**. The **INR target range** with mechanical valves is **2.5 - 3.5** (this is higher than the normal 2 - 3 range).

Types of Mechanic Heart Valves

Starr-Edwards valve
- Ball in cage valve
- Very successful but no longer being implanted
- Highest risk of thrombus formation

Tilting disc valve
- A single tilting disc

St Jude Valve
- Two tilting metal discs
- The two discs mean they are called **bileaflet valves**
- Least risk of thrombus formation

Mechanical Heart Valves

Major Complications
- **Thrombus** formation (blood stagnates and clots)
- **Infective endocarditis** (infection in prosthesis)
- **Haemolysis** causing anaemia (blood gets churned up in the valve)

Mechanical valves cause a click
- A click replaces S1 for metallic mitral valve
- A click replaces S2 for metallic aortic valve

Transcatheter Aortic Valve Implantation (TAVI)

This is a treatment for **severe aortic stenosis**, usually in patients that are high risk for an open valve replacement operation. It involves local or general anaesthetic, inserting a catheter in to the **femoral artery**, feeding a wire under **xray guidance** to the location of their aortic valve, then inflating a balloon to stretch the stenosed aortic valve and implanting a **bioprosthetic valve** in the location of the aortic valve.

Long term outcomes for TAVI are still not clear as it is a relatively new procedure. Therefore in younger, fitter patients open surgery is still the first line option.

Patient that have a TAVI do not typically require warfarin as the valve is **bioprosthetic**.

Infective Endocarditis

This occurs in around 2.5% of patients having a surgical valve replacement. The rate is slightly lower for TAVI at around 1.5%. Infective endocarditis in a prosthetic valve has quite a high mortality of around 15%. This is usually caused by one of three **gram positive cocci** organisms:

1. Staphylococcus
2. Streptococcus
3. Enterococcus

Patients with prosthetic valves used to be advised to take antibiotics for routine dental procedures to protect against infective endocarditis. This is no longer the case.

Atrial Fibrillation

Pathophysiology

Normally the **sinoatrial node** produces organised electrical activity that coordinates the contraction of the atria of the heart. **Atrial fibrillation** is where the contraction of the atria is uncoordinated, rapid and irregular. This due to **disorganised electrical activity** that overrides the normal, organised activity from the **sinoatrial node**. An ECG will show an **absence of p waves**. This reflects the lack of coordinated atrial electrical activity. This disorganised electrical activity in the atria also leads to irregular conduction of electrical impulses to the **ventricles**. This results in:

- **Irregularly irregular** ventricular contractions
- **Tachycardia**
- **Heart failure** due to **poor filling** of the ventricles during **diastole**
- Risk of **stroke**

There is a tendency for blood to collect in the **atria** and form blood clots. These clots can become **emboli**, travel to the brain and block the **cerebral arteries** causing an **ischaemic stroke**.

Presentation

Patients are often asymptomatic and atrial fibrillation is incidentally picked up when attending for other reasons.

Presenting symptoms can be:
- Palpitations
- Shortness of breath
- Syncope (dizziness or fainting)
- Symptoms of associated conditions (e.g. stroke, sepsis or thyrotoxicosis)

Irregularly irregular pulse

There are two differential diagnoses for an irregularly irregular pulse:
- **Atrial fibrillation**
- **Ventricular ectopics**

These can be differentiated using an ECG. An ECG should be performed on everyone with an irregularly irregular pulse.

Ventricular ectopics disappear when the heart rate gets over a certain threshold. Therefore a regular heart rate during exercise suggests a diagnosis of ventricular ectopics.

AF on an ECG

- Absent P waves
- Narrow QRS complex tachycardia
- Irregularly irregular ventricular rhythm

Valvular Versus Non-Valvular AF

Valvular AF is defined as patients with AF who also have moderate or severe **mitral stenosis** or a **mechanical heart valve**. The assumption is that the valvular pathology itself has lead to the atrial fibrillation. AF without valve pathology or with other valve pathology such as mitral regurgitation or aortic stenosis is classed as **non-valvular AF**.

Most common causes of AF (remember that AF affects mrs SMITH)

- **S**epsis
- **M**itral valve pathology (stenosis or regurgitation)
- **I**schaemic heart disease
- **T**hyrotoxicosis
- **H**ypertension

Principles of Treating AF

This is based on the most recent NICE guidelines from 2014 and has been adapted to make it easy to learn. Please read the full guideline before putting it into practice on real patients.

There are two principles to treating atrial fibrillation:
- **Rate** or **rhythm** control
- **Anticoagulation** to prevent stroke

Rate Control (vs Rhythm Control)

Normally the function of the **atria** is to pump blood in to the **ventricles**. In AF atrial contractions are not coordinated so the ventricles have to fill up by suction and gravity. This is considerably less efficient. The higher the heart rate, the less time is available for the ventricles to fill with blood, reducing the cardiac output. The aim is to get the heart rate below 100 to extend the time during diastole when the ventricles can fill with blood.

NICE guidelines (2014) suggest all patients with AF should have rate control as first line unless:
- There is reversible cause for their AF
- Their AF is of new onset (within the last 48 hours)
- Their AF is causing heart failure
- They remain symptomatic despite being effectively rate controlled

Options for Rate Control:
1. **Beta blocker** is first line (e.g. atenolol 50-100mg once daily)
2. **Calcium-channel blocker** (e.g. diltiazem) (not preferable in heart failure)
3. **Digoxin** (only in sedentary people. It needs monitoring and there is a risk of toxicity)

Rhythm Control

Rhythm control can be offered to patients where:
- There is a reversible cause for their AF
- Their AF is of new onset (within the last 48 hours)
- Their AF is causing heart failure
- They remain symptomatic despite being effectively rate controlled

The aim of rhythm control is to return the patient to **normal sinus rhythm**. This can be achieved through a single "**cardioversion**" event that puts the patient back in to sinus rhythm or **long term medical rhythm control** that sustains a normal rhythm.

Cardioversion:
Consider **cardioversion** in a candidate for rhythm control. There is a choice between immediate cardioversion or delayed cardioversion:
- **Immediate cardioversion** if the AF has been present for less than 48 hours or they are severely haemodynamically unstable.
- **Delayed cardioversion** if the AF has been present for more than 48 hours and they are stable.

In **delayed cardioversion** the patient should be **anticoagulated** for a minimum of 3 weeks prior to **cardioversion**. Anticoagulation is essential because during the 48 hours prior to cardioversion they may have developed a blood clot in the atria and reverting them back to sinus rhythm carries a high risk of mobilising that clot and causing a **stroke**. They should have **rate control** whilst waiting for cardioversion.

There are **two options** for *cardioversion*:
- *Pharmacological cardioversion*
- *Electrical cardioversion*

Pharmacological Cardioversion:
NICE guidelines (2014) say for *pharmacological cardioversion* first line is:
- *Flecanide*
- *Amiodarone* (the drug of choice in patients with structural heart disease)

Electrical Cardioversion:
The aim of *electrical cardioversion* is to rapidly shock the heart back into sinus rhythm. This involves **sedation** or *a general anaesthetic* and using a *cardiac defibrillator* machine to deliver controlled shocks in an attempt to restore sinus rhythm.

Long Term Medical Rhythm Control:
- *Beta blockers* are first line for rhythm control
- *Dronedarone* is second line for maintaining normal rhythm where patients have had successful cardioversion
- *Amiodarone* is useful in patients with heart failure or left ventricular dysfunction

Paroxysmal Atrial Fibrillation

Paroxysmal AF is when the AF comes and goes in episodes, usually not lasting more than 48 hours. Patients should still be anticoagulated based on their **CHADSVASc** score. They may be appropriate for a *"pill in the pocket"* approach. This is where they take a pill to terminated their atrial fibrillation only when they feel the symptoms of AF starting. To be appropriate for a *pill in the pocket* approach they need to have **infrequent episodes without any underlying structural heart disease**. They also need to be able to identify when they are in AF and understand when the treatment is appropriate.

Flecanide is the usual treatment for a "pill in the pocket" approach. Avoid *flecanide* in *atrial flutter* as it can cause 1:1 AV conduction and resulting in a significant tachycardia.

Anticoagulation

The uncontrolled and unorganised movement of the atria leads to blood stagnating in the left atrium, particularly in the *atrial appendage*. Eventually this stagnated blood leads to a *thrombus* (clot). This clot then mobilises (becomes an *embolus*) and travels with the blood. It travels from the *atria*, to the *ventricle*, to the *aorta* then up in the *carotid arteries* to the *brain*. It can then lodge in the *cerebral arteries* and cause an *ischaemic stroke*.

Anticoagulation acts to prevent *coagulation* (**thrombus formation**) by interfering with the clotting cascade. For perspective:
- WITHOUT anticoagulation, patients with AF have around a 5% risk of stroke **each year** (depending on **CHADSVASc** score).
- WITH anticoagulation, patients with AF have around a 1-2% risk of stroke **each year** (depending on **CHADSVASc** score). Anticoagulation **reduces the risk of stroke by about 2/3**.

Patients on anticoagulation have around a 3% risk of having a serious bleed each year depending on their **HAS-BLED** score. Generally bleeds are more reversible than strokes and have less long term consequences.

Warfarin

Warfarin is a **vitamin K antagonist**. Vitamin K is essential for the functioning of several clotting factors and warfarin blocks vitamin K. It prolongs the **prothrombin time**, which is the time it takes for blood to clot.

We measure **INR** (*international normalised ratio*), to assess **how anticoagulated** the patient is by **warfarin**. The **INR** is a calculation of how the **prothrombin time** of the **patient** compares with the **prothrombin time** of a **normal health adult**. An INR of 1 indicates a normal prothrombin time. An INR of 2 indicates that the patient has a prothrombin time twice that of a normal healthy adult (it takes them twice as long to form a blood clot).

Being started on warfarin is a reasonably large undertaking. It requires **close monitoring of their INR** and frequent **dose adjustments** to keep the INR in range. It is given once a day and usually at 6pm in hospital so that an INR can be obtained prior to the dose. The target INR for AF is 2 - 3.

Warfarin is affected by the **cytochrome P450** system in the **liver**. This system is involved in the metabolism of warfarin. The INR will be affected by other drugs that influence the activity of the P450 system. This includes many antibiotics. This means when starting new medications the INR needs close monitoring and the warfarin dose needs adjusting accordingly.

INR is also affected by many foods, particularly those that contain **vitamin K** such as **leafy green vegetables** and those that affect P450 such as **cranberry juice** and **alcohol**. This means it is important to monitor INR more closely when the patient changes medications or their diet.

Warfarin has a half-life of 1-3 days. It is also reversible with vitamin K in the event that the INR is very high or bleeding has occurred.

NOvel AntiCoagulants (NOACS) (i.e. Apixaban, Dabigatran and Rivaroxaban)

NOACS are now often referred to as **D**irect acting **O**ral **A**nti**C**oagulants (**DOACS**). They are currently on **patent**, which means the drugs companies that produce them can charge more money for them. For example it costs **£27 for apixaban** versus **£1 for warfarin** per month. This is often offset by the **cost of monitoring warfarin** and they will be coming off patent over the next few years, at which point they will become much cheaper.

Apixaban and **dabigatran** are taken twice daily, **rivaroxaban** is taken once daily. There is no way to reverse their effects however they have a lower bleeding risk and relatively short half life. NOACs have a 7-15 hour half-life, so reverse themselves in a short space of time. Apixaban has a half life of approximately 12 hours.

They have a number of potential advantages compared with warfarin:
- No monitoring is required
- No major interaction problems
- Equal or slightly better than warfarin at preventing strokes in AF
- Equal or slightly less risk of bleeding than warfarin

CHA2DS2-VASc

This is a tool for assessing whether a patient with **atrial fibrillation** should be started on **anticoagulation**. It is essentially a list of risk factors, and if you have one or more of these risk factors anticoagulation should be considered or started. The higher the score the higher the risk of developing a **stroke** or **TIA** and the greater the benefit from anticoagulation.

There is **no role for aspirin** in preventing stroke in AF. This used to be recommended, but not any longer.

CHA2DS2-VASc Score

- 0: no anticoagulation
- 1: consider anticoagulation
- **>1: offer anticoagulation**

CHA2DS2-VASc Mnemonic

- **C** - **C**ongestive heart failure
- **H** - **H**ypertension
- **A2** - **A**ge > 75 (Scores **2**)
- **D** - **D**iabetes
- **S2** - **S**troke or TIA previously (Scores **2**)
- **V** - **V**ascular disease
- **A** - **A**ge 65 - 74
- **S** - **S**ex (female)

HAS-BLED

HAS-BLED is an assessment tool for establishing a patient's risk of major bleeding **whilst on anticoagulation**. It can be used prior to initiating anticoagulation or as a monitoring tool in patients with a high risk of bleeding. It is not as essential to know inside out as the **CHADSVASc** but is useful to be aware of if you think a patient might have a higher risk of bleeding (for example those with at **risk of falls**). It is useful in practice for comparing the risk of stroke to the risk of bleeding to help patients and doctors make an informed decision about whether to start anticoagulation or not. Usually the **risk of stroke significantly outweighs the risk of bleeding**. Also, most bleeding can be treated, whereas a stroke often leads to significant long term morbidity and a lower quality of life.

The easiest way to calculate the HAS-BLED score is with an online calculator that will provide a risk of bleeding based on their score. It is scored based on:
- **H** - **H**ypertension
- **A** - **A**bnormal renal and liver function
- **S** - **S**troke
- **B** - **B**leeding
- **L** - **L**abile INRs (whilst on warfarin)
- **E** - **E**lderly
- **D** - **D**rugs or alcohol

Arrhythmias

As the name suggests, *arrhythmias* are abnormal heart rhythms. They result from an interruption to the normal electrical signals that coordinate the contraction of the heart muscle. There are several types of arrhythmia, each with different causes and management options.

Please read the Resuscitation Guidelines from the Resuscitation Council (UK) and attend their courses prior to treating patients. This section is a summary of these guidelines to improve your knowledge and understanding rather than guide treatment.

Four Cardiac Arrest Rhythms

These are the four possible rhythms that you will see in a pulseless unresponsive patient. They can be categorised into *shockable* (meaning **defibrillation** may be effective) and *non-shockable* (meaning **defibrillation** will not be effective and should not be used).

Shockable rhythms:
- *Ventricular tachycardia*
- *Ventricular fibrillation*

Non-shockable rhythms:
- *Pulseless electrical activity* (all electrical activity except VF/VT, including sinus rhythm without a pulse)
- *Asystole* (no significant electrical activity)

Tachycardia Treatment Summary

Unstable patient:
- Consider up to 3 synchronised shocks
- Consider an amiodarone infusion

In a stable patient:

Narrow complex (QRS < 0.12s)
- *Atrial fibrillation* – rate control with a beta blocker or diltiazem (calcium channel blocker)
- *Atrial flutter* – control rate with a beta blocker
- *Supraventricular tachycardias* – treat with vagal manoeuvres and adenosine

Broad complex (QRS > 0.12s)
- *Ventricular tachycardia* or unclear – amiodarone infusion
- If known **SVT with bundle branch block** treat as normal SVT
- If irregular may be variation of AF – seek expert help

Atrial Flutter

Normally the electrical signal passes through the atria once, stimulating a contraction then disappears through the AV node into the ventricles. Atrial flutter is caused by a "**re-entrant rhythm**" in either atrium. This is where the electrical signal re-circulates in a **self-perpetuating loop** due to an extra electrical pathway in the atria. The signal goes round and round the **atrium** without interruption. This stimulates **atrial contraction at 300 bpm**. The signal makes its way into the ventricles every second lap due to the long refractory period of the **AV node**, causing **150 bpm ventricular contraction**. It gives a "**sawtooth appearance**" on the ECG with P wave after P wave.

Associated Conditions:

- Hypertension
- Ischaemic heart disease
- Cardiomyopathy
- Thyrotoxicosis

Treatment is similar to atrial fibrillation:
- **Rate/rhythm control** with beta blockers or cardioversion
- Treat the reversible underlying condition (e.g. hypertension or thyrotoxicosis)
- **Radiofrequency ablation** of the re-entrant rhythm
- **Anticoagulation** based on CHA2DS2VASc score

Supraventricular Tachycardias (SVT)

Supraventricular tachycardia (SVT) is caused by the **electrical signal re-entering the atria** from the ventricles. Normally the electrical signal in the heart can only go from the atria to the ventricles. In SVT the electrical signal finds a way from the ventricles back into the atria. Once the signal is back in the atria it travels back through the **AV node** and causes another ventricular contraction. This causes a **self-perpetuating electrical loop** without an end point and results in fast **narrow complex tachycardia (QRS < 0.12)**. It looks like a QRS complex followed immediately by a T wave, QRS complex, T wave and so on.

Paroxysmal SVT describes a situation where SVT reoccurs and remits in the same patient over time.

There are three main types of SVT based on the source of the electrical signal:
- "**Atrioventricular nodal re-entrant tachycardia**" is when the re-entry point is back through the AV node.
- "**Atrioventricular re-entrant tachycardia**" is when the re-entry point is an accessory pathway (Wolff-Parkinson-White syndrome).
- "**Atrial tachycardia**" is where the electrical signal originates in the atria somewhere other than the **sinoatrial node**. This is not caused by a signal re-entering from the ventricles but instead from abnormally generated electrical activity in the atria. This ectopic electrical activity causes an atrial rate of >100bpm.

Acute Management of Stable Patients with SVT

When managing SVT take a stepwise approach trying each step to see whether it works before moving on. Make sure they are on **continuous ECG monitoring**.

- **Valsalva manoeuvre**. Ask the patient to blow hard against resistance, for example into a plastic syringe.
- **Carotid sinus massage**. Massage the carotid on one side gently with two fingers.
- **Adenosine** (see below)
- An alternative to adenosine is **verapamil** (**calcium channel blocker**)
- **Direct current cardioversion** may be required if the above treatment fails

Adenosine

Adenosine works by slowing cardiac conduction primarily though the **AV node**. It interrupts the **AV node / accessory pathway** during SVT and "resets" it back to sinus rhythm. It needs to be given as a rapid bolus to ensure it reaches the heart with enough impact to interrupt the pathway. It will often cause a brief period of **asystole** or **bradycardia** that can be scary for the patient and doctor, however it is quickly metabolised and sinus rhythm should return.

A few key points on administering adenosine:
- Avoid if patient has asthma, COPD, heart failure, heart block or severe hypotension
- Warn the patient about the scary feeling of dying or impending doom when injected
- Give it as a fast IV bolus into a large proximal cannula (e.g. grey cannula in the **antecubital fossa**)
- Initially **6mg**, then **12mg** and further **12mg** if no improvement between doses

Long Term Management of Patients with Paroxysmal SVT

When patients develop recurrent episodes of SVT then measures can be taken to prevent these episodes. The options are:
- Medication (**beta blockers**, **calcium channel blockers** or **amiodarone**)
- **Radiofrequency ablation**

Wolff-Parkinson-White Syndrome

Wolff-Parkinson-White syndrome is caused by an extra electrical pathway connecting the atria and ventricles. Normally there is only one pathway connecting the atria and ventricles called the **atrio-ventricular (AV) node.** The extra pathway that is present in **Wolff-Parkinson-White syndrome** is often called the **Bundle of Kent**.

The definitive treatment for **Wolff-Parkinson-White syndrome** is **radiofrequency ablation** of the **accessory pathway**.

ECG Changes:
- Short PR interval (< 0.12 seconds)
- Wide QRS complex (> 0.12 seconds)
- "**Delta wave**" (a slurred upstroke on the QRS complex)

Note: If the person has a combination of **atrial fibrillation** or **atrial flutter** and **WPW** there is a risk that the chaotic atrial electrical activity can pass through the accessory pathway into the ventricles causing a **polymorphic wide complex tachycardia**. Most **antiarrhythmic medications** (**beta blockers**, **calcium channel blockers**, **adenosine** etc) increase the risk of this by reducing conduction through the AV node and therefore promoting conduction through the accessory pathway. Therefore they are **contraindicated** in patients with WPW that develop atrial fibrillation or flutter.

Radiofrequency Ablation

Catheter ablation is performed in an electrophysiology laboratory, often called a "**cath lab**". It involves local or general anaesthetic, inserting a catheter into the **femoral veins** and feeding a wire through the **venous system** under **xray guidance** to the heart. Once in the heart it is placed against different areas to test the electrical signals at that point. This way the operator can hopefully find the location of any abnormal electrical pathways. The operator may try to induce the arrhythmia to make the abnormal pathways easier to find. Once identified, **radiofrequency ablation** (**heat**) is applied to burn the abnormal area of electrical activity. This leaves scar tissue that does not conduct the electrical activity. The aim is to remove the source of the arrhythmia.

This can be curative for certain cases of arrhythmia caused by abnormal electrical pathways, including:
- *Atrial fibrillation*
- *Atrial flutter*
- *Supraventricular tachycardias*
- *Wolff-Parkinson-White syndrome*

Torsades de Pointes

Torsades de pointes is a type of **polymorphic** (multiple shape) **ventricular tachycardia**. It translates from French as "twisting of the tips", describing the ECG characteristics. It looks like normal ventricular tachycardia on an ECG however there is an appearance that the QRS complex is twisting around the baseline. The height of the QRS complexes progressively get smaller, then larger then smaller and so on. It occurs in patients with a **prolonged QT interval**.

A prolonged QT interval is the ECG finding of prolonged **repolarisation** of the muscle cells in the heart after a contraction. **Depolarisation** is the electrical process that leads to the heart contraction. **Repolarisation** is a period of recovery before the heart muscle cells (**myocytes**) are ready to **depolarise** again. Waiting a longer time for **repolarisation** can result in random spontaneous **depolarisation** in some areas of the heart **myocytes**. These abnormal spontaneous **depolarisations** prior to **repolarisation** are known as "**afterdepolarisations**". These **depolarisations** spread throughout the ventricles, leading to a ventricular contraction prior to proper **repolarisation** occurring. When this occurs and the ventricles continue to stimulate recurrent contractions without normal repolarisation it is called **torsades de pointes**.

When a patient develops torsades de pointes it will either terminate spontaneously and revert back to sinus rhythm or progress to **ventricular tachycardia**. Usually they are self limiting but if they progress to VT it can lead to a cardiac arrest.

Causes of Prolonged QT
- **Long QT Syndrome** (inherited)
- Medications such as **antipsychotics**, **citalopram**, **flecainide**, **sotalol**, **amiodarone** and **macrolide antibiotics**
- Electrolyte disturbances such as **hypokalaemia**, **hypomagnesaemia** and **hypocalcaemia**

Acute Management of Torsades de Pointes
- Correct the cause (electrolyte disturbances or medications)
- Magnesium infusion (even if they have a normal serum magnesium)
- Defibrillation if VT occurs

Long Term Management of Prolonged QT Syndrome
- Avoid medications that prolong the QT interval
- Correct electrolyte disturbances
- Beta blockers (not sotalol)
- Pacemaker or implantable defibrillator

Ventricular Ectopics

Ventricular ectopics are **premature ventricular beats** caused by random electrical discharges from outside the atria. Patients often present complaining of random, brief palpitations ("an abnormal beat"). They are relatively common at all ages and in healthy patients however they are more common in patients with pre-existing heart conditions (e.g. ischaemic heart disease or heart failure).

They can be diagnosed on an ECG and appear as individual random, abnormal, broad QRS complexes on a background of a normal ECG.

Bigeminy
This is where the ventricular ectopics are occurring so frequently that they happen after every sinus beat. The ECG looks like a normal sinus beat followed immediately by an ectopic, then a normal beat, then ectopic and so on.

Management
- Check bloods for **anaemia**, **electrolyte disturbance** and **thyroid** abnormalities
- Reassurance and no treatment in otherwise healthy people
- Seek expert advice in patients with background heart conditions or other concerning features or findings such as chest pain, syncope, murmur or family history of sudden death.

AV Node Blocks (Heart Block)

First degree heart block

First degree heart block occurs where there is delayed atrioventricular conduction through the AV node. Despite this, every atrial impulse leads to a ventricular contraction, meaning every p waves results in a QRS complex. On an ECG this presents as a PR interval greater than 0.20 seconds (5 small or 1 big square).

Second Degree Heart Block

Second degree heart block is where some of the atrial impulses do not make it through the AV node to the ventricles. This means that there are instances where p waves do not lead to QRS complexes. There are three patterns of second degree heart block:

Wenckebach's phenomenon (Mobitz Type 1)
This is where the atrial imputes becomes gradually weaker until it does not pass through the AV node. After failing to stimulate a ventricular contraction the atrial impulse returns to being strong. This cycle then repeats.

On an ECG this will appear as an increasing PR interval until the p wave no longer conducts to ventricles. This culminates in an absent QRS complex after a p wave. The PR interval then returns to normal but progressively becomes longer again until another QRS complex is missed. This cycle repeats itself.

Mobitz Type 2
This is where there is intermitted failure or interruption of AV conduction. This results in missing QRS complexes. There is usually a set ratio of p waves to QRS complexes, for example 3 p waves to each QRS complex would be referred to as a 3:1 block. The PR interval remains normal. There is a **risk of asystole** with *Mobitz Type 2*.

2:1 Block
This is where there are 2 p waves for each QRS complex. Every second p wave is not a strong enough atrial impulse to stimulate a QRS complex. This can be caused by Mobitz Type 1 or Mobitz Type 2 and it is difficult to tell which.

Third Degree Heart Block

This is referred to as **complete heart block**. There is no observable relationship between p waves and QRS complexes. There is a significant **risk of asystole** with third degree heart block.

Treatment for Bradycardias and AV Node Blocks

Stable:
- Observe

Unstable or risk of asystole (i.e. Mobitz Type 2, complete heart block or previous asystole):
First line:
- *Atropine* 500mcg IV

No improvement:
- *Atropine* 500mcg IV (repeated up to 6 doses for a total to 3mg)
- Other *inotropes* (such as noradrenalin)
- *Transcutaneous cardiac pacing* (using a defibrillator)

In patients with high risk of **asystole** (i.e. **Mobitz Type 2**, **complete heart block** or previous **asystole**):
- **Temporary transvenous cardiac pacing** using an electrode on the end of a wire that is inserted into a vein and fed through the venous system to the right atrium or ventricle to stimulate them directly
- **Permanent implantable pacemaker** when available

Atropine is an **antimuscarinic** medication and works by **inhibiting** the **parasympathetic nervous system**. This leads to side effects of pupil dilatation, urinary retention, dry eyes and constipation.

Pacemakers

Pacemakers deliver controlled electrical impulses to specific areas of the heart to restore the normal electrical activity and improve the heart function. They consist of a **pulse generator** (the little pacemaker box) and **pacing leads** that carry electrical impulses to the relevant part of the heart. The box is implanted under the skin (most commonly in the **left anterior chest wall** or **axilla**) and the wires are implanted into the relevant chambers of the heart.

Modern pacemakers have a computer that monitors the natural electrical activity and tailors its function to that. Basically if it is already working perfectly, no intervention is provided by the pacemaker. The batteries last around **5 years**.

Pacemakers do not interact with day to day electrical activities but may be a contraindication for **MRI scans** (due to powerful magnets) and electrical interventions such as **TENS machines** and **diathermy** in surgery. Many modern pacemakers are "**MRI compatible**".

It is worth noting that it is essential that pacemakers are removed prior to cremation in deceased patients. On the "**cremation form**" one of the most important tasks is to confirm whether the deceased patient has a pacemaker and whether it has been removed. You may hear stories about pacemakers "blowing up" crematoriums (this is a dramatic exaggeration but they can explode when burned causing significant damage).

Indications for a Pacemaker

- *Symptomatic bradycardias*
- *Mobitz Type 2 AV block*
- *Third degree heart block*
- *Severe heart failure* (**biventricular pacemakers**)
- *Hypertrophic obstructive cardiomyopathy* (**ICDs**)

Single-chamber

Single-chamber pacemakers have **leads in a single chamber**, either in the **right atrium** or the **right ventricle**. They are placed in the **right atrium** if the **AV conduction** in the patient is normal and the issue is with the **SA node**. This way they stimulate **depolarisation** in the right atrium and this electrical activity then passes to the **left atrium** and through the **AV node** to the **ventricles** in the normal way. They are placed in the **right ventricle** if the **AV conduction** in the patient is abnormal and they stimulate the **ventricles** directly.

Dual-chamber

Dual-chamber pacemakers have leads in both the **right atrium** and **right ventricle**. This allows the **pacemaker** to synchronise the contractions of both **atria** and **ventricles**.

Biventricular (Triple-chamber) Pacemaker

Biventricular pacemakers have leads in **right atrium**, **right ventricle** and **left ventricle**.
These are usually in patients with heart failure. The objective is to synchronise the contractions in these chambers to try to optimise the heart function. They are also called **cardiac resynchronisation therapy** (**CRT**) **pacemakers**.

Implantable Cardioverter Defibrillators (ICDs)

Implantable cardioverter defibrillators continually monitor the heart and apply a **defibrillator shock** to **cardiovert** the patient back in to sinus rhythm if they identify a shockable **arrhythmia**.

ECG Changes with Pacemakers

It is quite common to be asked to state pacemaker type based on an ECG in exams. The pacemaker intervention can be seen as a **sharp vertical line** on **all leads** on the ECG trace. A line before each p-wave indicates a lead in the atria. A line before each QRS complex indicates a lead in the ventricles. Therefore:

- A line before either the P or QRS but not the other indicates a **single-chamber pacemaker**
- A line before both the P and QRS indicates a **dual-chamber pacemaker**

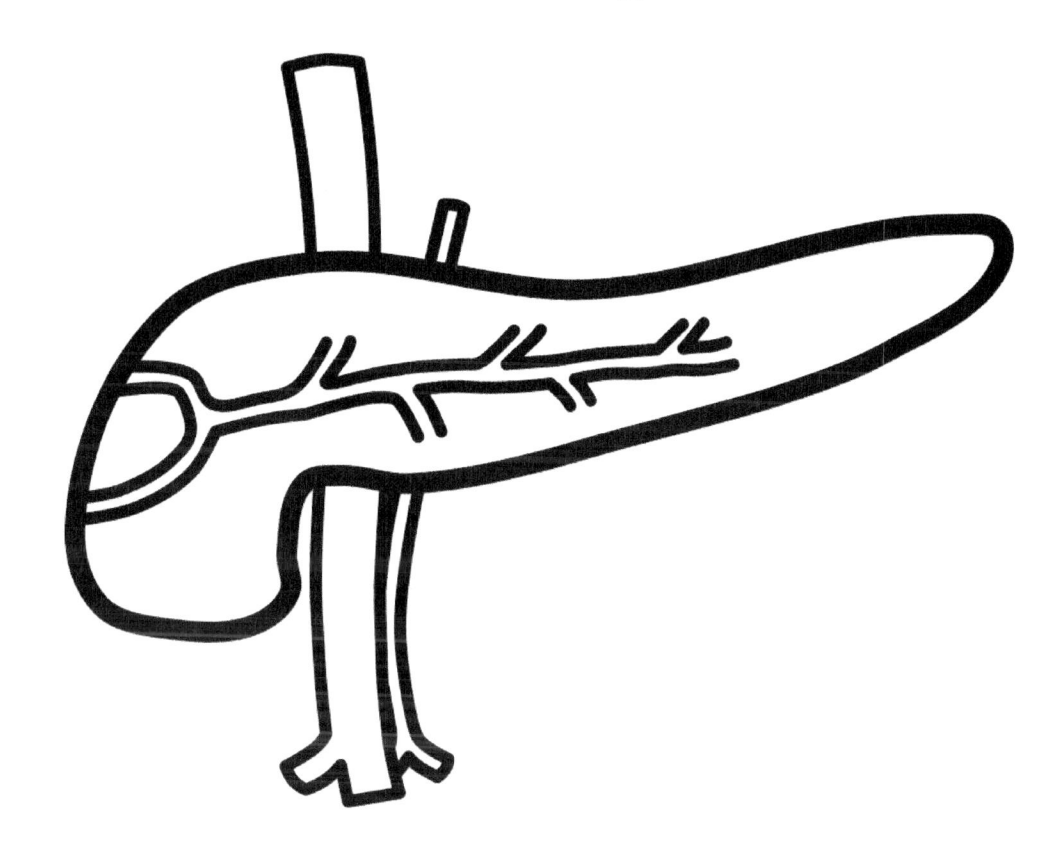

ENDOCRINOLOGY

2.1	Hormonal Axis Physiology	40
2.2	Cushing's Syndrome	42
2.3	Adrenal Insufficiency	44
2.4	Thyroid Function Tests	46
2.5	Hyperthyroidism	48
2.6	Hypothyroidism	50
2.7	Type 1 Diabetes	52
2.8	Type 2 Diabetes	56
2.9	Acromegaly	61
2.10	Hyperparathyroidism	62
2.11	Hyperaldosteronism	63
2.12	Syndrome of Inappropriate Anti-Diuretic Hormone (SIADH)	64
2.13	Diabetes Insipidus	66
2.14	Phaeochromocytoma	68

Hormonal Axis Physiology

The Hypothalamus and Pituitary

The **hypothalamus** sits above the **pituitary gland** and **stimulates it with various hormones**. The **pituitary gland** comprises of an **anterior** and a **posterior** section that release **separate hormones**.

The **anterior pituitary gland** releases:
- Thyroid stimulating hormone (TSH)
- Adrenocorticotropic hormone (ACTH)
- Follicle stimulating hormone (FSH) and luteinising hormone (LH)
- Growth hormone (GH)
- Prolactin

The **posterior pituitary** releases:
- Oxytocin
- Antidiuretic hormone (ADH)

The Thyroid Axis

The **hypothalamus** releases **thyrotropin-releasing hormone** (**TRH**). This **stimulates** the **anterior pituitary** to release **thyroid stimulating hormone** (**TSH**). This in turn **stimulates** the **thyroid gland** to release **triiodothyronine** (**T3**) and **thyroxine** (**T4**).

T3 and **T4** are sensed by the **hypothalamus** and **anterior pituitary**, and they **suppress** the release of **TRH** and **TSH**. This results in lower amounts of **T3** and **T4**. The lower levels of **T3** and **T4** offer **less suppression** of **TRH** and **TSH** and so more of these hormones are released, resulting in a rise of **T3** and **T4**. In this way, the level of thyroid hormone is closely regulated to keep it within normal limits. This is called **negative feedback**.

The Adrenal Axis

Cortisol is secreted by the **two adrenal glands**, which sit above each kidney. The release of **cortisol** is controlled by the **hypothalamus**. Cortisol is released in pulses and in response to a stressful stimulus (it is a "**stress hormone**"). It has **diurnal variation**, which basically means that it is high and low at **different times of the day**. Typically cortisol **peaks in the early morning**, triggering us to wake up and get going, and is at its **lowest late in the evening**, prompting us to relax and fall asleep.

The **hypothalamus** releases **corticotrophin release hormone** (**CRH**). This stimulates the **anterior pituitary** to release **adrenocorticotrophic hormone** (**ACTH**). This in turn stimulates the **adrenal gland** to release **cortisol**.

The **adrenal axis** is also controlled by **negative feedback**. **Cortisol** is sensed by the **hypothalamus** and **anterior pituitary**, and it **suppresses the release** of **CRH** and **ACTH**. This results in lower amounts of cortisol. In this way, cortisol is closely regulated to keep it within normal limits.

Cortisol has several actions within the body:
- Inhibits the immune system
- Inhibits bone formation
- Raises blood glucose
- Increases metabolism
- Increases alertness

Growth Hormone Axis

Growth hormone releasing hormone (**GHRH**) is released from the **hypothalamus**. This stimulates **growth hormone** (**GH**) release from the **anterior pituitary**. **Growth hormone** stimulates the release of **insulin-like growth factor 1** (**IGF-1**) from the **liver**.

Through this mechanism growth hormone works directly and indirectly on almost all cells of the body and has many functions. Most importantly **growth hormone**:
- Stimulates muscle growth
- Increases bone density and strength
- Stimulates cell regeneration and reproduction
- Stimulates growth of internal organs

Parathyroid Axis

Parathyroid hormone (**PTH**) is released from the **four parathyroid glands** (situated in four corners of the thyroid gland) in response to **low serum calcium**. It is also released in response to **low magnesium** and **high serum phosphate**. Its role is to **increase the serum calcium concentration**.

PTH increases the activity and number of **osteoclasts** in bone, causing reabsorption of calcium from the bone into the blood thereby increasing serum calcium concentration.

PTH also stimulates an **increase in calcium reabsorption in the kidneys** meaning that less calcium is excreted in the urine.

Additionally, it stimulates the kidneys to convert **vitamin D3** into **calcitriol**, which is the active form of **vitamin D** that promotes **calcium absorption** from food **in the small intestine**.

These **three effects** of **PTH** (increased calcium absorption from bone, the kidneys and the small intestine) all help to **raise the level of serum calcium**. When serum calcium is high this suppresses the release of PTH (via **negative feedback**) helping to reduce the serum calcium level.

Renin-Angiotensin System

Renin is a hormone secreted by the **juxtaglomerular cells** that sit in the **afferent** (and some in the **efferent**) **arterioles** in the **kidney**. They sense the **blood pressure** in these vessels. They secrete more renin in response to low blood pressure and secrete less renin in response to high blood pressure. Renin is an **enzyme** that acts to convert **angiotensinogen** (released by the **liver**) into **angiotensin I**. Angiotensin I converts to angiotensin II in the lungs with the help of an enzyme called **angiotensin-converting enzyme** (**ACE**).

Angiotensin II acts on blood vessels to cause **vasoconstriction**. This results in an increase in blood pressure. **Angiotensin II** also stimulates the release of **aldosterone** from the **adrenal glands**.

Aldosterone is a **mineralocorticoid steroid** hormone. It acts on the **nephrons** in the kidneys to:
- Increase **sodium reabsorption** from the **distal tubule**
- Increase **potassium secretion** from the **distal tubule**
- Increase **hydrogen secretion** from the **collecting ducts**

When sodium is reabsorbed in the kidneys water follows it by osmosis. This leads to an increase in **intravascular volume** and subsequently **blood pressure**.

Cushing's Syndrome

Cushing's syndrome is used to refer to the signs and symptoms that develop after **prolonged abnormal elevation of cortisol**. **Cushing's disease** is used to refer to the specific condition where a **pituitary adenoma** (tumour) secretes excessive **ACTH**. **Cushing's disease** causes a **Cushing's syndrome**, but **Cushing's Syndrome** is not always caused by **Cushing's disease**.

Cushing's Syndrome Features

There are a large number of features of Cushing's syndrome, so they don't easily fit in to the handy mnemonic. I find it easier to picture the patient as very round in the middle with thin, weak limbs and then imagine the effects of high levels of stress hormone.

Round in the middle with thin limbs:
- Round "moon" face
- Central obesity
- Abdominal striae
- "Buffalo hump" (fat pad on upper back)
- Proximal limb muscle wasting

High levels of stress hormone:
- Hypertension
- Cardiac hypertrophy
- Hyperglycaemia (type 2 diabetes)
- Depression
- Insomnia

Extra effects:
- Osteoporosis
- Easy bruising and poor skin healing

Causes of Cushing's Syndrome

- *Exogenous steroids* (in patients on long term high dose steroid medications)
- *Cushing's disease* (a *pituitary adenoma* releasing excessive *ACTH*)
- *Adrenal adenoma* (a hormone secreting adrenal tumour)
- *Paraneoplastic Cushing's*

Paraneoplastic Cushing's is when excess *ACTH* is released from a cancer (except in the pituitary) and stimulates excessive cortisol release. *ACTH* from somewhere other than the pituitary is called "*ectopic ACTH*". **Small cell lung cancer** is the most common cause of paraneoplastic Cushing's.

Dexamethasone Suppression Tests (DST)

The *dexamethasone suppression test* is the test of choice for diagnosing *Cushing's syndrome*. This involves initially giving the patient the "low dose" test. If the low dose test is normal, Cushing's can be excluded. If the low dose test is abnormal, then a high dose test is performed to differentiate between the underlying causes.

To perform the test the patient takes a dose of *dexamethasone* (a synthetic glucocorticoid steroid) at night (i.e. 10pm) and their *cortisol* and *ACTH* is measured in the morning (i.e. 9am). The intention is the find out whether the *dexamethasone* **suppresses** their normal morning spike of *cortisol*.

Low Dose Dexamethasone Suppression Test (1mg dexamethasone)

A normal response is for the dexamethasone to suppress the release of cortisol by effecting negative feedback on the *hypothalamus* and *pituitary*. The *hypothalamus* responds by **reducing the CRH** output. The *pituitary* responds by **reducing the ACTH** output. The lower CRH and ACTH levels result in a low cortisol level. When the cortisol level is not suppressed, this is the abnormal result seen in *Cushing's Syndrome*.

High Dose Dexamethasone Suppression Test (8mg dexamethasone)

The high dose dexamethasone suppression test is performed after an abnormal result on the low dose test.

In *Cushing's disease* (*pituitary adenoma*) the pituitary still shows some response to *negative feedback* and 8mg of dexamethasone is enough to **suppress cortisol**.

Where there is an *adrenal adenoma*, cortisol production is independent from the pituitary. Therefore, cortisol is **not** suppressed, however ACTH **is** suppressed due to negative feedback on the hypothalamus and pituitary gland.

Where there is *ectopic ACTH* (e.g. from a *small cell lung cancer*), neither cortisol or ACTH will be suppressed because the ACTH production is independent of the hypothalamus or pituitary gland.

	Cortisol	ACTH
Pituitary Adenoma	Suppressed	Suppressed
Adrenal Adenoma	Not Suppressed	Suppressed
Ectopic ACTH	Not Suppressed	Not Suppressed

Other Investigations

24 hour urinary free cortisol can be used as an alternative to the dexamethasone suppression test to diagnose Cushing's syndrome but it does not indicate the underlying cause and is cumbersome to carry out.

Other investigations:
- **FBC** (raised white cells) and **electrolytes** (potassium may be low if *aldosterone* is also secreted by an *adrenal adenoma*)
- **MRI brain** for *pituitary adenoma*
- **Chest CT** for *small cell lung cancer*
- **Abdominal CT** for *adrenal tumours*

Treatment

The main treatment is to remove the underlying cause (surgically remove the tumour)
- *Trans-sphenoidal* (through the nose) removal of pituitary adenoma
- Surgical removal of adrenal tumour
- Surgical removal of a tumour producing ectopic ACTH

If surgical removal of the cause is not possible another option is to remove both adrenal glands and give the patient replacement steroid hormones for life.

Adrenal Insufficiency

Adrenal insufficiency is where the **adrenal glands** do not produce enough steroid hormones, particularly **cortisol** and **aldosterone**. Steroids are essential for life. Therefore the condition is life threatening unless the hormones are replaced.

Addison's disease refers to the specific condition where the adrenal glands have been damaged, resulting in a reduction in the secretion of **cortisol** and **aldosterone**. This is also called *primary adrenal insufficiency*. The most common cause is *autoimmune*.

Secondary adrenal insufficiency is a result of inadequate **ACTH** stimulating the **adrenal glands**, resulting in low cortisol release. This is the result of loss or damage to the pituitary gland. This can be due to surgery to remove a pituitary tumour, infection, loss of blood flow or radiotherapy. There is also a condition called **Sheehan's syndrome** where massive blood loss during childbirth leads to pituitary gland necrosis.

Tertiary adrenal insufficiency is the result of inadequate **CRH** release by the **hypothalamus**. This is usually the result of patients being on **long term oral steroids** (for more than 3 weeks) causing suppression of the **hypothalamus**. When the **exogenous steroids** are suddenly withdrawn the hypothalamus does not "wake up" fast enough and **endogenous steroids** are not adequately produced. Therefore long term steroids should be tapered slowly to allow time for the adrenal axis to regain normal function.

Symptoms

- Fatigue
- Nausea
- Cramps

- Abdominal pain
- Reduced libido

Signs

- Bronze **hyperpigmentation** of the skin (**ACTH** stimulates **melanocytes** to produce **melanin**)
- **Hypotension** (particularly postural hypotension)

Investigations

Hyponatraemia (low sodium) is a key biochemical clue. Sometimes the only presenting feature of adrenal insufficiency is hyponatraemia.

Hyperkalaemia (high potassium) is also possible.

Early morning cortisol (8 - 9am) has a role but is often falsely normal.

The **short synacthen test** is the test of choice to diagnose adrenal insufficiency.

ACTH levels. In **primary adrenal failure** the **ACTH level is high** as the pituitary is trying very hard to stimulate the adrenal glands without any **negative feedback** in the absence of **cortisol**. In **secondary adrenal failure** the **ACTH level is low** as the reason the adrenal glands are not producing cortisol is that they are not being stimulated by ACTH.

Adrenal autoantibodies are present in 80% of autoimmune adrenal insufficiency: **adrenal cortex antibodies** and **21-hydroxylase antibodies**.

CT or **MRI adrenal glands** if suspecting an adrenal tumour, haemorrhage or other structural pathology. This is not routinely recommended by NICE for autoimmune adrenal insufficiency.

MRI pituitary gives further information about pituitary pathology.

Short Synacthen Test (ACTH stimulation test)

The **short synacthen test** is the test of choice for **adrenal insufficiency**. It is ideally performed in the morning when the adrenal glands are most "fresh". The test involves giving **synacthen**, which is **synthetic ACTH**. The blood cortisol is measured at baseline, 30 and 60 minutes after administration. The synthetic ACTH will stimulate healthy adrenal glands to produce cortisol and the cortisol level should at least double. A failure of cortisol to rise (**less than double the baseline**) indicates **primary adrenal insufficiency (Addison's disease)**.

Long Synacthen Test

The **long synacthen test** is rarely used anymore because we can now measure **ACTH** levels. It was used to distinguish between **primary adrenal insufficiency** and **adrenal atrophy** secondary to prolonged under stimulation in **secondary adrenal insufficiency**. It involves giving an infusion of **ACTH** over a long period.

- In **primary adrenal failure** there is no cortisol response as the adrenals no longer function.
- In **adrenal atrophy** (**secondary adrenal insufficiency**), the prolonged ACTH eventually gets the adrenals going again and cortisol rises.

Now we can simply measure **ACTH** and this indicates the underlying cause.

Treatment

Treatment of adrenal insufficiency is with replacement steroids titrated to signs, symptoms and electrolytes. **Hydrocortisone** is a glucocorticoid hormone and is used to replace **cortisol**. **Fludrocortisone** is a mineralocorticoid hormone and is used to replace **aldosterone** if aldosterone is also insufficient.

Patients are given a **steroid card** and an **emergency ID tag** to alert emergency services that they are dependent on steroids for life. Doses should not be missed as they are essential to life. **Doses are doubled** during an acute illness to match the normal steroid response to illness.

Addisonian Crisis (AKA Adrenal Crisis)

Addisonian crisis is the term used to describe an acute presentation of **severe Addisons**, where the absence of steroid hormones leads to a life threatening presentation. They present with:
- Reduced consciousness
- Hypotension
- Hypoglycaemia, hyponatraemia and hyperkalaemia
- Patients can be very unwell

It can be the **first presentation** of *Addison's disease* or triggered by infection, trauma or other acute illness in someone with established Addison's. It can present in someone on long term steroids suddenly stopping those steroids.

Do not wait to perform investigations and establish a definitive diagnosis before treating someone with suspected Addisonian crisis as it is life threatening and they need immediate treatment.

Management of Addisonian Crisis

- Intensive monitoring if unwell
- Parenteral steroids (i.e. IV hydrocortisone 100mg stat then 100mg every 6 hours)
- IV fluid resuscitation
- Correct hypoglycaemia
- Careful monitoring of electrolytes and fluid balance

Thyroid Function Tests

Thyroid Stimulating Hormone (TSH)

If you are concerned about possible **thyroid disease** you can use **TSH** alone as a screening test. When TSH is abnormal, then you can measure T3 and T4 to find out more information.

In **hyperthyroidism**, **TSH is suppressed** by the high thyroid hormones so you get a **low TSH level**. The exception is a **pituitary adenoma** that secretes TSH in which case it is high.

In *hypothyroidism*, **TSH is high** as it is trying to stimulate more thyroid hormone release. The exception is a *pituitary* or *hypothalamic* cause of the hypothyroid (secondary hyperthyroidism), in which case the TSH level will be low.

T3 and T4

In *hyperthyroidism* you expect **raised T3 and T4 and suppressed TSH**. In *hypothyroidism* you expect **low T3 and T4 and raised TSH**.

Thyroid Status	TSH	T3 and T4
Hyperthyroidism	Low	High
Primary Hypothyroidism	High	Low
Secondary Hypothyroidism	Low	Low

Antibodies

Antithyroid peroxidase (anti-TPO) antibodies are antibodies against the thyroid gland itself. They are the most relevant thyroid autoantibody in autoimmune thyroid disease. They are usually present in *Grave's disease* and *Hashimoto's thyroiditis*.

Antithyroglobulin antibodies are antibodies against *thyroglobulin*, a protein produced and extensively present in the thyroid gland. Measuring them is of limited use as they can be present in normal individuals. They are are usually present in *Grave's disease*, *Hashimoto's thyroiditis* and *thyroid cancer*.

TSH receptor antibodies are autoantibodies that mimic TSH, bind to the *TSH receptor* and stimulate thyroid hormone release. They are the cause of *Grave's disease* and so will be present in this condition.

Imaging

Thyroid Ultrasound
Ultrasound of the thyroid gland is useful in diagnosing *thyroid nodules* and distinguishing between *cystic* (fluid filled) and *solid nodules*. Ultrasound can also be used to guide biopsy of a thyroid lesion.

Radioisotope Scan
Radioisotope scans are used to investigate *hyperthyroidism* and *thyroid cancers*. *Radioactive iodine* is given orally or intravenously and travels to the thyroid where it is taken up by the cells. Iodine is normally used by thyroid cells to produce thyroid hormones. The more active the thyroid cells, the faster the radioactive iodine is taken up. A *gamma camera* is used to detect *gamma rays* emitted from the radioactive iodine. The more gamma rays that are emitted from an area the more radioactive iodine has been taken up. This gives really useful **functional information** about the thyroid gland:
- Diffuse high uptake is found in *Grave's Disease*
- Focal high uptake is found in *toxic multinodular goitre* and *adenomas*
- "Cold" areas (i.e. abnormally low uptake) can indicate *thyroid cancer*

Hyperthyroidism

Definitions

Hyperthyroidism is where there is over-production of thyroid hormone by the thyroid gland. **Thyrotoxicosis** refers to an abnormal and excessive quantity of thyroid hormone in the body.

Primary hyperthyroidism is due to thyroid pathology. It is the thyroid itself that is behaving abnormally and producing excessive thyroid hormone.

Secondary hyperthyroidism is the condition where the thyroid is producing excessive thyroid hormone as a result of overstimulation by **thyroid stimulating hormone**. The pathology is in the **hypothalamus** or **pituitary**.

Grave's disease is an *autoimmune* condition where **TSH receptor antibodies** cause a primary hyperthyroidism. These **TSH receptor antibodies** are abnormal **antibodies** produced by the immune system that **mimic TSH** and stimulate the **TSH receptors** on the thyroid. This is the **most common cause** of **hyperthyroidism**.

Toxic multinodular goitre (also known as **Plummer's disease**) is a condition where **nodules** develop on the thyroid gland that **act independently of the normal feedback system** and continuously produce **excessive thyroid hormone**.

Exophthalmos is the term used to describe bulging of eyeball out of the socket caused by **Grave's disease**. This is due to *inflammation*, swelling and **hypertrophy** of the tissue behind the eyeball that forces the eyeball forward.

Pretibial myxoedema is a dermatological condition where there are deposits of **mucin** under the skin on the anterior aspect of the leg (the **pre-tibial area**). This gives a discoloured, waxy, oedematous appearance to the skin over this area. It is **specific to Grave's disease** and is a **reaction to the TSH receptor antibodies**.

Universal Features of Hyperthyroidism

- Anxiety and irritability
- Sweating and heat intolerance
- Tachycardia
- Weight loss
- Fatigue
- Frequent loose stools
- Sexual dysfunction

Unique Features of Grave's Disease

These features all relate to the presence of **TSH receptor antibodies**.

- Diffuse goitre (without nodules)
- Graves eye disease
- Bilateral *exopthalmos*
- **Pretibial myxoedema**

Unique Features of Toxic Multinodular Goitre

- Goitre with firm nodules
- Most patients are aged over 50
- Second most common cause of thyrotoxicosis (after Grave's)

Solitary Toxic Thyroid Nodule

This is where a single abnormal thyroid nodule is acting alone to release thyroid hormone. The nodules are usually benign adenomas. They are treated with surgical removal of the nodule.

De Quervain's Thyroiditis

De Quervain's thyroiditis describes the presentation of a viral infection with fever, neck pain and tenderness, **dysphagia** and features of **hyperthyroidism**. There is a **hyperthyroid** phase followed by **hypothyroid** phase as the TSH level falls due to **negative feedback**. It is a self-limiting condition and supportive treatment with **NSAIDs** for pain and inflammation and **beta blockers** for symptomatic relief of hyperthyroidism is usually all that is necessary.

Thyroid Storm

Thyroid storm is a rare presentation of **hyperthyroidism**. It is also known as **"thyrotoxic crisis"**. It is a more severe presentation of hyperthyroidism with pyrexia, tachycardia and delirium. It requires admission for monitoring and is treated the same way as any other presentation of thyrotoxicosis, although they may need supportive care with fluid resuscitation, anti-arrhythmic medication and beta blockers.

Hyperthyroidism Management

Information here is summarised from NICE CKS 2016. Treatment is guided by a specialist.

Carbimazole
Carbimazole is the **first line** anti-thyroid drug. It is usually successful in treating patients with Grave's disease, leaving them with normal thyroid function after 4 to 8 weeks. Once the patient has normal thyroid hormone levels, they continue on maintenance carbimazole and either:
- The dose is carefully titrated to maintain normal levels (known as **"titration-block"**)
- The dose is sufficient to block all production and the patient takes levothyroxine titrated to effect (known as **"block and replace"**)

Complete remission and the ability to stop taking carbimazole is usually achieved within 18 months of treatment.

Propylthiouracil
Propylthiouracil is the **second line** anti-thyroid drug. It is used in a similar way to carbimazole. There is a small risk of severe hepatic reactions, including death, which is why carbimazole is preferred.

Radioactive Iodine
Treatment with **radioactive iodine** involves drinking a single dose of radioactive iodine. This is taken up by the thyroid gland and the emitted radiation destroys a proportion of the thyroid cells. The reduction in the number of cells results in a decrease in thyroid hormone production and thus remission from the hyperthyroidism. Remission can take 6 months and patients can be left **hypothyroid** afterwards and require **levothyroxine** replacement.

With radioactive iodine there are strict rules where the patient:
- Must not be pregnant and are not allowed to get pregnant within 6 months
- Must avoid close contact with children and pregnant women for 3 weeks (depending on the dose)
- Limit contact with anyone for several days after receiving the dose

Beta-blockers
Beta-blockers are used to block the adrenalin related symptoms of hyperthyroidism. **Propranolol** is a good choice because it non-selectively blocks adrenergic activity as opposed to more "selective" beta blockers that only act on the heart. They do not actually treat the underlying problem but control the symptoms whilst the definitive treatment takes time to work. They are particularly useful in patients with *thyroid storm*.

Surgery
A definitive option is to surgically remove the whole thyroid or toxic nodules. This effectively stops the production of thyroid hormone, however the patient will be left hypothyroid post thyroidectomy and require *levothyroxine* replacement for life.

Hypothyroidism

Hypothyroidism is the term used to describe inadequate output of thyroid hormones by the thyroid gland.

Causes

Hashimoto's Thyroititis
This is the most common causes of hypothyroidism in the developed world. It is caused by autoimmune inflammation of the thyroid gland. It is associated with **antithyroid peroxidase (anti-TPO) antibodies** and **antithyroglobulin antibodies**. Initially it causes a goitre after which there is atrophy of the thyroid gland.

Iodine Deficiency
This is the most common cause of hypothyroidism in the developing world. Iodine is added to foods such as table salt to prevent iodine deficiency.

Secondary to Treatment of Hyperthyroidism
All of the treatments for hyperthyroidism have the potential to cause hypothyroidism:
- Carbimazole
- Prophylthiouracil
- Radioactive iodine
- Thyroid surgery

Medications
Lithium inhibits the production of thyroid hormones in the thyroid gland and can cause a goitre and hypothyroidism. **Amiodarone** interferes with thyroid hormone production and metabolism, usually causing hypothyroidism but it can also cause thyrotoxicosis.

Central Causes (Secondary Hypothyroidism)
This is where the **pituitary gland** is failing to produce enough TSH. This is often associated with a lack of other pituitary hormones such as ACTH. This is called **hypopituitarism** and has many causes:

- Tumours
- Infection
- Vascular (e.g. Sheehan syndrome)
- Radiation

Presentation and Features

- Weight gain
- Fatigue
- Dry skin
- Coarse hair and hair loss
- Fluid retention (including oedema, pleural effusions and ascites)
- Amenorrhoea
- Constipation

Investigations

Primary hypothyroidism is caused by thyroid gland insufficiency. Thyroid hormones (i.e. free T3 and T4) will be low. TSH will be high because there is no negative feedback to the brain, so the pituitary produces lots of TSH to try and get the thyroid working.

Secondary hypothyroidism is caused by pituitary pathology that results in low production of TSH. Thyroid hormones will be low due to the low TSH.

Thyroid Status	Site of Pathology	TSH	T3 and T4
Primary Hypothyroidism	Thyroid Gland	High	Low
Secondary Hypothyroidism	Pituitary Gland	Low	Low

Management

Replacement of thyroid hormone with oral **levothyroxine** is the treatment of hypothyroidism. Levothyroxine is **synthetic T4**, and metabolises to **T3** in the body. The **dose is titrated** until TSH levels are normal. When starting levothyroxine, initially measure TSH levels monthly until stable, then once stable it can be checked less frequently unless they become symptomatic.

If the TSH level is high, the dose is too low and needs to be increased. If the TSH is low, the dose is too high and needs to be reduced.

Type 1 Diabetes

Basic Physiology

Eating carbohydrates causes in a rise in **blood glucose** (sugar) levels. As the body uses these carbohydrates for energy there is a fall in blood glucose levels. The body ideally wants to keep blood glucose concentration **between 4.4 and 6.1 mmol/l**.

Insulin is a hormone produced by the **pancreas** that reduces blood sugar levels. It is produced by the **beta cells** in the **Islets of Langerhans** in the **pancreas**. It is an **anabolic** hormone (a building hormone). It is always present in small amounts, but increases when blood sugar levels rise. **Insulin reduces blood sugar** in two ways: Firstly, it causes cells in the body to absorb glucose from the blood and use it as fuel. Secondly, it causes muscle and liver cells to absorb glucose from the blood and store it as **glycogen**. Insulin is essential in letting cells take glucose out of the blood and use it as fuel. **Without insulin, cells cannot take up and use glucose**.

Glucagon is a hormone also produced in the **pancreas** that increases blood sugar levels. It is produced by the **alpha cells** in the **Islets of Langerhans** in the **pancreas**. It is a **catabolic** hormone (a breakdown hormone). It is released in response to low blood sugar levels and stress. It tells the liver to break down stored **glycogen** into glucose. This process is called **glycogenolysis**. It also tells the liver to convert proteins and fats into glucose. This process is called **gluconeogenesis**.

Ketogenesis

Ketogenesis occurs when there is insufficient glucose supply and glycogens stores are exhausted, such as in prolonged fasting. The liver takes **fatty acids** and converts them to **ketones**. Ketones are water soluble fatty acids that can be used as fuel. They can cross the blood brain barrier and be used by the brain. Producing ketones is normal and not harmful in healthy patients when under fasting conditions or on very low carbohydrate, high fat diets. Ketones levels can be measured in the urine by "**dip-stick**" and in the blood using a **ketone meter**. People in **ketosis** have a characteristic **acetone** smell to their breath.

Ketone acids (ketones) are buffered in normal patients so the blood does not become **acidotic**. When underlying pathology (i.e. type 1 diabetes) causes extreme **hyperglycaemic ketosis** this results in a **metabolic acidosis** that is life threatening. This is called **diabetic ketoacidosis**.

Type 1 Diabetes

Type 1 diabetes mellitus (**T1DM**) is a disease where the **pancreas** stops being able to produce **insulin**. What causes the pancreas to stop producing insulin is unclear. There may be a genetic component. It may be triggered by certain viruses, such as the **Coxsackie B virus** and **enterovirus**. When there is no insulin being produced, the cells of the body cannot take glucose from the blood and use it for fuel. Therefore the cells think the body is being fasted and has no glucose supply. Meanwhile the level of glucose in the blood keeps rising, causing **hyperglycaemia**.

Pathophysiology of Diabetic Ketoacidosis (DKA)

Diabetic ketoacidosis occurs in type 1 diabetes where the person is not producing adequate insulin themselves and is not injecting adequate insulin to compensate for this. It occurs when they body does not have enough insulin to use and process glucose. The main problems are ketoacidosis, dehydration and potassium imbalance.

Ketoacidosis

As the cells in the body have no fuel and think they are starving they initiate the process of **ketogenesis** so that they have a usable fuel. Over time the patient gets higher and higher glucose and ketones levels. Initially the kidneys produce **bicarbonate** to counteract the ketone acids in the blood and maintain a normal pH. Over time the **ketone acids** use up the bicarbonate and the blood starts to become acidic. This is called **ketoacidosis**.

Dehydration

Hyperglycaemia overwhelms the kidneys and glucose starts being filtered into the urine. The glucose in the urine draws water out with it in a process called **osmotic diuresis.** This causes the patient to urinate a lot (**polyuria**). This results in severe dehydration. The dehydration stimulates the thirst centre to tell the patient to drink lots of water. This excessive thirst is called **polydipsia**.

Potassium Imbalance

Insulin normally drives **potassium** into cells. Without insulin potassium is not added to and stored in cells. **Serum potassium** can be high or normal as the kidneys continue to balance blood potassium with the potassium excreted in the urine, however **total body potassium is low** because no potassium is stored in the cells. When treatment with insulin starts patients can develop severe **hypokalaemia** (low serum potassium) very quickly and this can lead to fatal **arrhythmias**.

Presentation of DKA

This is a life threatening medical emergency. The pathophysiology described above leads to:
- Hyperglycaemia
- Dehydration
- Ketosis
- Metabolic acidosis (with a low bicarbonate)
- Potassium imbalance

The patient will therefore present with symptoms of these abnormalities:
- Polyuria
- Polydipsia
- Nausea and vomiting
- Acetone smell to their breath
- Dehydration and subsequent hypotension
- Altered Consciousness
- They may have symptoms of an underlying trigger (i.e. sepsis)

The most dangerous aspects of DKA are **dehydration**, **potassium imbalance** and **acidosis**. These are what will kill the patient. Therefore the priority is **fluid resuscitation** to correct the dehydration, electrolyte disturbance and acidosis. This is followed by an insulin infusion to get the cells to start taking up and using glucose and stop producing ketones.

Diagnosing DKA

Check the local DKA diagnostic criteria for your hospital. To diagnose DKA you require:
- Hyperglycaemia (i.e. blood glucose > 11 mmol/l)
- Ketosis (i.e. blood ketones > 3 mmol/l)
- Acidosis (i.e. pH < 7.3)

Treating DKA (FIG-PICK)

Follow local protocols carefully.

- **F - Fluids** - IV fluid resuscitation with normal saline (e.g. 1 litre stat, then 4 litres with added potassium over the next 12 hours)
- **I - Insulin** - Add an insulin infusion (e.g. Actrapid at 0.1 Unit/kg/hour)
- **G - Glucose** - Closely monitor blood glucose and add a dextrose infusion if below a certain level (e.g. < 14 mmol/l)
- **P - Potassium** - Closely monitor serum potassium (e.g. 4 hourly) and correct as required
- **I - Infection** - Treat underlying triggers such as infection
- **C - Chart** fluid balance
- **K - Ketones** - Monitor blood ketones (or bicarbonate if ketone monitoring is unavailable)

Establish the patient on their normal subcutaneous insulin regime prior to stopping the insulin and fluid infusion.

Remember as a general rule potassium should not be infused at a rate of more than 10 mmol per hour.

Long Term Management of Type 1 Diabetes

Patient education is essential. Monitoring and treatment is relatively complex. The condition is life-long and requires the patient to fully understand and engage with their condition. It involves the following components:
- Subcutaneous insulin regimes
- Monitoring dietary carbohydrate intake
- Monitoring blood sugar levels on waking, at each meal and before bed
- Monitoring for and managing complications, both short and long term

Insulin is usually prescribed as a combination of a **background, long acting insulin** given once a day and a **short acting insulin** injected 30 minutes before intake of carbohydrates (i.e. **at meals**). Insulin regimes are initiated by a diabetic specialist.

Injecting into the same spot can cause a condition called "*lipodystrophy*", where the subcutaneous fat hardens and patients do not absorb insulin properly from further injections into this spot. For this reason patients should cycle their injection sites. If a patient is not responding to insulin as expected, ask where they inject and check for lipodystrophy.

Short Term Complications

Short term complications relate to immediate insulin and blood glucose management:
- *Hypoglycaemia*
- *Hyperglycaemia* (and DKA)

Hypoglycaemia
Hypoglycaemia is a low blood sugar level. Most patients are aware when they are hypoglycaemic by their symptoms, however some patients can be unaware until severely hypoglycaemic. Typical symptoms are tremor, sweating, irritability, dizziness and pallor. More severe hypoglycaemia will lead to reduced consciousness, coma and death unless treated.

Hypoglycaemia needs to be treated with a combination of **rapid acting glucose** such as lucozade and **slower acting carbohydrates** such as biscuits and toast for when the rapid acting glucose is used up. Options for treating severe hypoglycaemia are **IV dextrose** and **intramuscular glucagon**.

Hyperglycaemia

If the patient is hyperglycaemic but not in DKA then they may require their insulin dose to be increased. Patients will get to know their own individual response to insulin and be able to administer a dose to correct the hyperglycaemia. For example, they may learn that 1 unit of novorapid reduces their sugar level by around 4 mmol/l. Be conscious that it can take several hours to take effect and repeated doses could lead to hypoglycaemia. If they meet the criteria for DKA they need admission for treatment of DKA.

Long Term Complications

Chronic exposure to **hyperglycaemia** causes damage to the **endothelial cells** of blood vessels. This leads to leaky, malfunctioning vessels that are unable to regenerate. High levels of sugar in the blood also causes **suppression of the immune system**, and provides an optimal environment for infectious organisms to thrive.

Macrovascular Complications
- **Coronary artery disease** is a major cause of death in diabetics
- Peripheral ischaemia causes poor healing, ulcers and "**diabetic foot**"
- Stroke
- Hypertension

Microvascular Complications
- Peripheral neuropathy
- Retinopathy
- Kidney disease, particularly **glomerulosclerosis**

Infection Related Complications
- Urinary tract infections
- Pneumonia
- Skin and soft tissue infections, particularly in the feet
- Fungal infections, particularly oral and vaginal candidiasis

Monitoring

HbA1c
When we check HbA1c we are counting **glycated haemoglobin**, which is how much glucose is attached to the haemoglobin molecule. This is considered to reflect the average glucose level over the last 3 months because red blood cells have a lifespan of around 3 to 4 months. We measure it **every 3 to 6 months** to track progression of the patient's diabetes and how effective the interventions are. It requires a blood sample sent to the lab, usually red top EDTA bottle.

Capillary Blood Glucose
This is measured using a little machine called a glucose meter that gives an immediate result. Patients with type 1 and type 2 diabetes rely on these machines for self-monitoring their sugar levels.

Flash Glucose Monitoring (e.g. FreeStyle Libre)
This uses a **sensor** on the skin that measures the glucose level of **interstitial fluid**. There is a **lag of 5 minutes** behind blood glucose. This sensor records the glucose readings at short intervals so you get a really good impression of what the glucose levels are doing over time. The user needs to use a "**reader**" to swipe over the **sensor** and it is the reader that shows the blood sugar readings. Sensors need replacing every 2 weeks for the **FreeStyle Libre** system. It is quite expensive and NHS funding is only available in certain areas at present. The 5 minute delay also means it is necessary to do capillary blood glucose checks if **hypoglycaemia** is suspected.

Type 2 Diabetes

Simplified Pathophysiology

Repeated exposure to **glucose** and **insulin** makes the cells in the body become **resistant** to the effects of insulin. It therefore requires more and more insulin to produce a response from the cells to get them to take up and use glucose. Over time, the **pancreas** (specifically the **beta cells**) becomes fatigued and damaged by producing so much insulin and they start to produce less. A continued onslaught of glucose on the body in light of insulin resistance and pancreatic fatigue leads to **chronic hyperglycaemia**. Chronic hyperglycaemia leads to **microvascular**, **macrovascular** and **infectious** complications as described in the **type 1 diabetes** section.

Risk Factors

Non-Modifiable
- Older age
- Ethnicity (Black, Chinese, South Asian)
- Family history

Modifiable
- Obesity
- Sedentary lifestyles
- High carbohydrate (particularly refined carbohydrate) diet

Presentation

Consider **type 2 diabetes** in any patient fitting the **risk factors** above. It is easy to screen for diabetes with a **HbA1C** and early treatment goes a long way to prevent the long term complications. It is possible to reverse diabetes with the proper diet and lifestyle, therefore knowing about it early is worthwhile.

Symptoms of diabetes that should prompt testing:
- Fatigue
- **Polydipsia** and **polyuria** (thirsty and urinating a lot)
- Unintentional weight loss
- Opportunistic infections
- Slow healing
- Glucose in urine (on dipstick)

Oral Glucose Tolerance Test (OGTT)

An oral glucose tolerance test (OGTT) is performed in the morning prior to having breakfast. It involves taking a baseline **fasting plasma glucose** result, giving a **75g glucose drink** and then measuring plasma glucose **2 hours later**. It tests the ability of the body to cope with a carbohydrate meal.

Pre-Diabetes

Pre-diabetes is an indication that the patient is heading towards diabetes. They do not fit the full diabetic diagnostic criteria but should be educated regarding diabetes and implement lifestyle changes to reduce their risk of becoming diabetic. They are not currently recommended to start treatment at this point.

Pre-Diabetes Diagnosis

Pre-diabetes can be diagnosed with a **HbA1c** or by "**impaired fasting glucose**" or "**impaired glucose tolerance**". **Impaired fasting glucose** means their body struggles to get their blood glucose levels into normal range even after a prolonged period without eating carbohydrates. **Impaired glucose tolerance** means their body struggles to cope with processing a carbohydrate meal.

- **HbA1c** - 42 47 mmol/mol
- **Impaired fasting glucose** - fasting glucose 6.1 – 6.9 mmol/l
- **Impaired glucose tolerance** - plasma glucose at 2 hours 7.8 – 11.1 mmol/l on an **OGTT**

Diabetes Diagnosis

Diabetes can be diagnosed if the patient fits the criteria on plasma glucose, an oral glucose tolerance test or HbA1c:
- **HbA1c** >48 mmol/mol
- **Random glucose** > 11 mmol/l
- **Fasting glucose** > 7 mmol/l
- **OGTT** > 11 mmol/l

Management

Patient education about their condition and the lifestyle changes they need to make is essential. It is important to advise the patient that it is possible to cure type 2 diabetes. This has been proven in clinical studies such as the DiRECT study, where they put patients on an 800 calorie per day diet and achieved a good rate of remission.

Dietary Modification
- Vegetables and oily fish
- Typical advice is low glycaemic, high fibre diet
- A low carbohydrate diet may in fact be more effective in treating and preventing diabetes but is not yet mainstream advice

Optimise Other Risk Factors
- Exercise and weight loss
- Stop smoking
- Optimise treatment for other illnesses, for example hypertension, hyperlipidaemia and cardiovascular disease

Monitoring for Complications
- Diabetic retinopathy
- Kidney disease
- Diabetic foot

Treatment Targets

See the section on type 1 diabetes for information on the methods for monitoring blood glucose and HbA1c.

SIGN Guidelines 2017 and NICE Guideline 2015 recommend the following HbA1c treatment targets:
- 48 mmol/mol for new type 2 diabetics
- 53 mmol/mol for diabetics that have moved beyond metformin alone

Medical Management

NICE Guidelines 2015 (updated 2017):

First line: *metformin* titrated up as tolerated. Initially 500mg once daily.

Second line add: *sulfonylurea*, *pioglitazone*, *DPP-4 inhibitor* or *SGLT-2 inhibitor*. The decision should be based on individual factors and drug tolerance.

Third line:
- Triple therapy with metformin and two of the second line drugs combined, or;
- Metformin plus insulin

SIGN Guidelines 2017 suggest the use of *SGLT-2 inhibitors* (e.g. empagliflozin) or *GLP-1 mimetics* (e.g. liraglutide) preferentially in patients with cardiovascular disease.

Metformin

Metformin is a "*biguanide*". It increases insulin sensitivity and decreases liver production of glucose. It is considered to be "**weight neutral**" and does not increase or decrease body weight.

Notable side effects of metformin:
- Diarrhoea and abdominal pain. This is dose dependent and reducing the dose often resolves the symptoms
- *Lactic acidosis*
- Does NOT typically cause hypoglycaemia

Pioglitazone

Pioglitazone is a "*thiazolidinedione*". It increases insulin sensitivity and decreases liver production of glucose.

Notable side effects of pioglitazone:
- Weight gain
- Fluid retention
- Anaemia
- Heart failure
- Extended use may increase the risk of bladder cancer
- Does NOT typically cause hypoglycaemia

Sulfonylurea

The most common sulfonyluria is "**gliclazide**". Sulfonylureas stimulate insulin release from the pancreas.

Notable side effects of sulfonylureas:
- Weight gain
- Hypoglycaemia
- **Increased risk** of **cardiovascular disease** and **myocardial infarction** when used as monotherapy

Incretins (relevant for DPP-4 inhibitors and GLP-1 mimetics)

Incretins are hormones produced by the GI tract. They are secreted in response to large meals and act to reduce blood sugar. They:
- Increase insulin secretion
- Inhibit glucagon production
- Slow absorption by the GI tract

The main incretin is "**glucagon-like peptide-1**" (**GLP-1**). **Incretins** are **inhibited** by an enzyme called "**dipeptidyl peptidase-4**" (**DPP-4**).

A recent meta-analysis (JAMA 2018) showed that GLP-1 mimetics were associated with a reduction in all cause mortality whereas DPP-4 inhibitors were not.

DPP-4 Inhibitors

The most common DPP-4 inhibitor is "**sitagliptin**". It inhibits the **DPP-4 enzyme** and therefore increases **GLP-1** activity.

Notable side effects of DPP-4 inhibitors:
- GI tract upset
- Symptoms of upper respiratory tract infection
- Pancreatitis

GLP-1 Mimetics

These medications mimic the action of GLP-1. Two common GLP-1 mimetics are "**exenatide**" and "**liraglutide**". **Exenatide** is given as a subcutaneous injection either twice daily by the patient or once weekly in a **modifiable-release** form. **Liraglutide** is given daily as a subcutaneous injection. They are sometimes used in combination with metformin and a sulfonylurea in overweight patients. Liraglutide is used as a weight loss medication in the US (but not in the UK).

Notable side effects of GLP-1 mimetics:
- GI tract upset
- Weight loss
- Dizziness
- Low risk of hypoglycaemia

SGLT-2 Inhibitors

SGLT-2 inhibitors end with the suffix "**-gliflozin**", such as **empagliflozin**, **canagliflozin** and **dapagliflozin**. The SGLT-2 protein is responsible for reabsorbing glucose from the urine into the blood in the **proximal tubules** of the **kidneys**. SGLT-2 inhibitors block the action of this protein and cause glucose to be excreted in the urine.

Empagliflozin has been shown to reduce the risk of cardiovascular disease, hospitalisation with heart failure and all cause mortality in type 2 diabetes (see the EMPA-REG study). **Canagliflozin** has been shown to reduce the risk of MI, stroke, death and hospitalisation with heart failure in type 2 diabetes (see the CANVAS trial). These reduced risks are likely related to the class rather than the individual medications but have not been proven for all SGLT-2 inhibitors.

Notable side effect of SGLT-2 inhibitors:
- **Glucoseuria** (glucose in the urine)
- Increased rate of urinary tract infections
- Weight loss
- **Diabetic ketoacidosis**, notably with only moderately raised glucose. This is a rare complication

Insulin

Here are a few examples of insulins and their duration of action. They will become more relevant when you start seeing them day to day on patient prescriptions. You will get to know them well.

Rapid-acting Insulins
These start working after around 10 minutes and last around 4 hours:
- Novorapid
- Humalog
- Apidra

Short-acting Insulins
These start working in around 30 minutes and last around 8 hours:
- Actrapid
- Humulin S
- Insuman Rapid

Intermediate-acting Insulins
These start working in around 1 hour and last around 16 hours:
- Insulatard
- Humulin I
- Insuman Basal

Long-acting Insulins
These start working in around 1 hour and lasts around 24 hours:
- Lantus
- Levemir
- Degludec (lasts over 40 hours)

Combinations Insulins
These contain a rapid acting and an intermediate acting insulin. In brackets is the proportion of long to short acting:
- Humalog 25 (25:75)
- Humalog 50 (50:50)
- Novomix 30 (30:70)

Acromegaly

Acromegaly is the clinical manifestation of excessive **growth hormone** (**GH**). **Growth hormone** is produced by the **anterior pituitary gland**. The most common cause is unregulated growth hormone secretion by a **pituitary adenoma**. This adenoma can be **microscopic** or can be a significantly sized tumour that causes compression of local structures. Rarely, acromegaly can also be secondary to a cancer, such as lung or pancreatic cancer, that secretes **ectopic growth hormone releasing hormone** (**GHRH**) or **growth hormone**.

The **optic chiasm** sits just above the **pituitary gland**. The **optic chiasm** is the point where the optic nerves coming from the eyes crossover to different sides of the head. A **pituitary tumour** of sufficient size will start to press on the **optic chiasm**. Pressure on the optic chiasm will lead to a stereotypical "**bitemporal hemianopia**" visual field defect. This describes loss of vision on the outer half of both eyes.

Presentation

Space Occupying Lesion
- Headaches
- Visual field defect ("**bitemporal hemianopia**")

Overgrowth of tissues
- Prominent forehead and brow ("frontal bossing")
- Large nose
- Large tongue ("macroglossia")
- Large hands and feet
- Large protruding jaw ("prognathism")
- Arthritis from imbalanced growth of joints

GH can cause organ dysfunction
- Hypertrophic heart
- Hypertension
- Type 2 diabetes
- Colorectal cancer

Treatment

Trans-sphenoidal (through the nose and sphenoid bone) surgical removal of the **pituitary tumour** is the definitive treatment of acromegaly secondary to **pituitary adenomas**. Where **acromegaly** is caused by **ectopic** hormones from a pancreatic or lung cancer, surgical removal of these cancers is the treatment.

There are medication that can be used to block growth hormone:
- **Pegvisomant** is a GH antagonist given daily by a subcutaneous injection
- **Somatostatin analogues** block GH release (e.g. **ocreotide**)
- **Dopamine agonists** block GH release (e.g. **bromocriptine**)

Somatostatin is known as "**growth hormone inhibiting hormone**". It is normally secreted by the brain, gastro-intestinal tract and pancreas in response to complex triggers. One of the functions of somatostatin is to **block GH release** from the pituitary gland. **Dopamine** also has an **inhibitory effect on GH release**, however not as potent as somatostatin.

Hyperparathyroidism

There are four **parathyroid glands** situated in four corners of the thyroid gland. The parathyroid glands, specifically the **chief cells** in the glands, produce **parathyroid hormone** in response to **hypocalcaemia** (low blood calcium).

Parathyroid hormone acts to **raise the blood calcium** level by:
- Increasing **osteoclast** activity in bones (reabsorbing calcium from bones)
- Increasing calcium absorption from the gut
- Increasing calcium absorption from the kidneys
- Increasing **vitamin D** activity

Vitamin D acts to increase calcium absorption from the intestines. **Parathyroid hormone** acts on **vitamin D** to convert it into active forms. Therefore, vitamin D and parathyroid hormone act together to raise blood calcium levels.

Primary Hyperparathyroidism

Primary hyperparathyroidism is caused by uncontrolled parathyroid hormone produced directly by a tumour of the parathyroid glands. This leads **hypercalcaemia**: an abnormally high level of calcium in the blood. This is treated by **surgically removing the tumour**.

Secondary Hyperparathyroidism

This is where insufficient **vitamin D** or **chronic renal failure** leads to low absorption of calcium from the intestines, kidneys and bones. This causes **hypocalcaemia**: a low level of calcium in the blood.

The **parathyroid glands** reacts to the low serum calcium by excreting more parathyroid hormone. Over time the total number of cells in the parathyroid glands increase as they respond to the increased need to produce parathyroid hormone. This is called **hyperplasia**. The glands become more bulky. The **serum calcium level will be low or normal** but the **parathyroid hormone will be high**. This is treated by correcting the vitamin D deficiency or performing a renal transplant to treat renal failure.

Tertiary Hyperparathyroidism

This happen when **secondary hyperparathyroidism** continues for a long period of time. It leads to **hyperplasia** of the glands. The **baseline** level of parathyroid hormone increases dramatically. Then, when the cause of the secondary hyperparathyroidism is treated the parathyroid hormone level remains inappropriately high. This high level of parathyroid hormone in the absence of the previous pathology leads to inappropriately high absorption of calcium in the intestines, kidneys and bones causing **hypercalcaemia**. This is treated by **surgically** removing part of the parathyroid tissue to return the parathyroid hormone to an appropriate level.

Hyperparathyroidism	Cause	PTH	Calcium
Primary	Tumour	High	High
Secondary	Low vitamin D or CKD	High	Low / Normal
Tertiary	Hyperplasia	High	High

Hyperaldosteronism

Physiology

In the *afferent arteriole* in the **kidney** there are special cells called *juxtaglomerular cells*. They sense the blood pressure in these vessels. When they sense a *low blood pressure* in the **arteriole** they secrete a hormone called **renin**. The **liver** secretes a protein called **angiotensinogen**. Renin acts to convert **angiotensinogen** to **angiotensin I**. **Angiotensin I** converts to **angiotensin II** in the **lungs** with the help of **angiotensin converting enzyme** (ACE). Angiotensin II stimulates the release of aldosterone from the adrenal glands.

Aldosterone is a *mineralocorticoid* steroid hormone. It acts on the kidney to:
- Increase sodium reabsorption from the **distal tubule**
- Increase potassium secretion from the **distal tubule**
- Increase hydrogen secretion from the **collecting ducts**

Primary Hyperaldosteronism (Conn's Syndrome)

Primary hyperaldosteronism is when the adrenal glands are directly responsible for producing too much aldosterone. **Serum renin** will be low as it is suppressed by the high blood pressure. There are several possible reasons for this:
- An *adrenal adenoma* secreting aldosterone (most common)
- Bilateral adrenal hyperplasia
- Familial hyperaldosteronism type 1 and type 2 (rare)
- Adrenal carcinoma (rare)

Secondary Hyperaldosteronism

Secondary hyperaldosteronism is where excessive **renin** stimulates the adrenal glands to produce more **aldosterone**. Serum renin will be high.

There are several causes of high renin levels and they occur when the blood pressure in the kidneys is disproportionately lower than the blood pressure in the rest of the body:
- **Renal artery stenosis**
- Renal artery obstruction
- Heart failure

Renal artery stenosis is a narrowing of the artery supplying the kidney. This is usually found in patients with atherosclerosis, as an atherosclerotic plaque causes narrowing of this vessel. This is similar to the narrowing of the coronary arteries in angina. This can be confirmed with a *doppler ultrasound*, *CT angiogram* or *magnetic resonance angiography* (*MRA*).

Investigations

The best screening tool for someone that you suspect has hyperaldosteronism is to check the renin and aldosterone levels and calculate a *renin:aldosterone ratio*:
- **High aldosterone** and **low renin** indicates *primary hyperaldosteronism*
- **High aldosterone** and **high renin** indicates *secondary hyperaldosteronism*

Other investigations that relate to the effects of aldosterone:
- Blood pressure (**hypertension**)
- Serum electrolytes (**hypokalaemia**)
- Blood gas analysis (**alkalosis**)

If a high aldosterone level is found then investigate for the cause:
- CT or MRI to look for an adrenal tumour
- Renal doppler ultrasound, CT angiogram or MRA for renal artery stenosis or obstruction

Management

Aldosterone antagonists
- **Eplerenone**
- **Spironolactone**

Treat the underlying cause
- Surgical removal of the adenoma
- **Percutaneous renal artery angioplasty** via the femoral artery to treat renal artery stenosis

TOM TIP: Hyperaldosteronism is worth remembering as the most common cause of secondary hypertension. If you have a patient with a high blood pressure that is not responding to treatment consider screening for hyperaldosteronism with a renin:aldosterone ratio. One clue that could prompt you to test for hyperaldosteronism might be a low potassium however be aware that potassium levels may be normal.

Syndrome of Inappropriate Anti-Diuretic Hormone (SIADH)

Pathophysiology

Anti-diuretic hormone (**ADH**) is produced in the **hypothalamus** and secreted by the **posterior pituitary gland**. It is also known as "**vasopressin**". ADH stimulates water reabsorption from the **collecting ducts** in the kidneys. SIADH is a condition where there is inappropriately large amounts of ADH.

This may be the result of the **posterior pituitary** secreting too much ADH or the ADH may be coming from somewhere else, for example a **small cell lung cancer**.

The excessive ADH results in excessive water reabsorption in the **collecting ducts**. This water dilutes the sodium in the blood so you end up with a low sodium concentration (**hyponatraemia**). The excessive water reabsorption is not usually significant enough to cause fluid overload, therefore you end up with a "**euvolaemic hyponatraemia**". The urine becomes more concentrated as less water is excreted by the kidneys, therefore patients with SIADH have a high **urine osmolality** and high **urine sodium**.

Symptoms are Non-Specific

- Headache
- Fatigue
- Muscle aches and cramps
- Confusion
- *Severe hyponatraemia* can cause seizures and reduced consciousness

SIADH has Many Causes:

- *Post-operative* from major surgery (remember this for your surgical jobs)
- Infection, particularly *atypical pneumonia* and lung abscesses
- Head injury
- Medications (thiazide diuretics, carbamazepine, vincristine, cyclophosphamide, antipsychotics, SSRIs and NSAIDSs)
- Malignancy, particularly *small cell lung cancer*
- Meningitis

Initial Diagnosis

In a way, SIADH is a diagnosis of exclusion as we do not have a reliable test to directly measure ADH activity. Clinical examination will show *euvolaemia*. U&Es will show *hyponatraemia*. *Urine sodium* and *osmolality* will be high.

Other causes of hyponatraemia need to be excluded:
- Negative *short synacthen test* to exclude *adrenal insufficiency*
- No history of diuretic use
- No diarrhoea, vomiting, burns, fistula or excessive sweating
- No excessive water intake
- No *chronic kidney disease* or *acute kidney injury*

Establish the Cause

Sometimes the cause will be clear, for example a new medication, a chest infection or recent major surgery. This can be confirmed by treating the underlying cause and assessing whether the hyponatraemia resolves.

Perform a chest xray as a first line investigation for pneumonia, lung abscess and lung cancer.

We have to suspect malignancy in someone with persistent hyponatraemia with no clear cause, particularly in someone with a history of smoking, weight loss or other features of malignancy. If malignancy is suspected the NICE CKS (March 2015) recommend a CT thorax, abdomen and pelvis and MRI brain to find the malignancy.

Management

The aim is to establish and treat the cause of the SIADH. It is most common for medications to be the cause so if possible it is best to stop the causative medication. It is essential to correct the sodium slowly to prevent *central pontine myelinolysis*. Aim for a change in sodium of less than 10 mmol/l per 24 hours.

Fluid restriction involves restricting their fluid intake to 500 mls to 1litre. This may be enough to correct the hyponatraemia without the need for medications.

Tolvaptan. "**Vaptans**" are **ADH receptor blockers**. They are very powerful and can cause a rapid increase in sodium. Therefore they are usually initiated by a specialist endocrinologist and require close monitoring, for example 6 hourly sodium levels.

Demeclocycline is a **tetracycline antibiotic** that inhibits ADH. It was used prior to the development of vaptans and is now rarely used for this purpose.

Central Pontine Myelinolysis

Central pontine myelinolysis (**CPM**) is also (and more accurately) known as "**osmotic demyelination syndrome**". It is usually a complication of long term **severe hyponatraemia** (< 120 mmols/l) being treated too quickly (> 10 mmol/l increase over 24 hours).

As blood sodium level fall, **water** will move by **osmosis** across the **blood-brain barrier** into the cells of the brain from the area of low concentration of solutes (the blood) to the area of high concentration of solutes (the brain). This causes the brain to swell. The brain adapts to this by **reducing the solutes** in the brain cells so that water is balanced across the **blood-brain barrier** and the brain does not become **oedematous**. This adaptation takes a few days. Therefore, if the **hyponatraemia** has been present and severe for a long time the brain cells will also have a **low osmolality**. This is not a problem until the blood sodium levels rapidly rise. When this happens water will rapidly shift out of the brain cells and into the blood. This causes **two phases** of symptoms:

First phase: this is due to the electrolyte imbalance. The patient presents as encephalopathic and confused. They may have a headache or nausea and vomiting. These symptoms often resolve prior to the onset of the second phase.

Second phase: this is due to the demyelination of the neurones, particularly in the pons. This occurs a few days after the rapid correction of sodium. This may present as **spastic quadriparesis**, **pseudobulbar palsy** and **cognitive and behavioural changes**. There is a significant risk of death.

Prevention is essential as treatment is only **supportive** once **CPM** occurs. A proportion of patients make a clinical improvement but most are left with some neurological deficit.

Diabetes Insipidus

Diabetes insipidus is a lack of **antidiuretic hormone** (**ADH**) or a lack of **response** to **ADH**. This prevents the kidneys from being able to concentrate the urine leading to **polyuria** (excessive amounts of urine) and **polydipsia** (excessive thirst). It can be classified as **nephrogenic** or **cranial**.

Primary polydipsia is when the patient has a normally functioning ADH system but is drinking excessive quantities of water leading to excessive urine production. They don't have **diabetes insipidus**.

Nephrogenic Diabetes Insipidus

Nephrogenic diabetes insipidus is when the collecting ducts of the kidneys **do not respond to ADH**. It can also be caused by:
- Drugs, particularly **lithium** used in **bipolar affective disorder**

- Mutations in the AVPR2 gene on the X chromosome that codes for the ADH receptor
- Intrinsic kidney disease
- Electrolyte disturbance (*hypokalaemia* and *hypercalcaemia*)

Cranial Diabetes Insipidus

Cranial diabetes insipidus is when the **hypothalamus** does not produce ADH for the pituitary gland to secrete. It can be idiopathic, without a clear cause or it can be caused by:

- Brain tumours
- Head injury
- Brain malformations
- Brain infections (*meningitis*, *encephalitis* and *tuberculosis*)
- Brain surgery or radiotherapy

Presentation

- *Polyuria* (excessive urine production)
- *Polydipsia* (excessive thirst)
- Dehydration
- Postural hypotension
- *Hypernatraemia*

Investigations

- Low urine osmolality
- High serum osmolality
- Water deprivation test

Water Deprivation Test

The **water deprivation test** is also known as the **desmopressin stimulation test**. This is the test of choice for diagnosing **diabetes insipidus**.

Method
Initially the patient should avoid taking in any fluids for 8 hours. This is referred to as **fluid deprivation**. Then, **urine osmolality** is measured and **synthetic ADH** (**desmopressin**) is administered. 8 hours later **urine osmolality** is measured again.

Results
In **cranial diabetes insipidus** the patient lacks ADH. The kidneys are still capable of responding to ADH. Therefore initially the **urine osmolality** remains low as it continues to be diluted by excessive water secretion in the kidneys. Then when synthetic ADH is given the kidneys respond by reabsorbing water and concentrating the urine, so the urine osmolality will be high.

In **nephrogenic diabetes insipidus** the patient is unable to respond to ADH. They are diluting their urine with the excessive water secretion by the kidneys. Therefore the **urine osmolality** will be low initially and remain low even after the synthetic ADH is given.

In *primary polydipsia* the 8 hours of water deprivation will cause the **urine osmolality** to be high even before the synthetic ADH is given. A high urine osmolality after 8 hours of water deprivation indicates no diabetes insipidus.

Diagnosis	After Deprivation	After ADH
Cranial Diabetes Insipidus	Low	High
Nephrogenic Diabetes Insipidus	Low	Low
Primary Polydipsia	High	High

Management

If possible, treat underlying cause. Mild cases can be managed conservatively without any intervention.

Desmopressin (synthetic ADH) can be used in:
- Cranial diabetes insipidus to replace ADH
- Nephrogenic diabetes insipidus in higher doses under close monitoring

Phaeochromocytoma

Pathophysiology

Adrenaline is produced by the "*chromaffin cells*" in the *adrenal glands*. A *phaeochromocytoma* is a tumour of the *chromaffin cells* that secretes unregulated and excessive amounts of adrenaline. Adrenaline is a *catecholamine* hormone and neurotransmitter that stimulates the *sympathetic nervous system* and is responsible for the "fight or flight" response. In patients with a *phaeochromocytoma* the adrenaline tends to be secreted in bursts giving periods of worse symptoms followed by more settled periods.

25% are familial and associated with *multiple endocrine neoplasia type 2* (*MEN 2*).

There is a **10% rule** to describe the patterns of tumour:
- 10% bilateral
- 10% cancerous
- 10% outside the adrenal gland

Diagnosis

- **24 hour** urine *catecholamines*
- Plasma free *metanephrines*

Measuring serum *catecholamines* is unreliable as this will naturally fluctuate and it will be difficult to interpret the result. Measuring 24 hour urine *catecholamines* gives an idea of how much *adrenaline* is being secreted by the tumour over the 24 hour period.

Adrenaline has a short half life of only a few minutes in the blood, whereas **metanephrines** (a breakdown product of adrenaline) have a longer half life. This makes the level of **metanephrines** less prone to dramatic fluctuations and a more reliable diagnostic tool.

Presentation

Signs and symptoms tend to fluctuate with peaks and troughs relating to periods when the tumour is secreting adrenaline. Symptoms related to excessive adrenaline:
- Anxiety
- Sweating
- Headache
- Hypertension
- Tremor
- Palpitations, tachycardia and **paroxysmal atrial fibrillation**

Management

- Alpha blockers (i.e. **phenoxybenzamine**)
- Beta blockers once established on alpha blockers
- **Adrenalectomy** to remove the tumour is the definitive management

Patients should have symptoms controlled medically prior to surgery to reduce the risk of the anaesthetic and surgery.

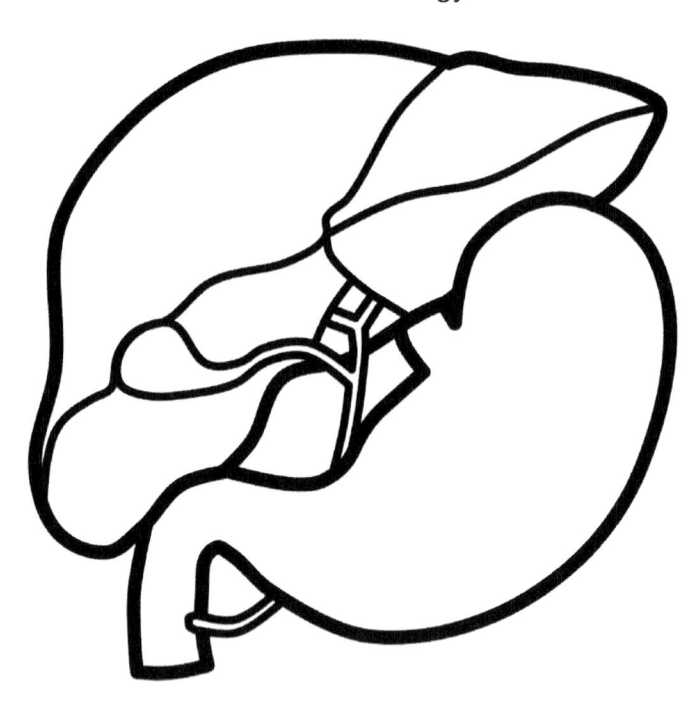

GASTROENTEROLOGY

3.1	Alcoholic Liver Disease	71
3.2	Liver Cirrhosis	74
3.3	Non Alcoholic Fatty Liver Disease	80
3.4	Hepatitis	81
3.5	Haemochromatosis	85
3.6	Wilsons Disease	86
3.7	Alpha 1 Antitrypsin Deficiency	87
3.8	Primary Biliary Cirrhosis	88
3.9	Primary Sclerosing Cholangitis	89
3.10	Liver Cancer	91
3.11	Liver Transplant	93
3.12	Gastro-Oesophageal Reflux Disease	94
3.13	Peptic Ulcers	96
3.14	Upper GI Bleed	97
3.15	Inflammatory Bowel Disease	99
3.16	Irritable Bowel Syndrome	101
3.17	Coeliac Disease	103

Alcoholic Liver Disease

The use of alcohol comes with several problems. Alcohol causes damage to various tissues in the body and can also lead to **alcohol dependence syndrome**. Here we will cover **alcoholic liver disease** and **alcohol dependence** and touch on some of the other harmful effects of alcohol consumption.

Alcoholic liver disease results from the effects of the long term excessive consumption of alcohol on the liver. The onset and progression of alcoholic liver disease varies between people, suggesting that there may be a **genetic predisposition** to having harmful effects of alcohol on the liver.

There is a stepwise process of progression of **alcoholic liver disease**:

1. **Alcohol related fatty liver**
Drinking leads to a build-up of fat in the liver. If drinking stops this process reverses in around 2 weeks.

2. **Alcoholic hepatitis**
Drinking alcohol over a long period causes inflammation in the liver sites. Binge drinking is associated with the same effect. Mild alcoholic hepatitis is usually reversible with permanent abstinence.

3. **Cirrhosis**
This is where the liver is made up of scar tissue rather than healthy liver tissue. This is irreversible. Stopping drinking can prevent further damage. Continued drinking has a very poor prognosis.

Recommended Alcohol Consumption

The latest recommendations (Department of Health, 2016) are to not regularly drink more than 14 units per week for both men and women. If drinking 14 units in a week, this should be spread evenly over 3 or more days and not more than 5 units in a single day.

The government guidelines also state that any level of alcohol consumption increases the risk of cancers, particularly breast, mouth and throat.

Pregnant women should avoid alcohol completely.

CAGE Questions

The CAGE questions can be used to quickly screen for harmful alcohol use:
- **C - C**UT DOWN? Ever thought you should?
- **A - A**NNOYED? Do you get annoyed at others commenting on your drinking?
- **G - G**UILTY? Ever feel guilty about drinking?
- **E - E**YE OPENER? Ever drink in the morning to help your hangover or nerves?

AUDIT Questionnaire

The **alcohol use disorders identification test** (**AUDIT**) was developed by the **World Health Organisation** to screen people for harmful alcohol use. It involves 10 questions with multiple choice answers and gives a score. A score of 8 or more gives an indication of harmful use.

Complications of Alcohol

- Alcoholic liver disease
- Cirrhosis and the complications of cirrhosis including hepatocellular carcinoma
- Alcohol dependence and withdrawal
- Wernicke-Korsakoff syndrome (WKS)
- Pancreatitis
- Alcoholic cardiomyopathy

Signs of Liver Disease

- Jaundice
- Hepatomegaly
- Spider naevi
- Palmar erythema
- Gynaecomastia
- Bruising (due to abnormal clotting)
- Ascites
- Caput medusae (engorged superficial epigastric veins)
- Asterixis ("flapping tremor" in decompensated liver disease)

Investigations

Bloods
- FBC shows raised MCV
- LFTs shows elevated ALT and AST (transaminases) and particularly raised **gamma-GT**. ALP will be elevated later in the disease. Low albumin due to reduced "**synthetic function**" of the liver. Elevated bilirubin in cirrhosis.
- Clotting shows elevated **prothrombin time** due to reduced "synthetic function" of the liver (reduced production of clotting factors)
- U+Es may be deranged in **hepatorenal syndrome**

Ultrasound
An ultrasound of the liver may show fatty changes early on described as "*increased echogenicity*". It can also demonstrate changes related to cirrhosis.

"**FibroScan**" can be used to check the elasticity of the liver by sending high frequency sound waves into the liver. It helps assess the degree of cirrhosis.

Endoscopy
Endoscopy can be used to assess for and treat oesophageal varices when portal hypertension is suspected.

CT and MRI scans
CT and MRI can be used to look for fatty infiltration of the liver, hepatocellular carcinoma, hepatosplenomegaly, abnormal blood vessel changes and ascites.

Liver Biopsy
Liver biopsy can be used to confirm the diagnosis of alcohol related hepatitis or cirrhosis. NICE recommend considering a liver biopsy in patients where steroid treatment is being considered.

General Management

- Stop drinking alcohol permanently
- Consider a detoxication regime
- Nutritional support with vitamins (particularly *thiamine*) and a high protein diet
- Steroids improve short term outcomes (over 1 month) in severe alcoholic hepatitis but infection and GI bleeding need to be treated first. Steroids do not improve outcomes over the long term.
- Treat complications of cirrhosis (portal hypertension, varices, ascites and hepatic encephalopathy)
- Referral for liver transplant in severe disease however they must abstain from alcohol for 3 months prior to referral

Alcohol Withdrawal

When someone is alcohol dependent there is a risk of them developing withdrawal symptoms when they stop drinking. These can range from mild and uncomfortable to *delirium tremens*, which is life threatening. Symptoms occur at different times after alcohol consumption ceases:

- 6-12 hours: tremor, sweating, headache, craving and anxiety
- 12-24 hours: *hallucinations*
- 24-48 hours: *seizures*
- 24-72 hours: *delerium tremens*

Delirium Tremens

Delirium tremens is a medical emergency associated with *alcohol withdrawal* with a mortality of 35% if left untreated. Alcohol stimulates *GABA receptors* in the brain. *GABA receptors* have a relaxing effect on the rest of the brain. Alcohol also inhibits *glutamate receptors* (also known as *NMDA receptors*) having a further inhibitory effect on the electrical activity of the brain.

Chronic alcohol use results in the *GABA system* becoming **up-regulated** and the *glutamate system* being **down-regulated** to balance the effects of alcohol. When alcohol is removed from the system, GABA under-functions and glutamate over-functions causing an extreme excitability of the brain with excessive *adrenergic* activity. This presents as:

- Acute confusion
- Severe agitation
- Delusions and hallucinations
- Tremor
- Tachycardia
- Hypertension
- Hyperthermia
- Ataxia (difficulties with coordinated movements)
- Arrhythmias

Managing Alcohol Withdrawal

The *CIWA-Ar* (clinical institute withdrawal assessment - alcohol revised) tool can be used to score the patient on their withdrawal symptoms and guide treatment.

Chlordiazepoxide ("*Librium*") is a benzodiazepine used to combat the effects of alcohol withdrawal. Diazepam is a less commonly used alternative. It is given orally as a reducing regime titrated to the required dose based on the local alcohol withdrawal protocol (e.g. 10 – 40 mg every 1 – 4 hours). This is continued for 5-7 days.

Intravenous high-dose B vitamins (*pabrinex*). This should be followed by regular lower dose oral *thiamine*. This is used to try and prevent Wernicke-Korsakoff syndrome.

Wernicke-Korsakoff Syndrome (WKS)

Alcohol excess leads to *thiamine* (*vitamin B1*) deficiency. Thiamine is poorly absorbed in the presence of alcohol. Alcoholics tend to have poor diets and rely on the alcohol for their calories. *Wernicke's encephalopathy* comes before *Korsakoffs syndrome*. These result from thiamine deficiency.

Features of Wernicke's encephalopathy
- Confusion
- Oculomotor disturbances (disturbances of eye movements)
- Ataxia (difficulties with coordinated movements)

Features of Korsakoffs syndrome
- Memory impairment (retrograde and anterograde)
- Behavioural changes

Wernicke's encephalopathy is a medical emergency and has a high mortality rate if untreated. *Korsakoffs syndrome* is often irreversible and results in patients requiring full time institutional care. Prevention and treatment involve thiamine supplementation and abstaining from alcohol.

Liver Cirrhosis

Liver cirrhosis is the result of **chronic inflammation** and damage to liver cells. When the liver cells are damaged they are replaced with scar tissue (*fibrosis*) and **nodules** of scar tissue form within the liver. This fibrosis affects the structure and blood flow through the liver, which causes increased **resistance** in the vessels leading in to the liver. This is called **portal hypertension**.

Causes

It is worth remembering the four most common causes of liver cirrhosis.
- Alcoholic liver disease
- Non alcoholic fatty liver disease
- Hepatitis B
- Hepatitis C

Cirrhosis also has a large number of rarer causes of liver damage that should also be considered as some of them are potentially reversible:
- Autoimmune hepatitis
- Primary biliary cirrhosis
- Haemochromatosis
- Wilsons disease
- Alpha-1 antitrypsin deficiency
- Cystic fibrosis
- Drugs (e.g. amiodarone, methotrexate, sodium valproate)

Signs of Cirrhosis

- Jaundice - caused by raised bilirubin
- Hepatomegaly - however the liver can shrink as it becomes more cirrhotic
- Splenomegaly - due to portal hypertension
- Spider naevi - these are telangiectasia with a central arteriole and small vessels radiating away
- Palmar erythema - caused by hyper dynamic circulation
- Gynaecomastia and testicular atrophy in males due to endocrine dysfunction
- Bruising - due to abnormal clotting
- Ascites
- Caput medusae - distended paraumbilical veins due to portal hypertension
- Asterixis - "flapping tremor" in decompensated liver disease

Investigations

Bloods
- Liver biochemistry is often normal, however in decompensated cirrhosis all of the markers (ALT, AST, ALP and bilirubin) become deranged.
- Albumin and prothrombin time are useful markers of the **synthetic function** of the liver. The albumin level drops and the prothrombin time increases as the synthetic function becomes worse.
- Hyponatraemia indicates fluid retention in severe liver disease.
- Urea and creatinine become deranged in hepatorenal syndrome.
- Further bloods can help establish the cause of the cirrhosis if unknown (such as viral markers and autoantibodies).
- Alpha-fetoprotein is a tumour marker for hepatocellular carcinoma and can be checked every 6 months as a screening test in patients with cirrhosis (along with an ultrasound scan).

Enhanced liver fibrosis (**ELF**) blood test. This is the **first line** recommended investigation for assessing fibrosis in **non-alcoholic fatty liver disease** but it is not currently available in many areas and cannot be used for diagnosing cirrhosis of other causes. It measures three markers (HA, PIIINP and TIMP-1) and uses an algorithm to provide a result that indicates the fibrosis of the liver:
- < 7.7 indicates **none to mild fibrosis**
- ≥ 7.7 to 9.8 indicates **moderate fibrosis**
- ≥ 9.8 indicates **severe fibrosis**

Ultrasound
In cirrhosis an ultrasound may show:
- Nodularity of the surface of the liver
- A "corkscrew" appearance to the hepatic arteries with increased flow as they compensate for reduced portal flow
- Enlarged portal vein with reduced flow
- Ascites
- Splenomegaly

Ultrasound is also used as a screening tool for hepatocellular carcinoma. NICE recommend screening patients with cirrhosis for HCC every 6 months.

FibroScan
"**FibroScan**" can be used to check the elasticity of the liver by sending high frequency sound waves into the liver and measuring how well they bounce back. It helps assess the degree of cirrhosis. This is called **transient elastography** and can be used to test for cirrhosis. NICE recommend retesting every 2 years in patients at risk of cirrhosis:

- Hepatitis C
- Heavy alcohol drinkers (men drinking > 50 units or women drinking > 35 units per week)
- Diagnosed alcoholic liver disease
- Non alcoholic fatty liver disease and evidence of fibrosis on the ELF blood test
- Chronic hepatitis B (they suggest yearly FibroScan for hep B)

Endoscopy

Endoscopy can be used to assess for and treat oesophageal varices when portal hypertension is suspected.

CT and MRI scans

CT and MRI can be used to look for hepatocellular carcinoma, hepatosplenomegaly, abnormal blood vessel changes and ascites.

Liver Biopsy

Liver biopsy can be used to confirm the diagnosis of cirrhosis.

Child-Pugh Score for Cirrhosis

Each factor is taken into account and given as score of 1, 2 or 3. The minimum score is 5 and the maximum score is 15. The score then indicates the severity of the cirrhosis and the prognosis.

Feature	Score 1	Score 2	Score 3
Bilirubin	<34	34-50	>50
Albumin	>35	28-35	<28
INR	<1.7	1.7-2.3	>2.3
Ascites	None	Mild	Moderate or severe
Encephalopathy	None	Mild	Moderate or severe

MELD Score

The MELD score is recommended by NICE to be used every 6 months in patients with compensated cirrhosis. It is a formula that takes into account the bilirubin, creatinine, INR and sodium and whether they are requiring dialysis. It gives a percentage estimated 3 month mortality and helps guide referral for liver transplant.

General Management

- Ultrasound and alpha-fetoprotein every 6 months for hepatocellular carcinoma
- Endoscopy every 3 years in patients without known varices
- High protein, low sodium diet
- MELD score every 6 months
- Consideration of a liver transplant
- Managing complications as below

Complications of Cirrhosis

The course of the disease is variable. 5 year survival is overall about 50% once cirrhosis has developed. The Child-Pugh score and the MELD score can be used as prognostic tools. There are several important complications of cirrhosis that we will go through below:
- Malnutrition
- Portal hypertension, varices an variceal bleeding
- Ascites and spontaneous bacterial peritonitis (SBP)
- Hepatorenal syndrome
- Hepatic encephalopathy
- Hepatocellular carcinoma

Malnutrition

Cirrhosis leads to malnutrition and muscle wasting. A simplified explanation is that it leads to increased use of muscle tissue as fuel and reduces the protein available in the body for muscle growth. Cirrhosis affects protein metabolism in the liver and reduces the amount of protein produced. It also disrupts the ability of the liver to store glucose as glycogen and release it when required. This results in the body using muscle tissue as fuel, leading to muscle wasting and weight loss.

Management
- Regular meals (every 2-3 hours)
- Low sodium diet to minimise fluid retention
- High protein and high calorie diet, particularly if underweight
- Avoid alcohol

Portal Hypertension and Varices

The **portal vein** comes from the **superior mesenteric vein** and the **splenic vein** and delivers blood to the liver. **Liver cirrhosis** increases the resistance of blood flow in the liver. As a result, there is increased back-pressure into the **portal system**. This is called **portal hypertension**. This back-pressure causes the vessels at the sites where the portal system **anastomoses** with the **systemic venous system** to become swollen and tortuous. These swollen, tortuous vessels are called **varices**. They occur at the:
- Gastro oesophageal junction
- Ileocaecal junction
- Rectum
- Anterior abdominal wall via the umbilical vein (**caput medusae**)

Varices do not cause symptoms or problems until they start bleeding. Due to the high blood flow through varices, once they start bleeding patients can **exsanguinate** (bleed out) very quickly.

Treatment of stable varices

- Propranolol reduces portal hypertension by acting as a non-selective beta blocker
- Elastic band ligation of varices
- Injection of sclerosant (less effective than band ligation)

Transjugular intra-hepatic portosystemic shunt (**TIPS**) is a technique where an interventional radiologist inserts a wire under xray guidance into the jugular vein, down the vena cava and into the liver via the hepatic vein. They then make a connection through the liver tissue between the **hepatic vein** and the **portal vein** and put a stent in place. This allows blood to flow directly from the portal vein to the hepatic vein and relieves the pressure in the portal system and varices. This is used if medical and endoscopic treatment of varices fail or if there are bleeding varices that cannot be controlled in other ways.

Bleeding Oesophageal Varices

Resuscitation
- **Vasopressin analogues** (i.e. **terlipressin**) cause vasoconstriction and slow bleeding in varices
- Correct any **coagulopathy** with **vitamin K** and **fresh frozen plasma** (which is full of clotting factors)
- Giving prophylactic **broad spectrum antibiotics** has been shown to reduce mortality
- Consider intubation and intensive care as they can bleed very quickly and become life threateningly unwell

Urgent Endoscopy
- Injection of **sclerosant** into the varices can be used to cause "**inflammatory obliteration**" of the vessel
- Elastic band ligation of varices

A **Sengstaken-Blakemore tube** is an inflatable tube inserted into the oesophagus to tamponade the bleeding varices. This is used when endoscopy fails.

Ascites

Ascites is basically fluid in the **peritoneal cavity**. The increased pressure in the portal system causes fluid to lead out of the capillaries in the liver and bowel into the peritoneal cavity. The drop in circulating volume caused by fluid loss into the peritoneal cavity causes a reduction in blood pressure entering the kidneys. The kidneys sense this lower pressure and release **renin**, which leads to increased **aldosterone** secretion (via the **renin-angiotensin-aldosterone system**). Increased aldosterone causes reabsorption of fluid and sodium in the kidneys, leading to fluid and sodium overload. Cirrhosis causes a **transudative**, meaning low protein content, ascites.

Management
- Low sodium diet
- Anti-aldosterone diuretics (spironolactone)
- Paracentesis (ascitic tap or ascitic drain)
- Prophylactic antibiotics against spontaneous bacterial peritonitis (ciprofloxacin or norfloxacin) in patients with less than 15g/litre of protein in the ascitic fluid
- Consider TIPS procedure in refractory ascites
- Consider liver transplantation in refractory ascites

Spontaneous Bacterial Peritonitis (SBP)

This occurs in around 10% of patients with ascites secondary to cirrhosis and can have a mortality of 10-20%. It involves an infection developing in the ascitic fluid and peritoneal lining without any clear cause (e.g. not secondary to an ascitic drain or bowel perforation).

Presentation
- Can be asymptomatic so have a low threshold for ascitic fluid culture
- Fever
- Abdominal pain
- Deranged bloods (raised WBC, CRP, creatinine or metabolic acidosis)

- Ileus (reduce movement in the intestines)
- Hypotension

Most common organisms
- Escherichia coli
- Klebsiella pnuemoniae
- Gram positive cocci (such as staphylococcus and enterococcus)

Management
- Take an ascitic culture prior to giving antibiotics
- Usually treated with an IV cephalosporin such as **cefotaxime**

Hepatorenal Syndrome

Hepatorenal syndrome occurs in **liver cirrhosis**. **Hypertension** in the **portal system** leads to stretching of the portal blood vessels causing dilatation. This leads to a loss of blood volume in other areas of the circulation, including the kidneys. Hypotension in the kidney leads to activation of the **renin-angiotensin system**. This causes renal **vasoconstriction**, which combined with low circulation volume leads to starvation of blood to the kidney. This leads to rapidly deteriorating kidney function. **Hepatorenal syndrome** is fatal within a week or so unless liver transplant is performed.

Hepatic Encephalopathy

This is also known as **portosystemic encephalopathy**. It is thought to be caused by the build up of toxins that affect the brain. One toxin that is particularly worth remembering is **ammonia**, which is produced by intestinal bacteria when they break down proteins. Ammonia is absorbed in the gut. There are two reasons that ammonia builds up in the blood in patients with cirrhosis: Firstly, the functional impairment of the liver cells prevents them metabolising the ammonia into harmless waste products. Secondly, collateral vessels between the portal and systemic circulation mean that the ammonia bypasses the liver altogether and enters the systemic system directly.

By giving **laxatives** we help clear the ammonia from the gut before it is absorbed. By giving **antibiotics** we reduce the number of bacteria in the gut producing ammonia.

Acutely, it presents with reduced consciousness and confusion. It can present more chronically with changes to personality, memory and mood.

Precipitating Factors
- Constipation
- Electrolyte disturbance
- Infection
- GI bleeding
- High protein diet
- Medications (particularly sedative medications)

Management
- Laxatives (i.e. lactulose) promote the excretion of ammonia. The aim is 2-3 soft motions daily. They may require enemas initially.
- Antibiotics (i.e. rifaximin) reduces the number of intestinal bacteria producing ammonia. Rifaximin is useful as it is poorly absorbed and so stays in the GI tract.
- Nutritional support. They may need nasogastric feeding.

Non Alcoholic Fatty Liver Disease

Non alcholic fatty liver disease (**NAFLD**) forms part of the "**metabolic syndrome**" group of chronic health conditions relating to processing and storing energy that increase the risk of heart disease, stroke and diabetes. It is estimated that up to 30% of adults have NAFLD. It is characterised by fat deposited in liver cells. These fat deposits can interfered with the functioning of the liver cells. NAFLD does not cause problems initially, however it can progress to **hepatitis** and **cirrhosis**.

Stages

1. Non-alcoholic fatty liver disease
2. Non-alcoholic steatohepatitis (NASH)
3. Fibrosis
4. Cirrhosis

Risk factors

NAFLD shares the same risk factors as for cardiovascular disease and diabetes.
- Obesity
- Poor diet and low activity levels
- Type 2 diabetes
- High cholesterol
- Middle age onwards
- Smoking
- High blood pressure

Investigating Abnormal Liver Function Tests

When someone presents with abnormal liver function tests without a clear cause you will often be advised to perform a **non-invasive liver screen**. This is used to assess for possible underlying causes of liver pathology and includes:
- Ultrasound liver
- **Hepatitis B** and **C** serology
- Autoantibodies (**autoimmune hepatitis**, **primary biliary cirrhosis** and **primary sclerosing cholangitis**)
- Immunoglobulins (**autoimmune hepatitis** and **primary biliary cirrhosis**)
- Caeruloplasmin (**Wilsons disease**)
- Alpha 1 anti-trypsin levels (**alpha 1 anti-trypsin deficiency**)
- Ferritin and transferrin saturation (**hereditary haemochromatosis**)

Autoantibodies
- Antinuclear antibodies (ANA)
- Smooth muscle antibodies (SMA)
- Antimitochondrial antibodies (AMA)
- Antibodies to liver kidney microsome type-1 (LKM-1)

Investigation in Non-Alcoholic Fatty Liver Disease

Liver ultrasound can confirm the diagnosis of hepatic steatosis (fatty liver). It does not indicate the severity, the function of the liver or whether there is liver fibrosis.

Enhanced liver fibrosis (**ELF**) blood test. This is the **first line** recommended investigation for assessing fibrosis but it is not currently available in many areas. It measures three markers (HA, PIIINP and TIMP-1) and uses an algorithm to provide a result that indicates the fibrosis of the liver:
- < 7.7 indicates **none to mild fibrosis**
- ≥ 7.7 to 9.8 indicates **moderate fibrosis**
- ≥ 9.8 indicates **severe fibrosis**

NAFLD fibrosis score is the **second line** recommended assessment for liver fibrosis where the ELF test is not available. It is based on an algorithm of age, BMI, liver enzymes, platelets, albumin and diabetes and is helpful in **ruling out** fibrosis. It is not helpful for assessing the severity when NAFLD is present.

Fibroscan is the third line investigation. It involves a special type of ultrasound that measures the stiffness of the liver and gives an indication of fibrosis. This is performed if the ELF blood test or NAFLD fibrosis score indicates fibrosis.

Management

- Weight loss
- Exercise
- Stop smoking
- Control of diabetes, blood pressure and cholesterol
- Avoid alcohol
- Refer patients with **liver fibrosis** to a liver specialist where they may treat with **vitamin E** or **pioglitazone**.

Hepatitis

Hepatitis describes *inflammation* in the *liver*. This can vary from chronic low level inflammation to acute and severe inflammation that leads to large areas of necrosis and liver failure.

Causes

- Alcoholic hepatitis
- Non alcoholic fatty liver disease
- Viral hepatitis
- Autoimmune hepatitis
- Drug induced hepatitis (e.g. paracetamol overdose)

Presentation

Hepatitis may be asymptomatic or could present with non-specific symptoms:
- Abdominal pain
- Fatigue
- Pruritis (itching)
- Muscle and joint aches
- Nausea and vomiting
- Jaundice
- Fever (viral hepatitis)

Typical biochemical findings are that **liver function tests** become deranged with high **transaminases** (AST and ALT) with proportionally less of a rise in ALP. This is referred to as a **hepatitic picture**. **Transaminases** are liver enzymes that are released into the blood as a result of inflammation of the liver cells. **Bilirubin** can also rise as a result of inflammation of the liver cells. High bilirubin causes **jaundice**.

Hepatitis A

Hepatitis A is the most common viral hepatitis worldwide but it is relatively rare in the UK with under 1000 cases in England and Wales in 2017. It is an **RNA virus**. It is transmitted via the **faecal-oral route**, usually in contaminated water or food. It presents with nausea, vomiting, anorexia and jaundice. It can cause **cholestasis** (slowing of bile flow through the biliary system) with dark urine and pale stools and moderate hepatomegaly. It resolves without treatment in around 1 to 3 months. Management is with basic analgesia. Vaccination is available to reduce the chance of developing the infection. It is a notifiable disease and Public Health need to be notified of all cases.

Hepatitis B

Hepatitis B is a **DNA virus**. It is transmitted by direct contact with blood or bodily fluids, such as during sexual intercourse or sharing needles (i.e. IV drug users or tattoos). It can also be passed through sharing contaminated household products such as toothbrushes or contact between minor cuts or abrasions. It can also be passed from mother to child during pregnancy and delivery. This is known as **vertical transmission**.

Most people fully recover from the infection within 2 months, however 10-15% go on to become chronic hepatitis B **carriers**. In these patients the virus DNA has integrated into their own DNA and they continue to produce the viral proteins.

Viral markers
Remember that antibodies are produced by the immune system against pathogen proteins. Antigens are proteins that are targeted by the antibodies, in this scenario they are part of the virus. The different antigens and antibodies can be difficult to understand. Check out the video on the Zero to Finals YouTube channel explaining this in a simple way.

- **Surface antigen** (**HBsAg**) – active infection
- **E antigen** (**HBeAg**) - marker of viral replication and implies high infectivity
- **Core antibodies** (**HBcAb**) – implies past or current infection
- **Surface antibody** (**HBsAb**) - implies vaccination or past or current infection
- **Hepatitis B virus DNA** (**HBV DNA**) - this is a direct count of the viral load

When screening for hepatitis B, test **HBcAb** (for previous infection) and **HBsAg** (for active infection). If these are positive then do further testing for **HBeAg** and **viral load** (**HBV DNA**).

HBsAb demonstrates an immune response to HBsAg. The HBsAg is given in the vaccine, so having a positive HBsAb may simply indicate they have been vaccinated and created an immune response to the vaccine. The HBsAb may also be present in response to an infection. The other viral markers are necessary to distinguish between previous vaccination or infection.

HBcAb can help distinguish acute, chronic and past infections. We can measure IgM and IgG versions of the HBcAb. IgM implies an active infection and will give a high titre with an acute infection and a low titre with a chronic infection. IgG indicates a past infection where the HBsAg is negative.

HBeAg is important. Where the HBeAg is present it implies the patient is in an *acute phase* of the infection where the virus is actively replicating. The level of HBeAg correlates with their *infectivity*. If the HBeAg is higher, they are highly infectious to others. When they HBeAg is negative but the HBeAb is positive, this implies they have been through a phase where the virus was replicating but the virus has now stopped replicating and they are less infectious.

Vaccination

Vaccination is available and involves injecting the hepatitis B surface antigen. Vaccinated patients are tested for HBsAb to confirm their response to the vaccine. The vaccine requires 3 doses at different intervals. Vaccination to hepatitis B is now included as part of the UK routine vaccination schedule (as part of the *6 in 1 vaccine*).

Management:
- Have a low threshold for screening patients that are at risk of hepatitis B
- Screen for other blood born viruses (hepatitis A and B and HIV) and other sexually transmitted diseases
- Refer to gastroenterology, hepatology or infectious diseases for specialist management
- Notify Public Health (it is a notifiable disease)
- Stop smoking and alcohol
- Education about reducing transmission and informing potential at risk contacts
- Testing for complications: FibroScan for cirrhosis and ultrasound for hepatocellular carcinoma
- Antiviral medication can be used to slow the progression of the disease and reduce infectivity
- Liver transplantation for end-stage liver disease

Hepatitis C

Basics
Hepatitis C is an *RNA virus*. It is spread by blood and body fluids. No vaccine is available. It is now curable with *direct acting antiviral* medications.

Disease Course
- 1 in 4 fights off the virus and makes a full recovery
- 3 in 4 it becomes chronic

Complications
- *Liver cirrhosis* and associated complications of cirrhosis
- *Hepatocellular carcinoma*

Testing
- Hepatitis C antibody is the screening test
- Hepatitis C RNA testing is used to confirm the diagnosis of hepatitis C, calculate viral load and assess for the individual genotype

Management
- Have a low threshold for screening patients that are at risk of hepatitis C
- Screen for other blood born viruses (hepatitis A and B and HIV) and other sexually transmitted diseases
- Refer to gastroenterology, hepatology or infectious diseases for specialist management
- Notify *Public Health* (it is a notifiable disease)
- Stop smoking and alcohol
- Education about reducing transmission and informing potential at risk contacts
- Testing for complications: *FibroScan* for cirrhosis and ultrasound for *hepatocellular carcinoma*

- Antiviral treatment with **direct acting antivirals** (DAAs) is tailored to the specific viral genotype. They successfully cure the infection in over 90% of patients. They are typically taken for 8 to 12 weeks
- Liver transplantation for end-stage liver disease

Hepatitis D

Hepatitis D is an **RNA virus**. It can only survive in patients who also have a hepatitis B infection. It attaches itself to the HBsAg to survive and cannot survive without this protein. There are very low rates in the UK. Hepatitis D increases the complications and disease severity of hepatitis B. There is no specific treatment for hepatitis D. It is a notifiable disease and **Public Health** need to be notified of all cases.

Hepatitis E

Hepatitis E is an **RNA virus**. It is transmitted by the **faecal oral** route. It is very rare in the UK. Normally it produces only a mild illness, the virus is cleared within a month and no treatment is required. Rarely it can progress to chronic hepatitis and liver failure, more so in patients that are immunocompromised. There is no vaccination. It is a notifiable disease and Public Health need to be notified of all cases.

Autoimmune Hepatitis

Autoimmune hepatitis is a rare cause of chronic hepatitis. We are not sure of the exact cause, however it could be associated with a genetic predisposition and triggered by environmental factors such as a viral infection that causes a T cell-mediated response against the liver cells. The T cells of the immune system recognise the liver cells as being harmful and alert the rest of the immune system to attack these cells.

There are **two types** that have different ages of onset and autoantibodies:
- Type 1: occurs in adults
- Type 2: occurs in children

In type 1, women around their late forties or fifties present around or after the menopause with fatigue and features of liver disease on examination. The presentation is less acute than type 1.

In type 2, patients in their teenage years or early twenties present with acute hepatitis with high transaminases and jaundice.

Investigations will show raised transaminases (ALT and AST) and IgG levels. It is associated with many autoantibodies.

Type 1 Autoantibodies:
- Anti-nuclear antibodies (ANA)
- Anti-smooth muscle antibodies (anti-actin)
- Anti-soluble liver antigen (anti-SLA/LP)

Type 2 Autoantibodies:
- Anti-liver kidney microsomes-1 (anti-LKM1)
- Anti-liver cytosol antigen type 1 (anti-LC1)

Diagnosis can be confirmed using a liver biopsy.

Treatment is with high dose steroids (**prednisolone**) that are tapered over time as other immunosuppressants, particularly **azathioprine**, are introduced. Immunosuppressant treatment is usually successful in inducing remission, however it is usually required life long. Liver transplant may be required in end stage liver disease, however the autoimmune hepatitis can recur in transplanted livers.

Haemochromatosis

Haemochromatosis is an iron storage disorder that results in excessive total body iron and deposition of iron in tissues. The **human haemochromatosis protein** (**HFE**) gene is located on **chromosome 6**. The majority of cases of haemochromatosis relate to mutations in this gene, however there are other genes that can cause the condition. The haemochromatosis genetic mutation is **autosomal recessive**. This gene is important in regulating iron metabolism.

Symptoms

Haemochromatosis usually presents after the age of 40 when the iron overload becomes symptomatic. It presents later in females due to menstruation acting to regularly eliminate iron from the body. It presents with:
- Chronic tiredness
- Joint pain
- Pigmentation (bronze colouration)
- Hair loss
- Erectile dysfunction
- Amenorrhoea
- Cognitive symptoms (memory and mood disturbance)

Diagnosis

The main diagnostic method is to perform a **serum ferritin** level. Ferritin is an **acute phase reactant**, meaning that it goes up with **inflammatory** conditions such as infection. Performing a **transferrin saturation** is helpful in distinguishing between a high ferritin caused by **iron overload** (in which case **transferrin saturation is high**) from a high ferritin due to other causes such as inflammation or non alcoholic fatty liver disease. If serum ferritin and transferrin saturation is high and there is no other reason then **genetic testing** can be performed to confirm haemochromatosis.

Liver biopsy with **Perl's stain** can be used to establish the iron concentration in the **parenchymal** cells. This used to be the gold standard for diagnosis but it has been replaced by genetic testing.

A **CT abdomen** scan can show a non-specific increase in **attenuation** of the liver.

MRI can give a more detailed picture of liver deposits of iron. It can also be used to look at iron deposits in the heart.

Complications

- Type 1 diabetes (iron affects the functioning of the pancreas)
- Liver cirrhosis
- Iron deposits in the pituitary and gonads lead to endocrine and sexual problems (hypogonadism, impotence, amenorrhea and infertility)
- **Cardiomyopathy** (iron deposits in the heart)

- **Hepatocellular Carcinoma**
- **Hypothyroidism** (iron deposits in the thyroid)
- **Chrondocalcinosis** (calcium deposits in joints) causing arthritis

Management

- **Venesection** (a weekly protocol of removing blood to decrease total iron)
- Monitoring serum ferritin
- Monitoring and treatment of complications

Wilson Disease

Wilson disease is the excessive accumulation of copper in the body and tissues. It is caused by a mutation in the "**Wilson disease protein**" on **chromosome 13**. The Wilson disease protein also has the catchy name "**ATP7B copper-binding protein**" and is responsible for various functions, including the removal of excess copper in the liver. Genetic inheritance is **autosomal recessive**.

Features

Most patients with Wilson disease present with one or more of:
- Hepatic problems (40%)
- Neurological problems (50%)
- Psychiatric problems (10%)

Copper deposition in the liver leads to **chronic hepatitis** and eventually liver **cirrhosis.** Copper deposition in the **central nervous system** can lead to **neurological** and **psychiatric** problems.

Neurological symptoms can be subtle and range from concentration and coordination difficulties to **dysarthria** (speech difficulties) and **dystonia** (abnormal muscle tone). Copper deposition in the **basal ganglia** leads to **Parkinsonism** (tremor, bradykinesia and rigidity). These Parkinsonism symptoms are symmetrical, differentiating them from the asymmetrical symptoms in Parkinson disease.

Psychiatric symptoms can vary from mild **depression** to full **psychosis** and the underlying cause of Wilson disease is often missed and treatment delayed.

Kayser-Fleischer rings in **cornea** (deposition of copper in **Descemet's corneal membrane**) can be present in patients in Wilson disease. These are brownish circles surrounding the iris. They can usually be seen by the naked eye but proper assessment is made using **slit lamp examination**.

Other features:
- Haemolytic anaemia
- Renal tubular damage leading to **renal tubular acidosis**
- **Osteopenia** (loss of bone mineral density)

Diagnosis

The initial investigation of choice is the **serum caeruloplasmin**. Caeruloplasmin is the protein that carries copper in the blood. It can be falsely normal or elevated in cancer or inflammatory conditions, therefore it is not specific to Wilson disease.

Liver biopsy to check the liver copper content is the definitive gold standard test for diagnosis. Diagnosis can also be established if the **24-hour urine copper assay** is sufficiently elevated. Alternatively there are **scoring systems** that take into account various features and laboratory tests to establish a diagnosis of Wilson disease.

Other investigations:
- Low serum copper
- Kayser-Fleischer rings
- MRI brain shows nonspecific changes

Management

Treatment is with copper chelation using:
- *Penicillamine*
- *Trientene*

Alpha 1 Antitrypsin Deficiency

Alpha 1 antitrypsin deficiency is an *inherited* deficiency of a *protease inhibitor* called *alpha 1 antitrypsin*. This leads to an excess of *protease enzymes* that attack the liver and lung tissue and cause liver cirrhosis and lung disease.

Pathophysiology

Elastase is an enzyme secreted by **neutrophils**. This enzyme digests connective tissues. **Alpha-1-antitrypsin (A1AT)** is present in tissues to inhibit the **neutrophil elastase** and protect tissues. A1AT is coded for on **chromosome 14**. In A1AT deficiency, there is an **autosomal recessive** defect in the gene for A1AT. This results in a lack of protection against neutrophil elastase, leading to connective tissue damage.

Two main organs are affected, the liver and the lungs. It leads to:
- *Liver cirrhosis* after 50 years old
- *Pulmonary basal emphysema* after 30 years old

Diagnosis

- Low **serum alpha 1 antitrypsin**. This is the screening test of choice.
- **Liver biopsy** shows cirrhosis and *acid-Schiff-positive staining globules* (this is a test to stain the breakdown products of the action of the proteases) in hepatocytes
- **Genetic testing** for the A1AT gene
- **High resolution CT thorax** diagnoses pulmonary emphysema

Management

- Stop smoking (smoking dramatically accelerates emphysema)
- Symptomatic management
- NICE recommend **against** the use of replacement **alpha 1 antitrypsin**, however the research and debate is ongoing regarding the possible benefits
- **Organ transplant** for end stage liver or lung disease
- Monitoring for complications (e.g. **hepatocellular carcinoma**)

Primary Biliary Cirrhosis

Pathophysiology

Primary biliary cirrhosis is a condition where the immune system attacks the **small bile ducts** in the liver. The first parts to be affected are the **intralobar ducts**, also known as the **Canals of Hering**. This causes obstruction of the outflow of bile, which is called **cholestasis**. The back-pressure of the bile obstruction and the overall disease process ultimately leads to fibrosis, cirrhosis and liver failure.

Bile acids, **bilirubin** and **cholesterol** are usually excreted through the bile ducts into the intestines. When there is obstruction to the outflow of these chemicals they build up in the blood as they are not being excreted. Raised bile acids cause itching and raised bilirubin causes jaundice. Raised cholesterol causes cholesterol deposits in the skin called **xanthelasma**. **Xanthoma** are larger nodular deposits of cholesterol in the skin or tendons. Cholesterol deposits in blood vessels increase the risk of cardiovascular disease.

Bile acids are normally responsible for helping the gut digest fats. Having a lack bile acids in the stool cause gastrointestinal disturbance, malabsorption of fat and **greasy stools**. Bilirubin normally causes the dark colour of stools, so a lack of bilirubin causes **pale stools**.

Presentation

- Fatigue
- Pruritus
- GI disturbance and abdominal pain
- Jaundice and pale, greasy stools
- **Xanthoma** and **xanthelasma**
- Signs of cirrhosis and failure (e.g. ascites, splenomegaly, spider naevi)

Associations

- Middle aged women
- Other autoimmune diseases (e.g. thyroid, coeliac)
- Rheumatoid conditions (e.g. systemic sclerosis, Sjogrens and rheumatoid arthritis)

Diagnosis

Liver Function Tests
- **Alkaline phososphatase** is first liver enzyme to be raised (as with most obstructive pathology)
- Other liver enzymes and bilirubin are raised later in the disease

Autoantibodies
- **Anti-mitochondrial antibodies** are the most specific to PBC and form part of the diagnostic criteria
- **Anti-nuclear antibodies** are present in about 35% of patients

Other blood tests:
- Raised ESR
- Raised IgM

Liver biopsy is used in diagnosing and staging the disease.

Treatment

- **Ursodeoxycholic acid** reduces the intestinal absorption of cholesterol
- **Colestyramine** is a bile acid sequestrate. It binds to bile acids to prevent absorption in the gut and can help with pruritus due to raised bile acids.
- Liver transplant in end stage liver disease
- Immunosuppression (e.g. with steroids) is considered in some patients

Disease Progression

Disease course and symptoms vary significantly. Some people live decades without symptoms. The most important end results of the disease are **advanced liver cirrhosis** and **portal hypertension**.

Some other issues and complications are:
- Symptomatic pruritus
- Fatigue
- Steatorrhoea (greasy stools due to lack of bile salts to digest fats)
- Distal ronal tubular acidosis
- Hypothyroidism
- Osteoporosis
- Hepatocellular carcinoma

Primary Sclerosing Cholangitis

Primary sclerosing cholangitis is a condition where the intrahepatic or extrahepatic ducts become strictured and fibrotic. This causes an obstruction to the flow of bile out of the liver and into the intestines. **Sclerosis** refers to the stiffening and hardening of the bile ducts, and **cholangitis** is inflammation of the bile ducts. Chronic bile obstruction eventually leads to liver inflammation (**hepatitis**), **fibrosis** and **cirrhosis**.

The cause is mostly unclear although there is likely to be a combination of genetic, autoimmune, intestinal microbiome and environmental factors. There is an established association with **ulcerative colitis**, with around 70% of cases being alongside pre-existing ulcerative colitis.

Risk Factors

- Male
- Aged 30-40
- Ulcerative colitis
- Family history

Presentation

- Jaundice
- Chronic right upper quadrant pain
- Pruritus
- Fatigue
- Hepatomegaly

Liver Function Tests

Liver function tests show a "**cholestatic**" picture. This means alkaline phosphatase is the most deranged LFT and may be the only abnormality at first.

There may be a rise in bilirubin as the strictures become more severe and prevent bilirubin from being excreted through the bile duct. Other LFTs (i.e. transaminases: ALT and AST) can also be deranged, particularly as the disease progresses to hepatitis.

Autoantibodies

No antibodies are highly sensitive or specific to PSC. They aren't very helpful in diagnosis but they can indicate where there is an autoimmune element to the disease that may respond to immunosuppression. The main autoantibodies are:
- Antineutrophil cytoplasmic antibody (p-ANCA) in up to 94%
- Antinuclear antibodies (ANA) in up to 77%
- Anticardiolipin antibodies (aCL) in up to 63%

Diagnosis

The gold standard investigation for diagnosis is an MRCP, which is short for magnetic resonance cholangiopancreatography. This involves an MRI scan of the liver, bile ducts and pancreas. In primary sclerosis cholangitis it may show bile duct lesions or strictures.

Associations and complications

- Acute bacterial cholangitis
- Cholangiocarcinoma develops in 10-20% of cases
- Colorectal cancer
- Cirrhosis and liver failure

- Biliary strictures
- Fat soluble vitamin deficiencies

Management

Liver transplant can be curative but is associated with its own problems (around 80% survival at 5 years).

- ERCP can be used to dilate and stent any strictures
- **Ursodeoxycholic acid** is used and may slow disease progression
- **Colestyramine** is a bile acid sequestrate. It binds to bile acids to prevent absorption in the gut and can help with pruritus due to raised bile acids.
- Monitoring for complications such as **cholangiocarcinoma**, **cirrhosis** and **oesophageal varices**

ERCP

ERCP (**endoscopic retrograde cholangio-pancreatography**) involves inserting a endoscope through the persons oesophagus, stomach and duodenum to the point in the duodenum where the bile ducts empty into the GI tract. They then go through the **sphincter of Oddi** into the **ampulla of Vater**. From the ampulla of Vater they can enter the bile ducts and inject contrast and use X rays to identify any strictures. These strictures can then be dilated and stented during the same procedure, providing improved flow through those ducts and an improvement in symptoms.

Liver Cancer

Primary liver cancer is cancer that originates in the liver. There are two main types: **hepatocellular carcinoma** (80%) and **cholangiocarcinoma** (20%).

Secondary liver cancer is cancer that originates outside the liver and **metastasises** to the liver. Metastasis to the liver can occur in almost any cancer that spreads. There is a poor prognosis when there is cancer with liver metastasis. The first stage is to search for the primary (e.g. full body CT scan and thorough history and examination of the skin and breasts). It is not uncommon to have liver metastases of unknown primary.

Risk factors

The main risk factor for **hepatocellular carcinoma** (**HCC**) is liver **cirrhosis** due to:
- Viral hepatitis (B and C)
- Alcohol
- Non alcoholic fatty liver disease
- Other chronic liver disease

Patients with chronic liver disease are screened for HCC.

Cholangiocarcinoma is associated with **primary sclerosing cholangitis**. However, only 10% of patients with **cholangiocarcinoma** had **primary sclerosing cholangitis**. Cholangiocarcinoma usually presents in patients more than 50 years old, unless related to **primary sclerosing cholangitis**.

Presentation

Liver cancer often remains asymptomatic for a long time and then presents late, making prognosis poor.

There are non specific symptoms associated with liver cancer:
- Weight loss
- Abdominal pain
- Anorexia
- Nausea and vomiting
- Jaundice
- Pruritus

Cholangiocarcinoma often presents with painless jaundice in a similar way to pancreatic cancer.

Investigations

- **Alpha-fetoprotein** is a tumour marker for **hepatocellular carcinoma**.
- **CA19-9** is a tumour marker for **cholangiocarcinoma**.
- Liver ultrasound can identify tumours.
- CT and MRI scans are used for diagnosis and staging of the cancer.
- ERCP can be used to take biopsies or brushings to diagnose cholangiocarcinoma.

Treatment of Hepatocellular Carcinoma

HCC has a very poor prognosis unless diagnosed early. Resection of early disease in a resectable area of the liver can be curative. Liver transplant when the HCC is isolated to the liver can be curative.

There are several **kinase inhibitors** that are licensed as medical treatment for HCC. They work by inhibiting the proliferation of cancer cells. Some examples of these are **sorafenib, regorafenib** and **lenvatinib**. They can potentially extend life by months.

HCC is generally considered resistant to chemotherapy and radiotherapy. In certain circumstances they are used as part of palliative treatment or clinical trials.

Treatment of Cholangiocarcinoma

Cholangiocarcinomas have a very poor prognosis unless diagnosed very early. Early disease can potentially be cured with surgical resection.

ERCP can be used to place a stent in the bile duct where the cholangiocarcinoma is compressing the duct. This allows for drainage of bile and usually improves symptoms.

Cholangiocarcinoma is also generally considered resistant to chemotherapy and radiotherapy.

Haemangioma

Haemangiomas are common benign tumours of the liver. They are often found incidentally. They cause no symptoms and have no potential to become cancerous. No treatment or monitoring is required.

Focal Nodular Hyperplasia

Focal nodular hyperplasia is a benign liver tumour made of fibrotic tissue. This is often found incidentally. It is usually asymptomatic and has no malignant potential. It can be related to oestrogen and is therefore more common in women and those on the oral contraceptive pill. No treatment or monitoring is required.

Liver Transplant

The most obvious source for a liver is from a healthy person who has just died. When an **entire** liver is transplanted from a deceased patient to a recipient it is known as a **orthotopic transplant**. This translates as straight (**ortho-**) in place (**-topic**).

The liver can regenerate as an organ. Therefore, it is possible to take a portion of the organ from a living donor, transplant it into a patient and have both regenerate to become two fully functioning organs. This is known as a **living donor transplant**.

It is also possible to split the organ of a deceased person into two and transplant it into two patients and have them regenerate to their normal size in each recipient. This is known as **split donation**.

Indications for liver transplant can be split into two categories: **acute liver failure** or **chronic liver failure**. **Acute liver failure** usually requires an immediate liver transplant, and these patients are placed on the top of the transplant list. The most common causes are acute viral hepatitis and paracetamol overdose.

Chronic liver failure patients can wait longer for their liver transplant and are put on a standard transplant list. It is normal for it to take around 5 months for a liver to become available.

Factors Suggesting Unsuitability for Liver Transplantation

- Significant co-morbidities (e.g. severe kidney or heart disease)
- Excessive weight loss and malnutrition
- Active hepatitis B or C or other infection
- End stage HIV
- Active alcohol use (generally 6 months of abstinence is required)

Surgery

The liver transplant surgery is carried out in a specialist transplant centre. It involves a "**rooftop**" or "**Mercedes Benz**" incision along the lower costal margin for open surgery. The liver is mobilised away from the other tissues and excised. The new liver, biliary system and blood supply is then implanted and connected.

Post Transplantation Care

Patients will require livelong **immunosuppression** (e.g. steroids, azathioprine and tacrolimus) and careful monitoring of these drugs. They are required to follow lifestyle advice and require monitoring and treatment for complications:
- Avoid alcohol and smoking
- Treating opportunistic infections
- Monitoring for disease recurrence (i.e. of hepatitis or primary biliary cirrhosis)
- Monitoring for cancer as there is a significantly higher risk in immunosuppressed patients

Monitoring for evidence of transplant rejection:
- Abnormal LFTs
- Fatigue
- Fever
- Jaundice

Gastro-Oesophageal Reflux Disease

Gastro-oesophageal reflux disease (**GORD**) is where acid from the stomach refluxes through the **lower oesophageal sphincter** and irritates the lining of the oesophagus.

The **oesophagus** has a **squamous epithelial lining** that makes it more sensitive to the effects of stomach acid. The stomach has a **columnar epithelial lining** that is more protected against stomach acid.

Presentation

Dyspepsia is a non-specific term used to describe indigestion. It covers the symptoms of GORD:
- Heartburn
- Acid regurgitation
- Retrosternal or epigastric pain
- Bloating
- Nocturnal cough
- Hoarse voice

Referral for Endoscopy

Endoscopy can be used to assess for peptic ulcers, oesophageal or gastric malignancy if there are concerning features.

Patients with evidence of a GI bleed (i.e. **melaena** or **coffee ground vomiting**) need admission and urgent endoscopy.

Patients with symptoms suspicious of cancer should have a two-week-wait referral so that endoscopy is performed within 2 weeks. The NICE guidelines have various criteria for when to refer urgently and when to refer routinely. The key **red flag** features indicating referral are:
- **Dysphagia** (difficulty swallowing) at any age gets a two week wait referral
- Aged over 55 (this is generally the cut off for urgent versus routine referrals)
- Weight loss
- Upper abdominal pain and reflux
- Treatment resistant dyspepsia
- Nausea and vomiting
- Low haemoglobin
- Raised platelet count

Management

Lifestyle advice
- Reduce tea, coffee and alcohol
- Weight loss
- Avoid smoking
- Smaller, lighter meals
- Avoid heavy meals before bed time
- Stay upright after meals rather than lying flat

Acid neutralising medication when required:
- Gaviscon
- Rennie

Proton pump inhibitors (reduce acid secretion in the stomach)
- Omeprazole
- Lansoprazole

Ranitidine
- This is an alternative to PPIs
- It is a H2 receptor antagonist (antihistamine)
- Reduces stomach acid

Surgery for reflux is called *laparoscopic fundoplication*. This involves tying the fundus of the stomach around the lower oesophagus to narrow the lower oesophageal sphincter.

Helicobacter Pylori

H. pylori is a *gram negative aerobic bacteria*. It lives in the stomach. It causes damage the epithelial lining of the stomach resulting in gastritis, ulcers and increasing the risk of stomach cancer. It avoids the acidic environment by forcing its way into the **gastric mucosa**. The breaks it creates in the mucosa exposes the **epithelial cells** underneath to acid.

It also produces **ammonia** to neutralise the stomach acid. The **ammonia** directly damages the **epithelial cells**. Other chemicals produced by the bacteria also damage the epithelial lining

We offer a test for *H. pylori* to anyone with dyspepsia. They need 2 weeks without using a PPI before testing for H. pylori for an accurate result.

Tests:
- **Urea breath test** using radiolabelled carbon 13
- **Stool antigen test**
- **Rapid urease test** can be performed during endoscopy.

A **rapid urease test** is also known as a **CLO test** (**Campylobacter-like organism test**). It is performed **during endoscopy** and involves taking a small biopsy of the stomach **mucosa**. **Urea** is added to this sample. If **H. pylori** are present, they produce **urease enzymes** that converts the **urea** to **ammonia**. The ammonia makes the solution more alkali giving a positive result on when the pH is tested.

Eradication

The eradication regime involves **triple therapy** with a **proton pump inhibitor** (e.g. omeprazole) plus **2 antibiotics** (e.g. amoxicillin and clarithromycin) for **7 days**.

The **urea breath test** can be used as a test of eradication after treatment. This is not routinely necessary.

Barretts Oesophagus

Constant reflux of acid results in the lower oesophageal epithelium changing in a process known as **metaplasia** from a **squamous** to a **columnar epithelium**. This change to columnar epithelium is called Barretts oesophagus. When this change happens patients typically get an **improvement** in reflux symptoms.

Barretts oesophagus is considered a "**premalignant**" condition and is a risk factor for the development of **adenocarcinoma** of the oesophagus (3-5% lifetime risk with Barretts). Patients identified as having **Barretts oesophagus** are monitored for **adenocarcinoma** by regular **endoscopy**. In some patients there is a progression from Barretts oesophagus (columnar epithelium) with no dysplasia to **low grade dysplasia** to **high grade dysplasia** and then to **adenocarcinoma**.

Treatment of **Barretts oesophagus** is with **proton pump inhibitors** (e.g. omeprazole). There is new evidence that treatment with regular aspirin can reduce the rate of adenocarcinoma developing however this is not yet in guidelines.

Ablation treatment during endoscopy using **photodynamic therapy**, **laser therapy** or **cryotherapy** is used to destroy the epithelium so that it is replaced with normal cells. This is not recommended in patients with no dysplasia but has a role in low and high grade dysplasia in preventing progression to cancer.

Peptic Ulcers

Peptic ulcers involve ulceration of the mucosa of the stomach (gastric ulcer) or the duodenum (duodenal ulcer). Duodenal ulcers are more common.

Pathophysiology

The stomach mucosa is prone to ulceration from:
- Breakdown of the protective layer of the stomach and duodenum
- Increase in stomach acid

There is a protective layer in the stomach comprised of **mucus** and **bicarbonate** secreted by the **stomach mucosa**. This **protective layer can be broken down** by:
- Medications (e.g. **steroids** or **NSAIDs**)
- **Helicobacter pylori**

Increased acid can result from:
- Stress
- Alcohol
- Caffeine
- Smoking
- Spicy foods

Presentation

- Epigastric discomfort or pain
- Nausea and vomiting
- Dyspepsia
- Bleeding causing haematemesis, "coffee ground" vomiting and melaena
- Iron deficiency anaemia (due to constant bleeding)

TOM TIP: In your MCQ exams, eating typically worsens the pain of gastric ulcers and improves the pain of duodenal ulcers.

Management

Peptic ulcers are diagnosed by **endoscopy**. During endoscopy a **rapid urease test** (**CLO test**) can be performed to check for **H. pylori**. Biopsy should be considered during endoscopy to **exclude malignancy** as cancers can look similar to ulcers during the procedure.

Medical treatment is the same as with **GORD**, usually with high dose **proton pump inhibitors**. Endoscopy can be used to monitoring the ulcer to ensure it heals and to assess for further ulcers.

Complications

Bleeding from the ulcer is a common and potentially life threatening complication.

Perforation resulting in an "*acute abdomen*" and **peritonitis**. This requires urgent surgical repair (usually laparoscopic).

Scarring and strictures of the muscle and mucosa. This can lead to a narrowing of the **pylorus** (the exit of the stomach) causing difficulty in emptying the stomach contents. This is known as **pyloric stenosis**. This presents with upper abdominal pain, distention, nausea and vomiting, particularly after eating.

Upper GI Bleed

Bleeding from the upper GI tract is a medical emergency that you will see often on the wards as a junior doctor. It involves some form of bleeding from the **oesophagus**, **stomach** or **duodenum**.

Causes

- Oesophageal varices
- Mallory-Weiss tear, which is a tear of the oesophageal mucous membrane
- Ulcers of the stomach or duodenum
- Cancers of the stomach or duodenum

Presentation

- **Haematemesis** (vomiting blood)
- "**Coffee ground vomit**". This is caused by vomiting digested blood that looks like coffee grounds.
- **Melaena**, which are tar like, black, greasy and offensive stools caused by digested blood
- Haemodynamic instability occurs in large blood loss, causing a low blood pressure, tachycardia and other signs of shock. Bear in mind that young, fit patients may compensate well with normal observations until they have lost a lot of blood.

The patient may have symptoms related to the underlying pathology:
- Epigastric pain and dyspepsia in peptic ulcers
- Jaundice for ascites in liver disease with oesophageal varices

Glasgow-Blatchford Score

The **Glasgow-Blatchford Score** is used as a scoring system used in suspected upper GI bleed on their initial presentation. It establishes their risk of having an upper GI bleed to help you make a plan (for example whether to discharge them or not).

Using an online calculator is the easiest way to calculate the score. A **score > 0 indicates high risk** for an upper GI bleed. It takes into account various features indicating an upper GI bleed:
- Drop in Hb
- Rise in urea
- Blood pressure
- Heart rate
- Melaena
- Syncopy

TOM TIP: The reason urea rises in upper GI bleeds is that the blood in the GI tract gets broken down by the acid and digestive enzymes. One of the breakdown products is urea and this urea is then absorbed in the intestines.

Rockall Score

The **Rockall Score** is used for patients that **have had an endoscopy**. It provides a percentage risk of rebleeding and mortality. Use an **online calculator** to calculate the score. It take in to account risk factors from the clinical presentation and endoscopy findings such as:
- Age
- Features of shock (e.g. tachycardia or hypotension)
- Co-morbidities
- Cause of bleeding (e.g. Mallory-Weiss tear or malignancy)
- Endoscopic stigmata of recent haemorrhage such as clots or visible bleeding vessels

Management (ABATED)

- **A** - **A**BCDE approach to immediate resuscitation
- **B** - **B**loods
- **A** - **A**ccess (ideally 2 large bore cannula)
- **T** - **T**ransfuse
- **E** - **E**ndoscopy (arrange urgent endoscopy within 24 hours)
- **D** - **D**rugs (stop **anticoagulants** and **NSAIDs**)

Send **bloods** for:
- **Haemoglobin** (FBC)
- **Urea** (U&Es)
- **Coagulation** (INR, FBC for platelets)
- **Liver disease** (LFTs)
- **Crossmatch** 2 units of blood

TOM TIP: "Group and save" is where the lab simply checks the patients blood group and keeps a sample of their blood saved incase they need to match blood to it. "Crossmatch" is where the lab actually finds blood, tests that it is compatible and keeps it ready in the fridge to be used if necessary.

Transfusion is based on the individual presentation:
- Transfuse **blood**, **platelets** and clotting factors (**fresh frozen plasma**) to patients with massive haemorrhage
- Transfusing more **blood** than necessary can be harmful
- **Platelets** should be given in active bleeding and **thrombocytopenia** (platelets < 50)
- **Prothrombin complex concentrate** can be given to patients taking **warfarin** that are actively bleeding

There are some additional steps if **oesophageal varices** are suspected, for example in patients with a history of chronic liver disease:
- **Terlipressin**
- Prophylactic **broad spectrum** antibiotics

The definitive treatment is **oesophagogastroduodenoscopy** (**OGD**) to provide interventions that stop the bleeding. This could involve variceal banding or cauterisation of the bleeding vessel.

NICE recommend **against** using a **proton pump inhibitor** prior to endoscopy, however you may find senior doctors that do this.

Inflammatory Bowel Disease

Inflammatory bowel disease is the umbrella term for two main diseases causing inflammation of the GI tract: **ulcerative colitis** and **Crohn's disease**. They both involve inflammation of the walls of the GI tract and are associated with periods of remission and exacerbation.

Crohn's versus Ulcerative Colitis

Crohn's and ulcerative colitis have features that are distinct from each other that are commonly tested in exams.

Crohn's (crows NESTS)
- **N** - **N**o blood or mucus (less common)
- **E** - **E**ntire GI tract
- **S** - "**S**kip lesions" on endoscopy
- **T** - **T**erminal ileum most affected and **T**ransmural (full thickness) inflammation
- **S** - **S**moking is a risk factor (don't set the nest on fire)

Crohn's is also associated with weight loss, strictures and fistulas.

Ulcerative Colitis (remember U - C - CLOSEUP)
- C - **C**ontinuous inflammation
- L - **L**imited to colon and rectum
- O - **O**nly superficial mucosa affected
- S - **S**moking is protective
- E - **E**xcrete blood and mucus
- U - **U**se *aminosalicylates*
- P - **P**rimary sclerosing cholangitis

Presentation

- Diarrhoea
- Abdominal pain
- Passing blood
- Weight loss

Testing

- Routine bloods for anaemia, infection, thyroid, kidney and liver function
- CRP indicates inflammation and active disease
- **Faecal calprotectin** is released by the intestines when inflamed. It is a useful screening test and is more than 90% sensitive and specific to IBD in adults.
- Endoscopy (OGD and colonoscopy) with biopsy is diagnostic
- Imaging with ultrasound, CT and MRI can be used to look for complications such as fistulas, abscesses and strictures

Management of Crohn's

This section is based on **NICE guidelines** last updated May 2016. Please see the full guidelines and talk to seniors before treating patients.

Inducing Remission
- First line: **Steroids** (e.g. oral prednisolone or IV hydrocortisone)

If steroids alone don't work, consider adding immunosuppressant medication under specialist guidance:
- Azathioprine
- Mercaptopurine
- Methotrexate
- Infliximab
- Adalimumab

Maintaining Remission
Treatment is tailored to individual patients based on risks, side effects, nature of the disease and patient wishes. It is reasonable not to take any medications whilst well.

First line:
- Azathioprine
- Mercaptopurine

Alternatives:
- Methotrexate
- Infliximab
- Adalimumab

Surgery

When the disease only affects the **distal ileum** it is possible to surgically resect this area and prevent further flares. Crohn's typically involves the entire GI tract. Surgery can also be used to treat **strictures** and **fistulas** secondary to Crohns disease.

Management of Ulcerative Colitis

This section is based on **NICE guidelines** last updated June 2013. Please see the full guidelines and talk to seniors before treating patients.

Inducing Remission

Mild to moderate disease
- First line: **aminosalicylate** (e.g. **mesalazine** oral or rectal)
- Second line: corticosteroids (e.g. prednisolone)

Severe disease
- First line: IV corticosteroids (e.g. hydrocortisone)
- Second line: IV ciclosporin

Maintaining Remission

- **Aminosalicylate** (e.g. **mesalazine** oral or rectal)
- Azathioprine
- Mercaptopurine

Surgery

Ulcerative colitis typically only affects the colon and rectum. Therefore, removing the colon and rectum (**panproctocolectomy**) will remove the disease. The patient is then left with either a permanent **ileostomy** or something called an **ileo-anal anastomosis** (**J-pouch**). This is where the ileum is folded back on itself and fashioned into a larger pouch that functions a bit like a rectum. This "**J-pouch**" is then attached to the anus and collects stools prior to the person passing the motion.

Irritable Bowel Syndrome

Irritable bowel syndrome is a "**functional bowel disorder**". This means there is no identifiable organic disease underlying the symptoms. The symptoms are a result of the abnormal functioning of an otherwise normal bowel.

It is often described as a **diagnosis of exclusion**, meaning that a diagnosis is only made when other pathology is excluded.

It is very common and occurs in up to 20% of the population. It affects women more than men and is more common in younger adults.

Symptoms

- Diarrhoea
- Constipation
- Fluctuating bowel habit
- Abdominal pain
- Bloating
- Worse after eating
- Improved by opening bowels

Criteria for Diagnosis (NICE Guidelines)

Other pathology should be excluded:
- Normal FBC, ESR and CRP blood tests
- **Faecal calprotectin** negative to exclude inflammatory bowel disease
- Negative coeliac disease serology (**anti-TTG antibodies**)
- Cancer is not suspected or excluded if suspected

Symptoms should suggest IBS:
Abdominal pain and/or discomfort:
- Relieved on opening bowels, or
- Associated with a change in bowel habit

AND 2 of:
- Abnormal stool passage
- Bloating
- Worse symptoms after eating
- Mucus with stools

Management

Making a positive diagnosis and providing reassurance that there is no serious pathology present is important.

General healthy diet and exercise advice:
- Adequate fluid intake
- Regular small meals
- Reduced processed foods
- Limit caffeine and alcohol
- Low "**FODMAP**" diet guided by a dietician
- Trial of **probiotic** supplements for 4 weeks

First Line Medication:
- **Loperamide** for diarrhoea
- Laxatives for constipation. Avoid **lactulose** as it can cause bloating. **Linaclotide** is a specialist laxative for patients with IBS not responding to first line laxatives
- Antispasmodics for cramps e.g. **hyoscine butylbromide** (**Buscopan**)

Second Line Medication:
- Tricyclic antidepressants (i.e. **amitriptyline** 5-10mg at night)

Third Line Medication:
- SSRIs antidepressants

Cognitive Behavioural Therapy (**CBT**) is also an option to help patients psychologically manage the condition and reduce distress associated with symptoms.

Coeliac Disease

Coeliac disease is an autoimmune condition where exposure to **gluten** causes an autoimmune reaction that causes **inflammation** in the **small intestine**. It usually develops in early childhood but can start at any age.

In coeliac disease **auto-antibodies** are created in response to exposure to **gluten** that target the **epithelial cells** of the intestine and lead to inflammation. There are two antibodies to remember: **anti-tissue transglutaminase** (**anti-TTG**) and **anti-endomysial** (**anti-EMA**). These antibodies relate to disease activity and will rise with more active disease and may disappear with effective treatment.

Inflammation affects the small bowel, particularly the **jejunum**. It causes **atrophy** of the **intestinal villi**. The intestinal cells have villi on them that help with absorbing nutrients from the food passing through the intestine. The inflammation causes malabsorption of nutrients and the symptoms of the disease.

Presentation

Coeliac disease is often **asymptomatic**, so have a low threshold for testing for coeliac disease in patients where it is suspected. Symptoms can include:
- **Failure to thrive** in young children
- Diarrhoea
- Fatigue
- Weight loss
- Mouth ulcers
- Anaemia secondary to iron, B12 or folate deficiency
- **Dermatitis herpetiformis** (an itchy blistering skin rash typically on the abdomen)

Rarely coeliac disease can present with **neurological symptoms**:
- Peripheral neuropathy
- Cerebellar ataxia
- Epilepsy

TOM TIP: Remember for your exams that we test all new cases of type 1 diabetes for coeliac disease even if they don't have symptoms, as the conditions are often linked.

Genetic Associations

- HLA-DQ2 gene (90%)
- HLA-DQ8 gene

Auto-antibodies

- **Tissue transglutaminase antibodies (anti-TTG)**
- **Endomysial antibodies (EMAs)**
- **Deaminated gliadin peptides antibodies (anti-DGPs)**

TOM TIP: Anti-TTG and anti-EMA antibodies are IgA. Some patients have an IgA deficiency. When you test for these antibodies, it is important to test for total Immunoglobulin A levels because if total IgA is low the coeliac test will be negative even when they have coeliacs. In this circumstance, you can test for the IgG version of anti-TTG or anti-EMA antibodies or do an endoscopy with biopsies.

Diagnosis

Investigations must be carried out whilst the patient **remains on a diet containing gluten** otherwise it may not be possible to detect antibodies or inflammation in the bowel.

Check **total immunoglobulin A levels** to exclude **IgA deficiency** before checking for coeliac disease specific antibodies:
- Raised **anti-TTG antibodies** (first choice)
- Raised **anti-endomysial antibodies**

Endoscopy and intestinal biopsy show:
- "**Crypt hypertrophy**"
- "**Villous atrophy**"

Associations

Coeliac disease is associated with many other autoimmune conditions:
- Type 1 diabetes
- Thyroid disease
- Autoimmune hepatitis
- Primary biliary cirrhosis
- Primary sclerosing cholangitis

Complications of Untreated Coeliac Disease

- Vitamin deficiency
- Anaemia
- Osteoporosis
- Ulcerative jejunitis
- Enteropathy-associated T-cell lymphoma (EATL) of the intestine
- Non-Hodgkin lymphoma (NHL)
- Small bowel adenocarcinoma (rare)

Treatment

A **lifelong gluten free diet** is essentially curative. Relapse will occur on consuming gluten again. Checking coeliac antibodies can be helpful in monitoring the disease.

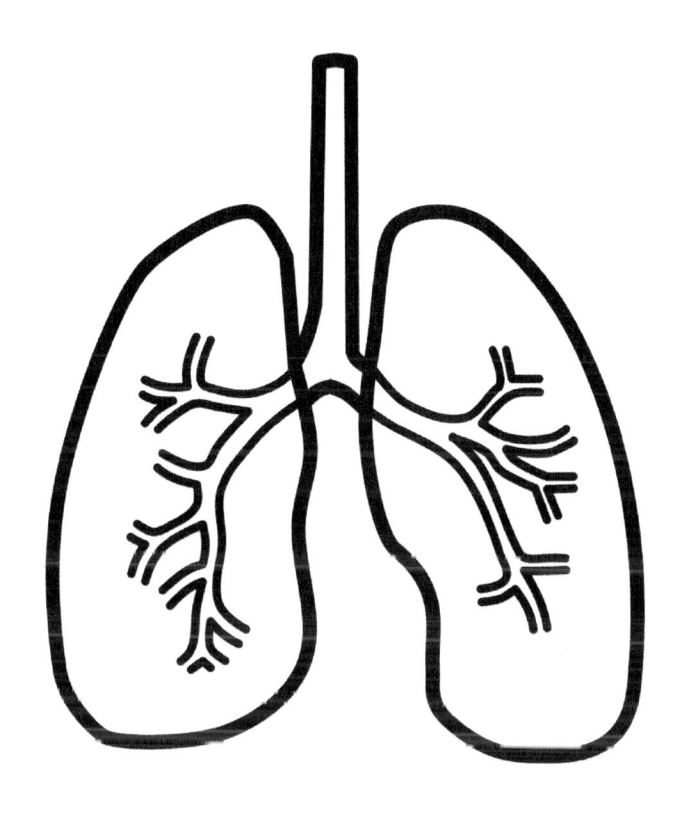

RESPIRATORY

4.1	Lung Cancer	106
4.2	Pneumonia	108
4.3	Lung Function Tests	111
4.4	Asthma	113
4.5	Acute Asthma	116
4.6	Chronic Obstructive Pulmonary Disease	117
4.7	Non Invasive Ventilation	121
4.8	Interstitial Lung Disease	122
4.9	Pleural Effusion	124
4.10	Pneumothorax	125
4.11	Pulmonary Embolism	126
4.12	Pulmonary Hypertension	129
4.13	Sarcoidosis	131
4.14	Obstructive Sleep Apnoea	134

Lung Cancer

Lung cancer is the third most common cancer in the UK behind **breast** and **prostate**. **Cigarette smoking** is the biggest cause and around 80% of lung cancers are thought to be preventable.

Histology

Non-small cell lung cancer
- *Squamous cell carcinoma* (35%)
- *Adenocarcinoma* (25%)

Small Cell Lung Cancer (SCLC) (20%)
Small cell lung cancer cells contain **neurosecretory granules** that can release **neuroendocrine hormones**. This makes SCLC responsible for multiple **paraneoplastic syndromes**.

Signs and Symptoms

- Shortness of breath
- Cough
- *Haemoptysis* (coughing up blood)
- Finger clubbing
- Recurrent pneumonia
- Weight loss
- Lymphadenopathy - often **supraclavicular** nodes are the first to be found on examination

Investigations

Chest xray is the first line investigation in suspected lung cancer. Findings suggesting cancer include:
- Hilar enlargement
- Peripheral opacity - a visible lesion in the lung field
- Pleural effusion - usually unilateral in cancer
- Collapse

Staging CT scan of chest, abdomen and pelvis to establish the stage and check for lymph node involvement and metastasis. This should be **contrast enhanced** using an injected contrast to give more detailed information about different tissues.

PET-CT (*positron emission tomography*) scans involve injecting a **radioactive tracer** (usually attached to glucose molecules) and taking images using a combination of a CT scanner and a gamma ray detector to visualise how metabolically active various tissues are. They are useful in identifying areas that the cancer has spread to by showing areas of increased metabolic activity.

Bronchoscopy with **endobronchial ultrasound** (**EBUS**) involves endoscopy with ultrasound equipment on the end of the scope. This allows detailed assessment of the tumour and ultrasound guided biopsy.

Histological diagnosis to check the type of cells in the cancer requires a biopsy. This can be either by bronchoscopy or percutaneously (through the skin).

Treatment options

All treatments are discussed at an MDT meeting involving various consultants and specialists, such as pathologists, surgeons, oncologists and radiologists. This is to make a joint decision about what is the most suitable options for the individual patient.

Surgery is offered first line in **non-small cell lung cancer** to patients that have disease isolated to a single area. The intention is to cure the cancer. **Lobectomy** (removing the lung lobe containing the tumour) is first line. **Segmentectomy** or **wedge resection** (taking a segment or wedge of lung to remove the tumour) is also an option.

Radiotherapy can also be curative in **non-small cell lung cancer** when diagnosed early enough.

Chemotherapy can be offered in addition to surgery or radiotherapy in certain patients to improve outcomes ("**adjuvant chemotherapy**") or as palliative treatment to improve survival and quality of life in later stages of **non-small cell lung cancer** ("**palliative chemotherapy**").

Treatment for small cell lung cancer is usually **chemotherapy** and **radiotherapy**. Prognosis is generally worse for small cell lung cancer compared with non-small cell lung cancer.

Endobronchial treatment with **stents** or **debulking** can be used as part of palliative treatment to relieve bronchial obstruction caused by lung cancer.

Extrapulmonary Manifestations

Lung cancer is associated with a lot of **extrapulmonary manifestations** and **paraneoplastic syndromes**. These are linked to different types and distributions of lung cancer. Exam questions commonly ask you to suggest the underlying cause of a paraneoplastic syndrome. Sometimes they can be the first evidence of a lung cancer in an otherwise asymptomatic patient.

Recurrent laryngeal nerve palsy presents with a hoarse voice. It is caused by the cancer pressing on or affecting the recurrent laryngeal nerve as it passes through the mediastinum.

Phrenic nerve palsy due to nerve compression. This causes diaphragm weakness and presents as shortness of breath.

Superior vena cava obstruction is a complication of lung cancer. It is caused by direct compression of the tumour on the superior vena cava. It presents with facial swelling, difficulty breathing and distended veins in the neck and upper chest. "**Pemberton's sign**" is where raising the hands over the head causes facial congestion and cyanosis. This is a medical emergency.

Horner's syndrome is a triad of partial **ptosis**, **anhidrosis** and **miosis**. It can be caused by a **Pancoast tumour** (tumour in the **pulmonary apex**) pressing on the **sympathetic ganglion**.

Syndrome of inappropriate ADH (**SIADH**) caused by **ectopic ADH** secretion by a **small cell lung cancer**. It presents with **hyponatraemia**.

Cushing's syndrome can be caused by **ectopic ACTH** secretion by a **small cell lung cancer**.

Hypercalcaemia caused by **ectopic parathyroid hormone** from a **squamous cell carcinoma**.

Limbic encephalitis. This is a paraneoplastic syndrome where the **small cell lung cancer** causes the immune system to make antibodies to tissues in the brain, specifically the limbic system, causing inflammation in these areas. This causes symptoms such as short term memory impairment, hallucinations, confusion and seizures. It is associated with **anti-Hu antibodies**.

Lambert-Eaton myasthenic syndrome.

Lambert-Eaton Myasthenic Syndrome

Lambert-Eaton myasthenic syndrome is a result of **antibodies** produced by the immune system against **small cell lung cancer** cells. These antibodies also target and damage **voltage-gated calcium channels** sited on the **presynaptic terminals** in **motor neurones**. This leads to weakness, particularly in the **proximal muscles** but can also affect **intraocular** muscles causing **diplopia** (double vision), **levator** muscles in the eyelid causing **ptosis** and **pharyngeal** muscles causing **slurred speech** and **dysphagia** (difficulty swallowing). This weakness gets worse with prolonged used of the muscles.

This syndrome has similar symptoms to **myasthenia gravis** although the symptoms tend to be more insidious and less pronounced in Lambert-Eaton syndrome. In older smokers with symptoms of **Lambert-Eaton syndrome** consider **small cell lung cancer**.

Mesothelioma

Mesothelioma is a lung malignancy affecting the **mesothelial cells** of the **pleura**. It is strongly linked to **asbestos inhalation**. There is a huge **latent period** between exposure to asbestos and the development of mesothelioma of up to 45 years. The prognosis is very poor. Chemotherapy can improve survival but it is essentially palliative.

Pneumonia

Pneumonia is simply an infection of the lung tissue. It causes inflammation of the lung tissue and production of sputum that fills the airways and alveoli. Pneumonia can be seen as **consolidation** on a **chest xray**.

Classification

If the pneumonia developed outside of hospital it is labelled **community acquired pneumonia**. If it develops more than 48h after hospital admission it is labelled **hospital acquired pneumonia**. If it develops as a result of **aspiration**, meaning after inhaling foreign material such as food, it is labelled **aspiration pneumonia**.

Presentation

- Shortness of breath
- Cough productive of sputum
- Fever
- Haemoptysis (coughing up blood)
- Pleuritic chest pain (sharp chest pain worse on inspiration)
- Delirium (acute confusion associated with infection)
- **Sepsis**

Signs

There may be a derangement in basic observations. These can indicate **sepsis** secondary to the pneumonia:
- Tachypnoea (raised respiratory rate)
- Tachycardia (raised heart rate)
- Hypoxia (low oxygen)
- Hypotension (shock)
- Fever
- Confusion

There are characteristic chest signs of pneumonia:
- **Bronchial breath sounds**. These are harsh breath sounds equally loud on inspiration and expiration. These are caused by consolidation of the lung tissue around the airway.
- **Focal coarse crackles**. These are air passing through sputum in the airways similar to using a straw to blow air through a drink.
- **Dullness to percussion** due to lung tissue collapse and/or consolidation.

Severity Assessment

NICE recommend using the scoring system CRB-65 out of hospital and CURB-65 in hospital. The only difference is that out of hospital you do not count urea. When you see someone out of hospital with a CRB-65 score of anything other than 0 NICE suggest considering referring to the hospital.

- **C** - **C**onfusion (new disorientation in person, place or time)
- **U** - **U**rea > 7
- **R** - **R**espiratory rate ≥ 30
- **B** - **B**lood pressure < 90 systolic or ≤ 60 diastolic.
- **65** - Age ≥ **65**

The **CURB 65** score predicts **mortality** (score 1 = under 5%, score 3 = 15%, score 4/5 = over 25%). The scoring system is there to help **guide** whether to admit the patient to hospital:
- Score 0/1: Consider treatment at home
- Score ≥ 2: Consider hospital admission
- Score ≥ 3: Consider intensive care assessment

Common Causes

- Streptococcus pneumoniae (50%)
- Haemophilus influenzae (20%)

Other Causes and Associations

- **Moraxella catarrhalis** in immunocompromised patients or those with chronic pulmonary disease
- **Pseudomonas aeruginosa** in patients with cystic fibrosis or bronchiectasis
- **Staphylococcus aureus** in patients with cystic fibrosis

Atypical Pneumonia

The definition of **atypical pneumonia** is pneumonia caused by an organism that cannot be **cultured** in the normal way or detected using a **gram stain**. They don't respond to penicillins. They can be treated with **macrolides** (e.g. clarithomycin), **fluoroquines** (e.g. levofloxacin) and **tetracyclines** (e.g. doxycycline).

Legionella pneumophila (**Legionnaires' disease**). This is typically caused by infected water supplies or air conditioning units. It can cause **hyponatraemia** (low sodium) by causing an **SIADH**. The typical exam patient has recently had a cheap hotel holiday and presents with hyponatraemia.

Mycoplasma pneumoniae. This causes a milder pneumonia and can cause a rash called **erythema multiforme** characterised by varying sized "**target lesions**" formed by **pink rings** with **pale centres**. It can also cause **neurological symptoms** in young patient in the exams.

Chlamydophila pneumoniae. The presentation might be a school aged child with a mild to moderate chronic pneumonia and wheeze. Be cautious though as this presentation is very common without chlamydophilia pneumoniae infection.

Coxiella burnetii AKA "**Q fever**". This is linked to exposure to animals and their bodily fluids. The MCQ patient is a farmer with a flu like illness.

Chlamydia psittaci. This is typically contracted from contact with infected birds. The MCQ patient is a parrot owner.

TOM TIP: You can remember the 5 causes of atypical pneumonia with the mnemonic: "Legions of psittaci MCQs"
- *Legions - Legionella pneumophila*
- *Psittaci - Chlamydia psittaci*
- *M - Mycoplasma pneumoniae*
- *C - Chlamydophila pneumoniae*
- *Qs - Q fever (coxiella burnetii)*

Fungal Pneumonia

Pneumocystis jiroveci (**PCP**) pneumonia occurs in patients that are **immunocompromised**. It is particularly important in patients with poorly controlled or new **HIV** with a **low CD4 count**. It usually presents subtly with a dry cough **without sputum**, shortness of breath **on exertion** and **night sweats**. Treatment is with **co-trimoxazole** (trimethoprim/sulfamethoxazole), which is known by the brand name "**Septrin**". Patients with low CD4 counts are prescribed **prophylactic** oral **co-trimoxazole** to protect against **PCP**.

Investigations

Patients in the community with CRB 0 or 1 pneumonia do not necessarily need investigations. NICE suggest considering a "**point of care**" test in primary care for CRP level to help guide management, however this is not widely available. If they arrive in hospital they will probably get a minimum of:
- Chest xray
- FBC (raised white cells)
- U&Es (for urea)
- CRP (raised in inflammation and infection)

Patients with moderate or severe cases should also have:
- Sputum cultures
- Blood cultures
- **Legionella and pneumococcal urinary antigens** (send a urine sample for antigen testing)

Inflammatory markers such as **white blood cells** and **CRP** are roughly raised in proportion to the severity of the infection. The trend can be helpful in monitoring the progress of the patient towards recovery. For example, repeating WBC and CRP after 3 days of antibiotics may show a downward trend suggesting the antibiotics are working. CRP commonly shows a delayed response so may be low on first presentation then spike very high a day or two later despite the patient improving on treatment. WBC typically responds faster than CRP and give a more "up to date" picture.

Patients that are *immunocompromised* **may not show an inflammatory response** and may not have raised inflammatory markers despite severe infection.

Antibiotics

Always follow your **local area guidelines**. These are developed by looking at the bacteria in the local area for their *antibiotic resistance*. They are specific to the local population. Moderate or severe pneumonia or septic patients usually start with IV antibiotics. These are then changed to oral antibiotics guided by clinical improvement or improvement in their inflammatory markers.

Typical antibiotic course lengths are:
- Mild CAP: 5 day course of oral antibiotics (amoxicillin or macrolide)
- Moderate to severe CAP: 7-10 day course of dual antibiotics (amoxicillin and macrolide)

Complications

- Sepsis
- Pleural effusion
- Empyema
- Lung abscess
- Death

Lung Function Tests

Lung function tests are used to help establish a diagnosis in lung disease. They are particularly helpful in **obstructive** and **restrictive** lung disease where there will be recognisable findings on the tests. This section gives a simple overview of lung function tests. There is a lot more to learn if you are interested.

Outcome Measures

Spirometry is the test used to establish objective measures of lung function. It involves different breathing exercises into a machine that measures volumes of air and flow rates and produces a report. **Reversibility testing** involves giving a bronchodilator (i.e. salbutamol) prior to repeating the spirometry to see the impact this has on the results.

FEV1

FEV1 means *forced expiratory volume* **in 1 second**. This is the volume of air a person can exhale as fast as they can in 1 second. This is a measure how easily air can flow out of the lungs. It will be reduced if there is any air flow **obstruction**.

FVC

FVC means *forced vital capacity*. This is the total amount of air a person can exhale after a full inhalation. This is a measure of the total volume of air that the person can take in to their lungs. It will be reduced if there is any **restriction** on the capacity of their lungs.

Obstructive Disease

Obstructive lung disease can be diagnosed when the **FEV1** is less than 75% of the **FVC** (**FEV1:FVC ratio < 75%**). This suggests that there is some obstruction slowing the passage of air getting out of the lungs. The person may have a relatively good lung volume but air is only able to move in and out of the lungs slowly, due to **obstruction**.

In **asthma**, the obstruction is a narrowed airway due to **bronchoconstriction**. In **COPD** there is **chronic** airway and lung damage causing obstruction. You can test for **reversibility** of this obstruction by giving a **bronchodilator** (i.e. salbutamol). The obstructive picture is typically reversible in asthma but not COPD.

Restrictive Disease

If **FEV1** and **FVC** are **equally reduced** and the **FEV1:FVC ratio > 75%**, this suggests *restrictive lung disease*.

Restrictive lung disease involves a restriction in the ability of the lungs to expand and fill with air. The lungs are restricted from effectively expanding. This can be differentiated from **obstructive lung disease**, where there is obstruction of air flow through the airways in to and out of the lungs.

This restriction of lung expansion leads to inadequate ventilation of the alveoli and therefore inadequate oxygenation of the blood.

Restrictive lung disease will cause the **FEV1/FVC** ratio to be normal or raised because there is no obstructive pathology present that would be affecting air flow through the airways. The **FVC** will be reduced because there is a restriction of the overall expansion and thus maximum capacity of the lungs.

Causes
Restrictive lung disease is caused by anything that will affect how well the chest wall and lungs can forcefully expand to draw air in:
- Interstitial lung disease such as pulmonary fibrosis
- Sarcoidosis
- Obesity
- Motor neurone disease
- Scoliosis

Peak Flow

"**Peak flow**" is a measure of the "peak", or fastest point, of a persons expiratory flow of air. It can be referred to as **peak expiratory flow rate** (**PEFR**). It is measured using a **peak flow meter**. It is a simple way of demonstrating how much obstruction to airflow is present in the patient's lungs. It is useful in **obstructive lung disease**, particularly **asthma**, to measure how well the asthma is controlled and how severe an acute exacerbation is.

The technique is to stand tall, take a deep breath in, make a good seal around the device with the lips and blow as fast and hard as possible into the device. Take **three attempts** and record the best result.

It varies dramatically based on the size and age of the patient. To put the result into context it is usually recorded as a **percentage of predicted**. The predicted peak flow can be obtained based on sex, height and age using a reference chart.

For example, an asthmatic patient with a predicted peak flow of 400 that only manages a score of 200 on their best attempt of 3 currently has a peak flow at 50% of predicted.

Asthma

Asthma is a **chronic inflammatory condition** of the airways that causes episodic exacerbations of **bronchoconstriction**. Bronchoconstriction is where the **smooth muscles** of the airways (the bronchi) contract, causing a reduction in the diameter of the airways. Narrowing of the airways causes an **obstruction** to airflow going in and out of the lungs.

In asthma there is **reversible airway obstruction** that typically responds to **bronchodilators** such as **salbutamol**. This bronchoconstriction is caused by airway **hypersensitivity** and can be triggered by environmental factors.

Typical Triggers

- Infection
- Night time or early morning
- Exercise
- Animals
- Cold, damp or dusty air
- Strong emotions

Presentation Suggesting a Diagnosis of Asthma

- Episodic symptoms
- Diurnal variability. Typically worse at night.
- Dry cough with wheeze and shortness of breath
- A history of other **atopic conditions** such as eczema, hayfever and food allergies
- Family history
- **Bilateral widespread "polyphonic" wheeze** heard by a **healthcare professional**

Presentation Indicating a Diagnosis other than Asthma

- Wheeze related to coughs and colds more suggestive of **viral induced wheeze**
- Isolated or productive cough
- Normal investigations
- No response to treatment
- Unilateral wheeze. This suggests a focal lesion or infection.

Diagnosis

There is a difference in the guidelines on diagnosis. The **British Thoracic Society** (**BTS**) and **SIGN guidelines** from 2016 advise making a clinical diagnosis when there is a high clinical suspicion of asthma and testing when there is an intermediate or low clinical suspicion. The newer **NICE guidelines** from 2017 advise against making a diagnosis without **definitive testing**.

BTS/Sign Guidelines on Diagnosis
- High probability of asthma clinically: Try treatment
- Intermediate probability of asthma: Perform spirometry with reversibility testing
- Low probability of asthma: Consider referral and investigating for other causes

NICE Guidelines on Diagnosis

NICE recommend assessment and testing at a "**diagnostic hub**" to establish a diagnosis. They specifically advise not to make a diagnosis clinically and require investigations.

First line investigations:
- *Fractional exhaled nitric oxide*
- *Spirometry with bronchodilator reversibility*

If there is diagnostic uncertainty after first line investigations these can be followed up with further testing:
- **Peak flow variability** measured by keeping a diary of peak flow measurements several times per day for 2 to 4 weeks
- **Direct bronchial challenge test** with **histamine** or **methacholine**

Long Term Management

There are key treatments for long term management of asthma that you should be familiar with:

Short acting beta 2 adrenergic receptor agonists, for example salbutamol. These work quickly but the effect only lasts for an hour or two. Adrenalin acts on the smooth muscles of the airways to cause relaxation. This results in dilatation of the bronchioles and improves the bronchoconstriction present in asthma. They are used as "**reliever**" or "**rescue**" medication during acute exacerbations of asthma when the airways are constricting.

Inhaled corticosteroids (**ICS**), for example **beclometasone**. These reduce the inflammation and reactivity of the airways. These are used as "**maintenance**" or "**preventer**" medications and are taken regularly even when well.

Long-acting beta 2 agonists (**LABA**), for example **salmeterol**. These work in the same way as short acting beta 2 agonists but have a much longer action.

Long-acting muscarinic antagonists (**LAMA**), for example **tiotropium**. These block the **acetylcholine receptors**. Acetylecholine receptors are stimulated by the **parasympathetic nervous system** and cause contraction of the bronchial smooth muscles. Blocking these receptors leads to **bronchodilation**.

Leukotriene receptor antagonists, for example **montelukast**. **Leukotrienes** are produced by the immune system and cause **inflammation**, **bronchoconstriction** and **mucus secretion** in the airways. Leukotriene receptor antagonists work by blocking the effects of leukotrienes.

Theophylline. This works by relaxing bronchial smooth muscle and reducing inflammation. Unfortunately it has a **narrow therapeutic window** and can be toxic in excess, so monitoring plasma theophylline levels in the blood is required. This is done 5 days after starting treatment and 3 days after each dose changes.

Maintenance and Reliever Therapy (**MART**). This is a combination inhaler containing a low dose inhaled corticosteroid and a fast acting LABA. This replaces all other inhalers and the patient uses this **single inhaler** both regularly as a "**preventer**" and also as a "**reliever**" when they have symptoms.

Confusingly the new **NICE guidelines** are slightly different to the **SIGN/BTS guidelines**. The medications they recommend are the same but they differ slightly in the stepwise ladder of which medications to introduce at what point. Most importantly they both start with a **short acting beta 2 agonist** followed by a **low dose inhaled corticosteroid**. The next step is then either a **leukotriene receptor antagonist** or an inhaled **LABA**.

The principles of using the stepwise ladder are to:
- Start at the most appropriate step for the severity of the symptoms
- Review at regular intervals based on severity
- Step up and down the ladder based on symptoms
- Aim to achieve no symptoms or exacerbations on the lowest dose and number of treatments. This is often difficult in practice.
- Always check inhaler technique and adherence at review

BTS/SIGN Stepwise Ladder (adapted from the 2016 guidelines)

1. Add a short-acting beta 2 agonist inhaler (e.g. **salbutamol**) as required for infrequent wheezy episodes.
2. Add a regular low dose corticosteroid inhaler.
3. Add **LABA** inhaler (e.g. salmeterol). Continue the **LABA** only if the patient has a good response.
4. Consider a trial of an oral **leukotriene receptor antagonist** (i.e. **montelukast**), **oral beta 2 agonist** (i.e. oral **salbutamol**), oral **theophylline** or an inhaled **LAMA** (i.e. **tiotropium**).
5. Titrate the inhaled corticosteroid up to "high dose". Combine additional treatments from step 4. Refer to a specialist.
6. Add oral steroids at the lowest dose possible to achieve good control.

NICE Guidelines (adapted from the 2017 guidelines)

1. Add a short-acting beta 2 agonist inhaler (e.g. **salbutamol**) as required for infrequent wheezy episodes.
2. Add a regular low dose **inhaled corticosteroid**.
3. Add an oral **leukotriene receptor antagonist** (i.e. **montelukast**).
4. Add **LABA** inhaler (e.g. **salmeterol**). Continue the **LABA** only if the patient has a good response.
5. Consider changing to a **maintenance and reliever therapy** (**MART**) regime.
6. Increase the inhaled corticosteroid to a "moderate dose".
7. Consider increasing the inhaled corticosteroid dose to "high dose" or oral **theophylline** or an inhaled **LAMA** (e.g. **tiotropium**).
8. Refer to a specialist.

Additional Management

- Each patient should have an individual asthma self-management programme
- Yearly flu jab
- Yearly asthma review
- Advise exercise and avoid smoking

Acute Asthma

An **acute exacerbation of asthma** is characterised by a rapid deterioration in symptoms. This could be triggered by any of the typical asthma triggers such as infection, exercise or cold weather.

Presentation

- Progressively worsening shortness of breath
- Use of accessory muscles
- Fast respiratory rate (tachypnoea)
- Symmetrical expiratory wheeze on auscultation
- The chest can sound "tight" on auscultation with reduced air entry

Grading Acute Asthma

Moderate
- PEFR 50 – 75% predicted

Severe
- PEFR 33-50% predicted
- Resp rate >25
- Heart rate >110
- Unable to complete sentences

Life-threatening
- PEFR <33%
- Sats <92%
- Becoming tired
- No wheeze. This occurs when the airways are so tight there is no air entry at all. This is ominously described as a "**silent chest**".
- Haemodynamic instability (i.e. shock)

Treatment

As a junior doctor you should not underestimate the danger of acute asthma. Patients can deteriorate quickly and it can be life threatening. Generally don't hesitate to keep adding treatment and escalate early to seniors and HDU or ICU if they are not improving or there are signs of severe asthma.

If asthma is severe, treatment decisions such as **aminophylline**, **IV salbutamol** and **IV magnesium** are normally made under senior guidance.

Moderate:
- Nebulised **beta-2 agonists** (i.e. salbutamol 5mg repeated as often as required)
- Nebulised **ipratropium bromide**
- **Steroids**. Oral prednisolone or IV hydrocortisone. These are usually continued for 5 days.
- Antibiotics if there is convincing evidence of bacterial infection

Severe:
- Oxygen if required to maintain sats 94-98%
- **Aminophylline** infusion
- Consider IV salbutamol

Life threatening:
- IV **magnesium sulphate** infusion
- Admission to HDU or ICU
- **Intubation** in the worst cases. This decision should be made early because it is very difficult to intubate with severe bronchoconstriction.

ABGs in Asthma:

Initially patients will have a **respiratory alkalosis** as **tachypnoea** causes a drop in CO_2. A normal pCO_2 or **hypoxia** is a concerning sign as it means they are tiring, it indicates life threatening asthma. A **respiratory acidosis** due to high CO_2 is a very bad sign in asthma.

Monitoring

To monitor the response to treatment you can use:
- Respiratory rate
- Respiratory effort
- Peak flow
- Oxygen saturations
- Chest auscultation

Additional Notes on Treatment

Monitor **serum potassium** when on **salbutamol** as it causes potassium to be absorbed from the blood into the cells. Salbutamol also causes **tachycardia** (fast heart rate).

Optimise asthma control after an acute attack. Discharge patients with an "**asthma action plan**" that provides them with a clear plan for everything they need to know about their asthma in one place. Consider prescribing a "rescue pack" of steroids for the person to initiate in the future if they have another exacerbation of asthma. NICE suggest referral to a respiratory specialist after 2 attacks in 12 months.

Chronic Obstructive Pulmonary Disease

Chronic obstructive pulmonary disease (**COPD**) is a non-reversible, long term deterioration in air flow through the lungs caused by damage to lung tissue. This lung damage is almost always the result of smoking. The damage to the lung tissues causes an obstruction to the flow of air through the airways making it more difficult to ventilate the lungs and making them prone to developing infections.

Unlike asthma, this obstruction is not significantly reversible with bronchodilators such as salbutamol. Patients are susceptible to **exacerbations** during which there is worsening of their lung function. Exacerbations are often triggered by infections and these are called **infective exacerbations**.

Presentation

Suspect COPD in a long term smoker presenting with chronic shortness of breath, cough, sputum production, wheeze and recurrent respiratory infections, particularly in winter.

Always consider differential diagnoses such as lung cancer, fibrosis or heart failure. COPD does NOT cause clubbing. It is unusual for it to cause **haemoptysis** (coughing up blood) or chest pain. These symptoms should be investigated for a different cause.

MRC (Medical Research Council) Dyspnoea Scale

This is a 5 point scale that NICE recommend for assessing the impact of their breathlessness:

Grades:
- Grade 1 - Breathless on strenuous exercise
- Grade 2 - Breathless on walking up hill
- Grade 3 - Breathlessness that slows walking on the flat
- Grade 4 - Stop to catch their breath after walking 100 meters on the flat
- Grade 5 - Unable to leave the house due to breathlessness

Diagnosis

Diagnosis is based on **clinical presentation** plus **spirometry**.

Spirometry will show an "**obstructive picture**". This means the overall lung capacity is not as bad as their ability to quickly blow air out of their lungs. The overall lung capacity is measured by **forced vital capacity** (**FVC**) and their ability to quickly blow air out is measured by the **forced expiratory volume in 1 second** (**FEV1**). Being able to blow air out is limited by the damage to their airways causing airway obstruction. Therefore in COPD:

- **FEV1/FVC ratio < 0.7**

The obstructive picture does not show a dramatic response to **reversibility testing** with **beta-2 agonists** such as **salbutamol** during spirometry testing. If there is a large response to reversibility testing them consider asthma as an alternative diagnosis.

Severity

The **severity** of the airflow obstruction can be graded using the **FEV1**:
- Stage 1: FEV1 >80% of predicted
- Stage 2: FEV1 50-79% of predicted
- Stage 3: FEV1 30-49% of predicted
- Stage 4: FEV1 <30% of predicted

Other Investigations

There are a number of other investigations that can be considered to help with diagnosis and management and to exclude other conditions:

- **Chest xray** to exclude other pathology such as lung cancer.
- **Full blood count** for polycythaemia or anaemia. Polycythaemia (raised haemoglobin) is a response to chronic hypoxia.
- **Body mass index** (BMI) as a baseline to later assess weight loss (e.g. cancer or severe COPD) or weight gain (e.g. steroids).
- **Sputum culture** to assess for chronic infections such as pseudomonas.
- **ECG** and **echocardiogram** to assess heart function.
- **CT thorax** for alternative diagnoses such as fibrosis, cancer or bronchiectasis.
- **Serum alpha-1 antitrypsin** to look for alpha-1 antitrypsin deficiency. Deficiency leads to early onset and more severe disease.
- **Transfer factor for carbon monoxide** (**TLCO**) is decreased in COPD. It can give an indication about the severity of the disease and may be increased in other conditions such as asthma.

Long Term Management

It is essential for people to stop smoking. Continuing to smoke will progressively worsen lung function and prognosis. They can be referred to smoking cessation services for support.

Patients should have the **pneumococcal** and **annual flu** vaccine.

STEP 1:
Short acting bronchodilators: **beta-2 agonists** (salbutamol or terbutaline) or **short acting antimuscarinics** (ipratropium bromide).

STEP 2:
If they do **not** have asthmatic or steroid responsive features they should have a combined **long acting beta agonist** (**LABA**) plus a **long acting muscarinic antagonist** (**LAMA**). "**Anoro Ellipta**", "**Ultibro Breezhaler**" and "**DuaKlir Genuair**" are examples of combination inhalers.

If they have **asthmatic or steroid responsive features** they should have a combined **long acting beta agonist** (**LABA**) plus an **inhaled corticosteroid** (**ICS**). "**Fostair**", "**Symbicort**" and "**Seretide**" are examples of combination inhalers. If these don't work they can step up to a combination of a **LABA, LAMA** and **ICS**. "**Trimbo**" and "**Trelegy Ellipta**" are examples of LABA, LAMA and ICS combination inhalers.

In more severe cases additional options are:
- Nebulisers (salbutamol and/or ipratropium)
- Oral theophylline
- Oral mucolytic therapy to break down sputum (e.g. carbocisteine)
- Long term prophylactic antibiotics (e.g. azithromycin)
- Long term oxygen therapy at home

Long term oxygen therapy is used for severe COPD that is causing problems such as **chronic hypoxia**, **polycythaemia**, **cyanosis** or **heart failure** secondary to pulmonary hypertension (**cor pulmonale**). It can't be used if they smoke, as oxygen plus cigarettes is a significant fire hazard.

Exacerbation of COPD

An exacerbation of COPD presents as acute worsening of symptoms such as cough, shortness of breath, sputum production and wheeze. It is usually triggered by a viral or bacterial infection.

Arterial Blood Gas

Remember that CO_2 makes blood acidotic by breaking down into **carbonic acid** (H_2CO_3). Low pH (acidosis) with a raised pCO_2 suggests they are acutely **retaining** (not able to get rid of) CO_2 and their blood has become acidotic. This is a **respiratory acidosis**.

Raised bicarbonate indicates they **chronically retain** CO_2 and their kidneys have responded by producing more **bicarbonate** to balance the acidic CO_2 and maintain a normal pH. In an acute exacerbation, the kidneys can't keep up with the rising level of CO_2 so they become acidotic despite having a higher bicarbonate than someone without COPD.

It is important to distinguish the **type of respiratory failure**:
- **Low pO_2** indicates hypoxia and respiratory failure
- **Normal pCO_2** with **low pO_2** indicates **type 1 respiratory failure** (only **one** is affected)
- **Raised pCO_2** with **low pO_2** indicates **type 2 respiratory failure** (**two** are affected)

Other Investigations

- **Chest xray** to look for pneumonia or other pathology
- **ECG** to look for arrhythmias or evidence of heart strain
- **FBC** to look for infection (raised white cells)
- **U&E** to check electrolytes, which can be affected by infections and medications
- **Sputum culture** if significant infection is present
- **Blood cultures** if septic

Oxygen Therapy in COPD:
Too much oxygen in someone that is prone to retaining CO_2 can depress their respiratory drive. This slows their breathing rate and effort and leads to them retaining more CO_2. Therefore, in someone who retains CO_2 the amount of oxygen that is given needs to be carefully balanced to optimise their pO_2 whilst not increasing their pCO_2. This is guided by oxygen saturations and repeat ABGs.

Venturi masks are designed to deliver a specific percentage concentration of oxygen. They allow some of the oxygen to leak out the side of the mask and normal air to be inhaled along with oxygen. The percentage of inhaled oxygen can be carefully controlled to balance how much oxygen they get. Environmental air contains 21% oxygen. Venturi masks deliver 24% (blue), 28% (white), 31% (orange), 35% (yellow), 40% (red) and 60% (green) oxygen.

A general rule regarding target oxygen saturations in COPD is:
- If retaining CO_2 aim for oxygen saturations of **88-92%** titrated by **venturi mask**
- If not retaining CO_2 and their bicarbonate is normal (meaning they do not normally retain CO_2) then give oxygen to aim for oxygen saturations **above 94%**

Medical Treatment:
Typical treatment if they are well enough to remain at home:
- **Prednisolone** 30mg once daily for 7-14 days
- Regular **inhalers** or home **nebulisers**
- **Antibiotics** if there is evidence of infection

In hospital:
- **Nebulised bronchodilators** (e.g. salbutamol 5mg/4h and ipratropium 500mcg/6h)
- **Steroids** (e.g. 200mg hydrocortisone or 30-40mg oral prednisolone)

- **Antibiotics** if evidence of infection
- **Physiotherapy** can help clear sputum

Options in severe cases not responding to first line treatment:
- IV **aminophylline**
- **Non-invasive ventilation** (**NIV**)
- **Intubation** and **ventilation** with admission to intensive care
- **Doxapram** can be used as a respiratory stimulant where NIV or intubation is not appropriate

Non Invasive Ventilation

Non-invasive ventilation is used to support the lungs in respiratory failure secondary to **obstructive lung disease**. It is an alternative to full intubation and ventilation. Intubation and ventilation involves giving the patient a general anaesthetic, putting a plastic tube into the trachea and ventilating the lungs artificially. Non-invasive ventilation involves using a full face mask or a tight fitting nasal mask to blow air forcefully into the lungs and ventilate them without having to intubate the patient. It is not pleasant, however it is much less invasive than intubation and ventilation and acts as a useful middle point between basic oxygen and intubation.

Non invasive ventilation can either be **BiPAP** or **CPAP**.

BiPAP

BiPAP stands for **bilevel positive airway pressure**. This involves a cycle of high and low pressure to correspond to the patients inspiration and expiration. BiPAP is used where there is **type 2 respiratory failure**, typically due to COPD. The criteria for initiating BiPAP are:

- **Respiratory acidosis** (pH < 7.35, $PaCO_2$ >6) **despite** adequate medical treatment.

The decision to initiate it would be made by a registrar or above. The main **contraindications** are an **untreated pneumothorax** or any structural abnormality or pathology affecting the face, airway or GI tract. Patients should have a chest xray prior to NIV to exclude pneumothorax where this does not cause a delay. A plan should be in place in case the NIV fails so that everyone agrees whether the patient should proceed to intubation and ventilation and ICU or whether palliative care is more appropriate.

IPAP (**inspiratory positive airway pressure**) is the pressure during inspiration. This is where air is forced into the lungs.

EPAP (**expiratory positive airway pressure**) is the pressure during expiration. This provides some pressure during expiration so that the airways don't collapse. It helps air to escape the lungs in patients with obstructive lung disease.

The initial pressures are estimated based on the patients body mass. Pressures are measured in cm of water. Potential starting points for an average male patient might be:
- IPAP 16-20cm H_2O
- EPAP 4-6cm H_2O

Repeat an ABG 1 hour after every change and 4 hours after that until stable. The IPAP is increased by 2-5 cm increments until the acidosis resolves.

CPAP

CPAP stands for **continuous positive airway pressure**. It provides continuous air blown into the lungs that keeps the airways expanded so that air can more easily travel in and out. It is used to maintain the patient's airway in conditions where it is prone to collapse.

Indications for CPAP:
- Obstructive sleep apnoea
- Congestive cardiac failure
- Acute pulmonary oedema

Interstitial Lung Disease

Interstitial lung disease is an umbrella term to describe conditions that affect the lung **parenchyma** (the lung tissue) causing **inflammation** and **fibrosis**. **Fibrosis** involves the replacement of the normal elastic and functional lung tissue with scar tissue that is stiff and does not function effectively.

Diagnosis

Diagnosis of interstitial lung disease requires a combination of clinical features and **high resolution CT** scan of the thorax. HRCT shows a "**ground glass**" appearance with interstitial lung disease. When diagnosis is unclear **lung biopsy** can be used to take samples of the lung tissue and confirm the diagnosis on **histology**.

Management

Generally there is a poor prognosis and limited management options in interstitial lung disease as the damage is irreversible. Generally the treatment is supportive. Options are:
- Remove or treat the underlying cause
- Home oxygen where they are hypoxic at rest
- Stop smoking
- Physiotherapy and pulmonary rehabilitation
- Pneumococcal and flu vaccine
- **Advanced care planning** and palliative care where appropriate
- Lung transplant is an option but the risks and benefits need careful consideration

Idiopathic Pulmonary Fibrosis

This is a condition where there is progressive **pulmonary fibrosis** with no clear cause. It presents with an insidious onset of shortness of breath and dry cough over more than 3 months. It usually affects adults over 50 years old. Examination can show **bibasal fine inspiratory crackles** and **finger clubbing**. Prognosis is poor with a life expectancy of 2-5 years from diagnosis.

Two medications are licensed that can slow the progression of the disease:
- **Pirfenidone** is an antifibrotic and anti-inflammatory
- **Nintedanib** is a monoclonal antibody targeting **tyrosine kinase**

Drug Induced Pulmonary Fibrosis

There are several drugs that can cause pulmonary fibrosis. Key medication that are worth remembering are:
- Amiodarone
- Cyclophosphamide
- Methotrexate
- Nitrofurantoin

Secondary Pulmonary Fibrosis

Pulmonary fibrosis can occur secondary to other conditions:
- Alpha-1 antitripsin deficiency
- Rheumatoid arthritis
- Systemic lupus erythematosus (SLE)
- Systemic sclerosis

Hypersensitivity Pneumonitis (AKA Extrinsic Allergic Alveolitis)

Hypersensitivity pneumonitis is a *type III hypersensitivity reaction* to an environmental allergen. It causes *parenchymal inflammation* and destruction in people that are sensitive to that *allergen*. *Bronchoalveolar lavage* involves collecting cells from the airways during *bronchoscopy* by washing the airways with fluid then collecting that fluid for testing. This shows *raised lymphocytes* and *mast cells* in hypersensitivity pneumonitis.

Management is by removing the allergen, giving oxygen where necessary and steroids.

Examples of specific causes:
- *Bird-fanciers lung* is a reaction to bird droppings
- *Farmers lung* is a reaction to mouldy spores in hay
- *Mushroom workers' lung* is a reaction to specific mushroom antigens
- *Malt workers lung* is a reaction to mould on barley

Cryptogenic Organising Pneumonia

Cryptogenic organising pneumonia was previously known as *bronchiolitis obliterans organising pneumonia*. It involves a focal area of inflammation of the lung tissue. This can be idiopathic or triggered by infection, inflammatory disorders, medications, radiation or environmental toxins or allergens.

Presentation is very similar to infectious pneumonia with shortness of breath, cough, fever and lethargy. It also presents similarly to pneumonia on a chest xray with a focal consolidation.

Diagnosis is often delayed due to the similarities to infective pneumonia. Lung biopsy is the definitive investigation. Treatment is with systemic corticosteroids.

Asbestosis

Asbestosis is lung fibrosis related to the inhalation of asbestos. Asbestos is *fibrogenic*, meaning it causes lung fibrosis. It is also *oncogenic*, meaning it causes cancer. The effects of asbestos usually take several decades to develop. Asbestos inhalation causes several problems:

- Lung fibrosis
- Pleural thickening and pleural plaques
- Adenocarcinoma
- Mesothelioma

Suffers are eligible for compensation if they develop asbestos related health conditions (except isolated pleural plaques). All patients that die with known exposure to asbestos need to be referred to the coroner.

Pleural Effusion

A pleural effusion is a collection of fluid in the **pleural cavity**. This can be **exudative** meaning there is a high protein count (**more than 3g/l**) or **transudative** meaning there is a relatively lower protein count (**less than 3g/l**). Whether it is **exudative** or **transudative** helps determine the cause.

Causes

Exudative causes are related to **inflammation**. The inflammation results in protein leaking out of the tissues into the pleural space (**ex-** meaning moving out of). Think of the causes of **inflammation**:
- **Lung cancer**
- **Pneumonia**
- **Rheumatoid arthritis**
- **Tuberculosis**

Transudative causes relate to fluid moving across into the pleural space (**trans-** meaning moving across). Think of the causes of **fluid** shifting:
- **Congestive cardiac failure**
- **Hypoalbuminaemia**
- **Hypothroidism**
- **Meig's syndrome** (right sided pleural effusion with ovarian malignancy)

Presentation

- Shortness of breath
- Dullness to percussion over the effusion
- Reduced breath sounds
- Tracheal deviation away from the effusion if it is massive

Investigations

Chest xray shows:
- **Blunting** of the **costophrenic angle**
- Fluid in the lung **fissures**
- Larger effusions will have a **meniscus**. This is a curving upwards where it meets the chest wall and mediastinum.
- Tracheal and mediastinal **deviation** if it is a massive effusion

Respiratory

Taking a sample of the pleural fluid by aspiration or chest drain is required to analyse it for protein co glucose, LDH and microbiology testing.

Treatment

Conservative management may be appropriate as small effusions will resolve with treatment of the underlying cause. Larger effusions often need aspiration or drainage.

Pleural aspiration involves sticking a needle through the chest wall into the effusion and aspirating the fluid. This can temporarily relieve the pressure but the effusion may recur and repeated aspiration may be required.

Chest drain can be used to drain the effusion and prevent it recurring.

Empyema

Empyema is where there is an infected pleural effusion. Suspect an empyema in a patient who has an improving pneumonia but new or ongoing fever. Pleural aspiration shows pus, **acidic pH** (pH < 7.2), low glucose and high LDH. Empyema is treated by chest drain to remove the pus and antibiotics.

Pneumothorax

Pneumothorax occurs when air gets into the plural space separating the lung from the chest wall. It can occur spontaneously or secondary to trauma, medical interventions ("*iatrogenic*") or lung pathology. The typical patient in exams is a tall, thin young man presenting with sudden breathlessness and pleuritic chest pain, possibly whilst playing sports.

Causes

- Spontaneous
- Trauma
- Iatrogenic, for example due to lung biopsy, mechanical ventilation or central line insertion
- Lung pathology such as infection, asthma or COPD

Investigations

Erect chest xray is the investigation of choice for a simple pneumothorax. It shows an area between the lung tissue and the chest wall where there are no lung markings. There will be a line demarcating the edge of the lung where the lung markings ends and the pneumothorax begins.

Measuring the size of the pneumothorax on a chest xray can be done according to the **BTS guidelines** from 2010. This involves measuring **horizontally** from the lung edge to the inside of the chest wall at the level of the **hilum**.

CT thorax can detect a pneumothorax that is too small to see on a chest xray. It can also be used to accurately assess the size of the pneumothorax.

Respiratory

Management

This is based on the 2010 guidelines from the British Thoracic Society:
- If no SOB and there is a < 2cm rim of air on the chest xray then no treatment is required as it will spontaneously resolve. Follow up in 2 - 4 weeks is recommended.
- If SOB and/or there is a > 2cm rim of air on the chest xray then it will require aspiration and reassessment.
- If aspiration fails twice it will require a chest drain.
- Unstable patients or bilateral or secondary pneumothoraces generally require a chest drain.

Tension Pneumothorax

Tension pneumothorax is caused by trauma to chest wall that creates a **one way valve** that lets air in but not out of the pleural space. The one way valve means that during inspiration air is drawn in to the pleural space and during expiration the air is trapped in the pleural space. Therefore, more air keeps getting drawn in to the pleural space with each breath and cannot escape. This is dangerous as it creates pressure inside the thorax that will push the **mediastinum** across, kink the big vessels in the mediastinum and cause **cardiorespiratory arrest**.

Signs of Tension Pneumothorax
- Tracheal deviation away from side of the pneumothorax
- Reduced air entry on the affected side
- Increased resonant to percussion on the affected side
- Tachycardia
- Hypotension

Management of Tension Pneumothorax
The management sentence you need to learn and recite in your exams is: "**Insert a large bore cannula into the second intercostal space in the midclavicular line**."

If a tension pneumothorax is suspected do not wait for any investigations. Once the pressure is relieved with a cannula then a **chest drain** is required for definitive management.

Chest Drain

Chest drains are inserted in the "**triangle of safety**". This triangle is formed by:
- The **5th intercostal space** (or the inferior nipple line)
- The **mid axillary line** (or the lateral edge of the **latissimus dorsi**)
- The **anterior axillary line** (or the lateral edge of the **pectoris major**)

The needle is inserted just above the rib to avoid the **neurovascular bundle** that runs just below the rib. Once the chest drain is inserted, obtain a chest xray to check the positioning.

Pulmonary Embolism

Pulmonary embolism (**PE**) is a condition where a blood clot (**thrombus**) forms in the **pulmonary arteries**. This is usually the result of a **deep vein thrombosis** (**DVT**) that developed in the legs and travelled (**embolised**) through the venous system and the right side of the heart to the pulmonary arteries. Once in the pulmonary arteries the thrmobus will block the blood flow to the lung tissue and create strain on the right side of the heart. DVTs and PEs are collectively known as **venous thromboembolism (VTE)**.

Risk Factors

There are a number of factors for developing a DVT or PE. In many of these situations we give patients prophylactic treatment with **low molecular weight heparin** to reduce the risk.
- Immobility
- Recent surgery
- Long haul flights
- Pregnancy
- Hormone therapy with oestrogen
- Malignancy
- Polycythaemia
- Systemic lupus erythematosus
- Thrombophilia

TOM TIP: In your exams when a patient is presenting with possible features of a DVT or PE, ask about risk factors such as periods of immobility, surgery and long haul flights to score extra points from your examiners.

VTE Prophylaxis

Every patient admitted to hospital should be assessed for their risk of **venous thromboembolism (VTE)**. If they are at increased risk of VTE they should receive prophylaxis with a **low molecular weight heparin** such as **enoxaparin** unless contraindicated. Contraindications include active bleeding or existing anticoagulation with **warfarin** or a **NOAC**. **Anti-embolic compression stockings** are also used unless contraindicated. The main contraindication for compression stockings is significant **peripheral arterial disease**.

Presentation

Pulmonary embolism can present with subtle signs and symptoms. In patients with potential features of a PE, risk factors for PE and no other explanation for their symptoms, have a low threshold for suspecting a PE. Presenting features include:
- Shortness of breath
- Cough with or without blood (**haemoptysis**)
- Pleuritic chest pain
- Hypoxia
- Tachycardia
- Raised respiratory rate
- Low grade fever
- Haemodynamic instability causing hypotension

There may also be signs and symptoms of a deep vein thrombosis such as unilateral leg swelling and tenderness.

Wells Score

The **Wells score** predicts the risk of a patient presenting with symptoms actually having a DVT or pulmonary embolism. It takes in to account risk factors such as recent surgery and clinical findings such as **tachycardia** (heart rate >100) and **haemoptysis**.

Diagnosis

NICE recommend assessing for alternative causes with a:
- History
- Examination
- Chest xray

Perform a **Wells score** and proceed based on the outcome:
- **Likely**: perform a CT pulmonary angiogram
- **Unlikely**: perform a d-dimer and if positive perform a CTPA

D-dimer is a sensitive (95%) but not specific blood test for VTE. This makes it useful for excluding VTE where there is a low suspicion. It is almost always raised if there is a DVT, however other conditions can also cause a raised d-dimer:
- Pneumonia
- Malignancy
- Heart failure
- Surgery
- Pregnancy

There are two main options for establishing a definitive diagnosis: **CT pulmonary angiogram** or **ventilation–perfusion** (**VQ**) scan.

CT pulmonary angiogram (**CTPA**) involves a chest CT scan with an **intravenous contrast** that highlights the pulmonary arteries to demonstrate any blood clots. This is usually the first choice for investigating a pulmonary embolism as it tends to be more readily available, provides a more definitive assessment and gives information about alternative diagnoses such as pneumonia or malignancy.

Ventilation-perfusion (**VQ**) **scan** involves using **radioactive isotopes** and a **gamma camera** to compare the **ventilation** with the **perfusion** of the lungs. They are used in patients with renal impairment, contrast allergy or at risk from radiation, where a CTPA is unsuitable. First, the isotopes are inhaled to fill the lungs and a picture is taken to demonstrate **ventilation**. Next a contrast containing isotopes is injected and a picture is taken to demonstrate **perfusion**. The two pictures are compared. With a pulmonary embolism there will be a deficit in perfusion as the thrombus blocks blood flow to the lung tissue. This area of lung tissue will be ventilated but not perfused.

TOM TIP: Patients with a pulmonary embolism often have a respiratory alkalosis when an ABG is performed. This is because the high respiratory rate causes them to "blow off" extra CO_2. As a result of the low CO_2, the blood becomes alkalotic. It is one of the few causes of a respiratory alkalosis, the other main cause being hyperventilation syndrome. Patients with a PE will have a low pO_2 whereas patients with hyperventilation syndrome will have a high pO_2.

Management

Supportive Management
- Admission to hospital
- Oxygen as required
- Analgesia if required
- Adequate monitoring for any deterioration

Initial Management

The initial management is with treatment dose **low molecular weight heparin** (**LMWH**). This should be started immediately before confirming the diagnosis in patients where DVT or PE is suspected and there is a delay in getting the scan. Examples are *enoxaparin* and *dalteparin*.

Switching to Long Term Anticoagulation

The options for long term anticoagulation in VTE are *warfarin*, a **NOAC** or **LMWH**.

Warfarin is a vitamin K antagonist. The target INR for warfarin is between 2 and 3. When switching to warfarin continue LMWH for 5 days or the INR is between 2 and 3 for 24 hours on warfarin (whichever is longer).

NOACs (or **DOACs**) are essentially oral anticoagulants that are not warfarin. They are an alternative option for anticoagulation that does not require monitoring. Originally they were called "**novel oral anticoagulants**" but this has been changed to "**non-vitamin K oral anticoagulants**" because they are no longer novel. This is changing to DOACs, standing for "**direct-acting oral anticoagulants**". The main three options are *apixaban*, *dabigatran* and *rivaroxaban*.

LMWH long term is first line treatment in pregnancy or cancer.

Continue anticoagulation for:
- *3 months* if there is an obvious reversible cause (then review)
- *Beyond 3 months* if the cause is unclear, there is recurrent VTE or there is an irreversible underlying cause such as thrombophilia. This is often 6 months in practice.
- *6 months* in active cancer (then review)

Thrombolysis

Where there is a **massive PE** with **haemodynamic compromise** there is a treatment option called **thrombolysis**. **Thrombolysis** involves injecting a **fibrinolytic** medication (they break down **fibrin**) that rapidly dissolves clots. There is a significant risk of bleeding which can make it dangerous. It is only used in patients with a massive PE where the benefits outweigh the risks. Some examples of thrombolytic agents are **streptokinase**, **alteplase** and **tenecteplase**.

There are two ways **thrombolysis** can be performed:
- *Intravenously* using a peripheral cannula.
- Directly into the **pulmonary arteries** using a central catheter. This is called **catheter-directed thrombolysis**.

In **catheter directed thrombolysis** a catheter is inserted into the venous system, through the right side of the heart and into the pulmonary arteries. The operator can then administer the **thrombolytic agent** directly into the location of the thrombus. Special equipment can also be used to physically break down the thrombus and aspirate it. There is a risk of damaging the pulmonary arteries doing this.

Pulmonary Hypertension

Pulmonary hypertension is increased *resistance* and *pressure* of blood in the *pulmonary arteries*. Increasing the pressure and resistance in the pulmonary arteries causes strain on the right side of the heart trying to pump blood through the lungs. This also causes a back pressure of blood into the systemic venous system.

Causes

The causes of pulmonary hypertension can split into 5 groups:
- **Group 1** - *Primary pulmonary hypertension* or connective tissue disease such as *systemic lupus erythematous* (*SLE*)
- **Group 2** - Left heart failure usually due to myocardial infarction or systemic hypertension
- **Group 3** - Chronic lung disease such as *COPD*
- **Group 4** - Pulmonary vascular disease such as *pulmonary embolism*
- **Group 5** - Miscellaneous causes such as *sarcoidosis*, *glycogen storage disease* and *haematological disorders*

Signs and Symptoms

Shortness of breath is the main presenting symptom. Other signs and symptoms are:
- Syncope
- Tachycardia
- Raised JVP
- Hepatomegaly
- Peripheral oedema

Investigations

ECG Changes
The right sided heart strain causes ECG changes such as:
- *Right ventricular hypertrophy* seen as large R waves on the right sided chest leads (V1-3) and S waves on the left sided chest leads (V4-6)
- *Right axis deviation*
- *Right bundle branch block*

Chest Xray Changes
- Dilated pulmonary arteries
- Right ventricular hypertrophy

Other investigations
- A raised NT-proBNF blood test result indicates right ventricular failure
- Echo can be used to estimate pulmonary artery pressure

Management

The prognosis is quite poor with a 30-40% 5 year survival from diagnosis. This can increase to 60-70% where specific treatment is possible.

Primary pulmonary hypertension can be treated with:
- IV prostanoids (e.g. epoprostenol)
- Endothelin receptor antagonists (e.g. macitentan)
- Phosphodiesterase-5 inhibitors (e.g. sildenafil)

Secondary pulmonary hypertension is managed by treating the underlying cause, such as pulmonary embolism or SLE.

Supportive treatment for complications such as respiratory failure, arrhythmias and heart failure.

Sarcoidosis

Sarcoidosis is a *granulomatous* inflammatory condition. **Granulomas** are **nodules of inflammation** full of **macrophages**. The cause of these granulomas developing is unknown.

It is usually associated with chest symptoms but also has multiple **extra-pulmonary manifestations** such as **erythema nodosum** and **lymphadenopathy**. Symptoms can vary dramatically from asymptomatic (in up to 50%) to severe and life threatening.

There are two spikes in incidence, in young adulthood and again around age 60. Women are affected more often and it occurs more frequently in black people compared with other ethnic groups.

TOM TIP: The typical MCQ exam patient is a 20-40 year old black female presenting with a dry cough and shortness of breath. They may have nodules on their shins suggesting erythema nodosum.

Organs Affected

Sarcoidosis can affect almost any organ in the body. The most commonly affected are the lungs, so sarcoidosis is usually managed by respiratory physicians.

Lungs (affecting over 90%)
- Mediastinal lymphadenopathy
- Pulmonary fibrosis
- Pulmonary nodules

Systemic Symptoms
- Fever
- Fatigue
- Weight loss

Liver (affecting around 20%)
- Liver nodules
- Cirrhosis
- Cholestasis

Eyes (affecting around 20%)
- Uveitis
- Conjunctivitis
- Optic neuritis

Skin (affecting around 15%)
- Erythema nodosum (tender, red nodules on the shins caused by inflammation of the subcutaneous fat)
- Lupus pernio (raised, purple skin lesions commonly on cheeks and nose)
- Granulomas can develop in scar tissue

Heart (affecting around 5%)
- Bundle branch block
- Heart block
- Myocardial muscle involvement

Kidneys (affecting around 5%)
- Kidney stones (due to hypercalcaemia)
- Nephrocalcinosis
- Interstitial nephritis

Central Nervous System (affecting around 5%)
- Nodules
- Pituitary involvement (diabetes insipidus)
- Encephalopathy

Peripheral Nervous System (affecting around 5%)
- Bells palsy
- Mononeuritis multiplex

Bones (affecting around 2%)
- Arthralgia
- Arthritis
- Myopathy

Lofgren's Syndrome

This is a specific presentation of sarcoidosis. It is characteristic by a triad of:
- Erythema nodosum
- Bilateral hilar lymphadenopathy
- Polyarthralgia (joint pain in multiple joints)

Differential Diagnosis

- Tuberculosis
- Lymphoma
- Hypersensitivity pneumonitis
- HIV
- Toxoplasmosis
- Histoplasmosis

Blood Tests

- Raised **serum ACE**. This is often used as a screening test.
- **Hypercalcaemia** (raised calcium) is a key finding
- Raised **serum soluble interleukin-2 receptor**
- Raised CRP
- Raised immunoglobulins

Imaging

- Chest xray shows **hilar lymphadenopathy**
- High resolution CT thorax shows **hilar lymphadenopathy** and **pulmonary nodules**
- **MRI** can show **CNS involvement**
- **PET scan** can show active inflammation in affected areas

Histology

The **gold standard** for confirming the diagnosis of sarcoidosis is by histology from a biopsy. This is usually done by doing bronchoscopy with ultrasound guided biopsy of mediastinal lymph nodes.

The histology shows characteristic **non-caseating granulomas** with **epithelioid cells.**

Tests for other organ involvement

- **U&Es** for kidney involvement
- **Urine dipstick** or urine **albumin-creatinine ratio** to look for **proteinuria**, indicating nephritis
- **LFTs** for liver involvement
- **Ophthalmology** review for eye involvement
- **ECG** and **echocardiogram** for heart involvement
- **Ultrasound** abdomen for liver and kidney involvement

Treatment

- **No treatment** is considered as first line in patients with no or mild symptoms as it often resolves spontaneously
- **Oral steroids** are usually first line where treatment is required and are given for between 6 and 24 months. Patients should be given **bisphosphonates** to protect against osteoporosis whilst on such long term steroids.
- Second line options are **methotrexate** or **azathioprine**
- **Lung transplant** is rarely required in severe pulmonary disease

Prognosis

Sarcoidosis spontaneously resolves within 6 months in around 60% of patients. In a small number of patients it progresses and **pulmonary fibrosis** and **pulmonary hypertension** develop, potentially requiring a lung transplant. Death in sarcoidosis is usually when it affects the heart (causing arrhythmias) or the central nervous system.

Obstructive Sleep Apnoea

Obstructive sleep apnoea is caused by collapse of the **pharyngeal airway** during sleep. It is characterised by **apnoea episodes** during sleep where the person will stop breathing periodically for up to a few minutes. This is usually reported by the partner as the patient is unaware of these episodes.

Risk Factors

- Middle age
- Male
- Obesity
- Alcohol
- Smoking

Features

- Apnoea episodes during sleep (reported by their partner)
- Snoring
- Morning headache
- Waking up unrefreshed from sleep
- Daytime sleepiness
- Concentration problems
- Reduced oxygen saturation during sleep

Severe cases can cause hypertension, **heart failure** and can increase the risk of **myocardial infarction** and **stroke**.

TOM TIP: If interviewing someone that you suspect has obstructive sleep apnoea ask about daytime sleepiness and their occupation. Daytime sleepiness is a key feature that should make you suspect obstructive sleep apnoea. Patients that need to be fully alert for work, for example heavy goods vehicle operators, require urgent referral and may need amended work duties whilst awaiting assessment and treatment.

Management

Referral to an **ENT specialist** or a **specialist sleep clinic** where they can perform sleep studies. This involves the patient sleeping in a laboratory whilst staff monitor their oxygen saturations, heart rate, respiratory rate and breathing to establish any apnoea episodes and the extent of their snoring.

The first step in management is to **correct reversible risk factors** by advising them to stop drinking alcohol, stop smoking and loose weight.

The next step is to use a **continuous positive airway pressure** (**CPAP**) machine that provides continuous pressure to maintain the patency of the airway.

Surgery is another option. This involves quite significant surgical restructuring of the soft palate and jaw. The most common procedure is called **uvulopalatopharyngoplasty** (**UPPP**).

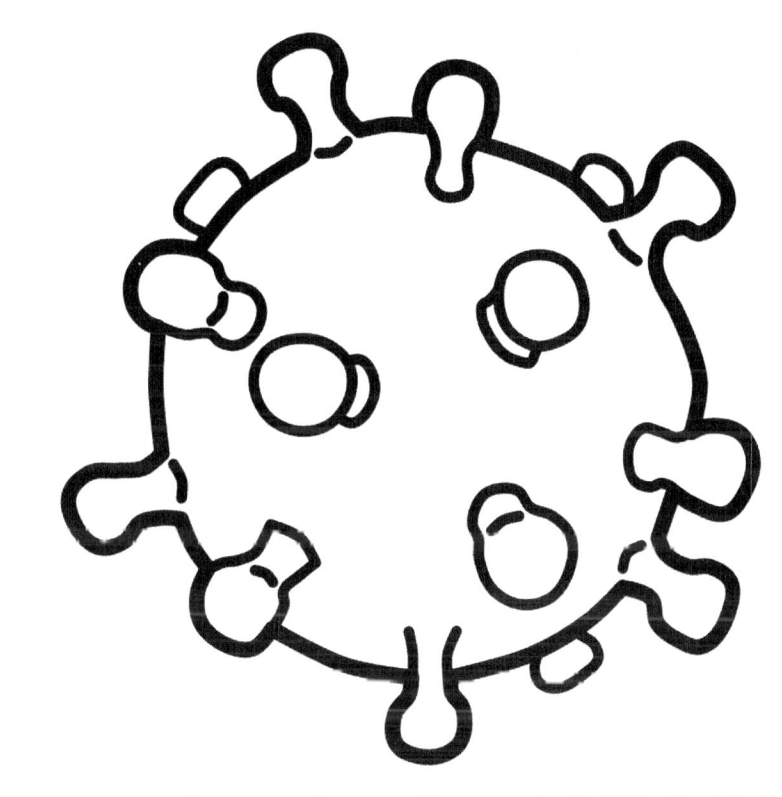

INFECTIOUS DISEASES

5.1	Bacteria	136
5.2	Antibiotics	138
5.3	Sepsis	141
5.4	Chest Infections	144
5.5	Urinary Tract Infections	145
5.6	Skin and Soft Tissue Infections	147
5.7	Ear, Nose and Throat Infections	148
5.8	Intra-Abdominal Infections	150
5.9	Septic Arthritis	151
5.10	Influenza	152
5.11	Gastroenteritis	154
5.12	Meningitis	157
5.13	Tuberculosis	160
5.14	HIV	164
5.15	Malaria	166

Bacteria

Bacteria are single celled organisms. They come in many shapes and sizes. Most bacteria are not harmful however some are **pathogenic** and cause infectious diseases. These pathogenic bacteria are the most relevant to learning medicine.

They can be categorised into **aerobic** and **anaerobic**, **gram positive** and **gram negative** and **atypical bacteria**. Learning where bacteria fall within these categories helps you work out which antibiotics will be effective against them.

Aerobic bacteria require oxygen whereas **anaerobic** bacteria do not. **Gram positive** bacteria have a thick **peptidoglycan cell wall** that stains with **crystal violet** stain. **Gram negative** bacteria don't have this thick peptidoglycan cell wall and don't stain with crystal violet stain but will stain with other stains. **Atypical bacteria** cannot be stained or cultured in the normal way.

Bacteria can also be classified based on their shapes. Rod shaped bacteria are called **bacilli** and circular shaped bacteria are called **cocci**.

Basic Anatomy and Physiology

There are some key components to learn about as they are the target of antibiotic treatment:

The **cell wall** is a structure that surrounds the outer cell membrane and is found on gram positive bacteria.

Nucleic acid is essential component of bacterial DNA.

Ribosomes are where bacteria proteins are synthesised within the bacterial cell.

Folic acid is essential for synthesis and regulation of DNA within the bacteria. Folic acid cannot be directly imported into the cell and requires a chain of intermediates to get in. This chain starts with **para-aminobenzoic acid** (**PABA**), which is directly absorbed across the cell membrane into the cell. **PABA** is converted to **dihydrofolic acid** (**DHFA**), which is converted inside the cell to **tetrahydrofolic acid** (**THFA**), then **folic acid**.

Gram Stain

A **gram stain** is used as a quick way to check a sample under the microscope to look for bacteria. It involves two main steps:

Add a **crystal violet stain**, which binds to molecules in the thick peptidoglycan **cell wall** in **gram positive** bacteria turning them **violet**.

Then add a **counterstain** (such as **safranin**) which binds to the **cell membrane** in bacteria that don't have a cell wall (**gram negative** bacteria) turning them **red/pink**.

Gram Positive Cocci

- Staphylococcus
- Streptococcus
- Enterococcus

Gram Positive Rods

Use the mnemonic "*corney Mike's list of basic cars*":
- Corney - **Corneybacteria**
- Mike's - **Mycobacteria**
- List of - **Listeria**
- Basic - **Bacillus**
- Cars - **Nocardia**

Gram Positive Anaerobes

Use the mnemonic "**CLAP**":
- **C** - **C**lostridium
- **L** - **L**actobacillus
- **A** - **A**ctinomyces
- **P** - **P**ropionibacterium

Gram Negative Bacteria

If the bacteria is not listed above then it is probably gram negative. Common gram negative organisms are:
- *Neisseria meningitidis*
- *Neisseria gonorrhoea*
- *Haemophilia influenza*
- *E. coli*
- *Klebsiella*
- *Pseudomonas aeruginosa*
- *Moraxella catarrhalis*

Atypical Bacteria

The **definition** of *atypical bacteria* is that they cannot be *cultured* in the normal way or detected using a *gram stain*. Atypical bacteria are most often implicated in pneumonia.

The atypical bacteria that cause *atypical pneumonia* can be remembered using the mnemonic "**legions of psittaci MCQs**":
- Legions - **Legionella pneumophila**
- Psittaci - **Chlamydia psittaci**
- M - **Mycoplasma pneumoniae**
- C - **Chlamydophila pneumoniae**
- Qs - **Q fever** (*coxiella burneti*)

Methicillin-Resistant Staphylococcus Aureus (MRSA)

MRSA refers to **staphylococcus aureus** bacteria that have become resistant to beta-lactam antibiotics such as penicillins, cephalosporins and carbapenems.

They are a problem in healthcare settings where antibiotics are commonly used. Think about MRSA in patients that have had hospital admissions or come from a nursing home or other healthcare institution.

People are often colonised with MRSA bacteria and have them living harmlessly on their skin and respiratory tract. If these bacteria become part of an infection they can be difficult to treat. Patients being admitted for surgery or inpatient treatment are screened for MRSA infection by taking nose and groin swabs, so that extra measures can be taken to try to eradicate them and stop their spread. Eradication usually involves a combination of **chlorhexidine** body washes and antibacterial nasal creams.

Antibiotic treatment options for MRSA are:
- Doxycycline
- Clindamycin
- Vancomycin
- Teicoplanin
- Linezolid

Extended Spectrum Beta Lactamase Bacteria (ESBLs)

ESBLs are bacteria that have developed resistance to **beta-lactam** antibiotics. They produce **beta lactamase enzymes** that destroy the beta-lactam ring on the antibiotic. They can be resistant to a very broad range of antibiotics.

ESBLs tend to be *e. coli* or *klebsiella* and typically cause urinary tract infections but can also cause other infections, such as pneumonia.

They are usually sensitive to *carbapenems* such as *meropenem* or *imipenem*.

Antibiotics

Antibiotics are used to treat bacterial infections. They work in various ways to either stop the reproduction and growth of bacteria (*bacteriostatic*) or kill the bacteria directly (*bactericidal*). Antibiotics need to be used carefully as over-use or inappropriate use can lead to **resistance** of bacteria to those antibiotics and increasing difficulty in treating infections.

Local Resistance and Guidelines

The bacteria in different **populations** develop **resistance** to different antibiotics. For example, the *e. coli* in one area of the country might be particularly resistant to **trimethoprim** whereas in another area of the country they may be resistant to **nitrofurantoin** but sensitive to **trimethoprim**. Therefore it is necessary to have local policies that guide what antibiotics to use in different scenarios.

TOM TIP: In your OSCEs questions about treating infections can always be answered with "treat with antibiotics according to the local antibiotic policy".

Antibiotics That Inhibit Cell Wall Synthesis

Antibiotics with a beta-lactam ring
- Penicillin
- Carbapenems such as meropenem
- Cephalosporins

Antibiotics without a beta-lactam ring
- Vancomycin
- Teicoplanin

Antibiotics that Inhibit Folic Acid Metabolism

Bacteria produce their own folic acid in a series of steps. This chain starts with *para-aminobenzoic acid* (**PABA**), which is directly absorbed across the cell membrane in to the cell. **PABA** is then converted to *dihydrofolic acid* (**DHFA**), then *tetrahydrofolic acid* (**THFA**) and finally *folic acid*.

Antibiotics can be used to disrupt steps along this chain:
- *Sulfamethoxazole* blocks the conversion of DHFA to THFA
- *Trimethoprim* blocks the conversion of THFA to folic acid

Co-trimoxazole is a combination of sulfamethoxazole and trimethoprim.

Metronidazole

The **reduction** of metronidazole into its active form only occurs in **anaerobic cells**. When partially reduced, metronidazole inhibits **nucleic acid synthesis**. This is why metronidazole is effective against anaerobes and not aerobes.

Antibiotics that inhibit protein synthesis by targeting the ribosome

- *Macrolides* such as erythromycin, clarithromycin and azithromycin
- *Clindamycin*
- *Tetracyclines* such as doxycycline
- *Gentamicin*
- *Chloramphenicol*

Penicillin Allergy

"Penicillin allergy" is very common. True penicillin allergy can lead to anaphylaxis and death so should not be taken lightly. The problem is that true allergy is more rare than reported allergy and being labelled as penicillin allergic stops patients from getting many potentially life saving antibiotics.

Around 10% of patients report penicillin allergy, however only around 10% of patients that report penicillin allergy have a true allergy to penicillin.

It is often believed that 10% of patients with penicillin allergy will have a reaction to *cephalosporins* and *carbapenems*. In reality this is probably closer to 1%.

TOM TIP: When taking an allergy history always ask what reaction patients have with that medication. If they report diarrhoea for example, this is a side effect rather than an allergy and means if necessary (for example in life threatening sepsis) they can still receive that medication.

Antibiotic Coverage

Use this table to think about how you could treat different presentations of patients with infections. It is not an exact science but helpful when starting out. For example, think about what antibiotics would be appropriate for a patient with a chest infection and why.

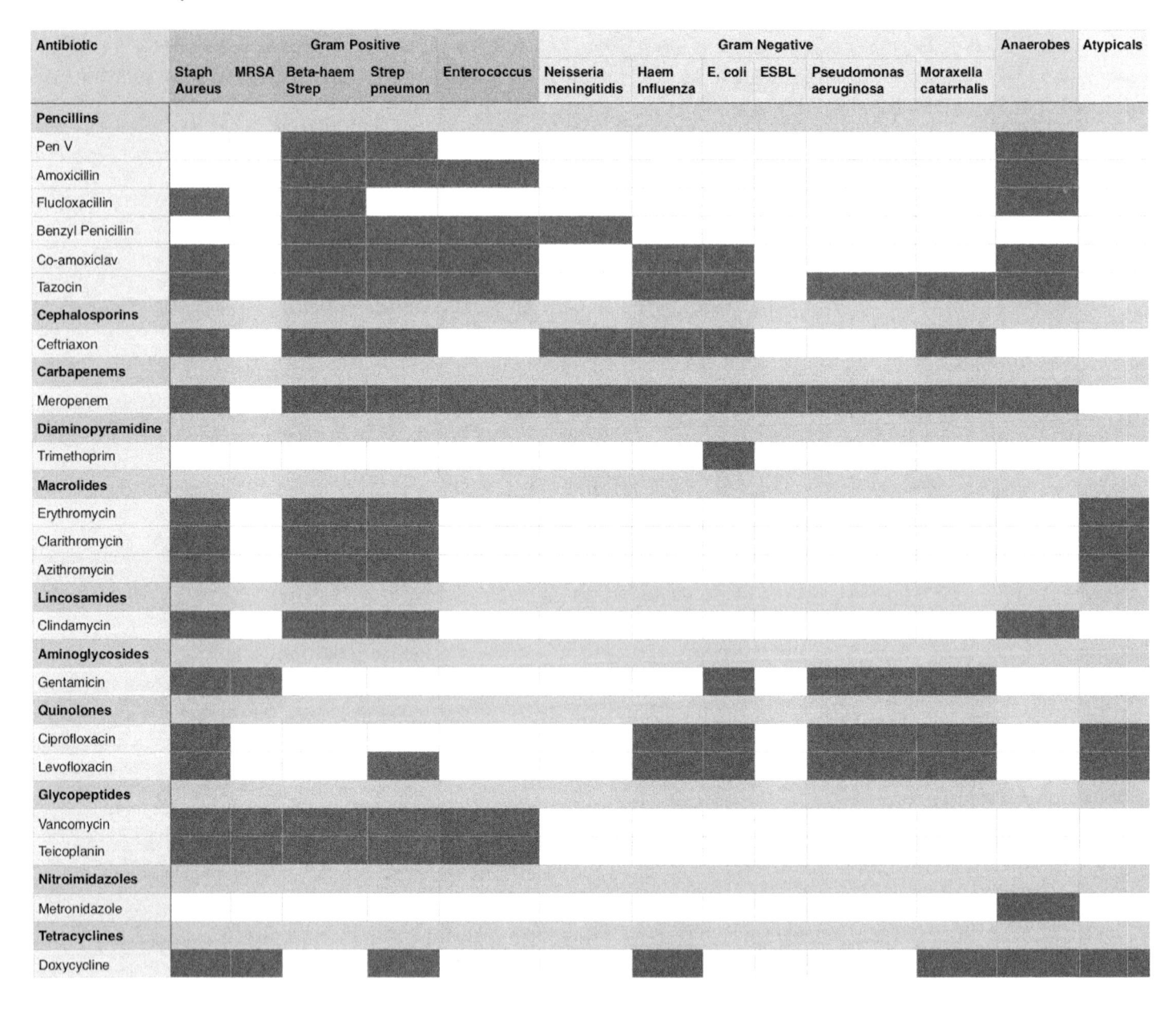

Antibiotic	Gram Positive					Gram Negative						Anaerobes	Atypicals
	Staph Aureus	MRSA	Beta-haem Strep	Strep pneumon	Enterococcus	Neisseria meningitidis	Haem Influenza	E. coli	ESBL	Pseudomonas aeruginosa	Moraxella catarrhalis		
Penicillins													
Pen V			■									■	
Amoxicillin			■	■	■							■	
Flucloxacillin	■		■									■	
Benzyl Penicillin			■	■	■	■						■	
Co-amoxiclav	■		■	■	■	■	■	■			■	■	
Tazocin	■		■	■	■	■	■	■		■	■	■	
Cephalosporins													
Ceftriaxon	■		■	■		■	■	■			■		
Carbapenems													
Meropenem	■		■	■	■	■	■	■	■	■	■	■	
Diaminopyramidine													
Trimethoprim								■					
Macrolides													
Erythromycin	■		■	■									■
Clarithromycin	■		■	■									■
Azithromycin	■		■	■									■
Lincosamides													
Clindamycin	■		■	■								■	
Aminoglycosides													
Gentamicin	■		■				■	■		■	■		
Quinolones								■		■	■		■
Ciprofloxacin	■						■	■		■	■		■
Levofloxacin	■			■			■	■		■	■		■
Glycopeptides													
Vancomycin	■	■	■	■	■								
Teicoplanin	■	■	■	■	■								
Nitroimidazoles													
Metronidazole												■	
Tetracyclines													
Doxycycline	■		■				■						■

When learning antibiotic coverage I used this stepwise process of escalating antibiotic treatment in a hospital patient to remember what antibiotics covered what bacteria. Each step covers all the bacteria in the previous step as well as new ones:

- Start with **amoxicillin** which covers **streptococcus**, **listeria** and **enterococcus**
- Switch to **co-amoxiclav** to additionally cover **staphylococcus**, **haemophilus** and **e. coli**
- Switch to **tazocin** to additionally cover **pseudomonas**
- Switch to **meropenem** to additionally cover **ESBLs**
- Add **teicoplanin** or **vancomycin** to cover **MRSA**
- Add **clarithromycin** or **doxycycline** to cover **atypical bacteria**

Sepsis

Sepsis is a condition where the body launches a large immune response to an infection that causes **systemic inflammation** and affects organ function.

Pathophysiology

The pathogens are recognised by **macrophages**, **lymphocytes** and **mast cells**. These cells release vast amounts of **cytokines** like **interleukins** and **tumor necrosis factor** to alert the immune system to the invader. These **cytokines** activate other parts of the immune system. This immune activation leads to further release of chemicals such as **nitrous oxide** that causes **vasodilation**. The immune response causes inflammation throughout the body.

Many of these **cytokines** cause the **endothelial lining** of blood vessels to become more **permeable**. This causes fluid to leak out of the blood into the **extracellular space**, leading to **oedema** and a reduction in **intravascular volume**. The **oedema** around blood vessels creates a space between the blood and the tissues, reducing the amount of oxygen that reaches the tissues.

Activation of the **coagulation system** leads to deposition of fibrin throughout the circulation, further compromising organ and tissue perfusion. It also leads to consumption of platelets and clotting factors as they are being used up to form the clots. This leads to **thrombocytopenia**, **haemorrhages** and an inability to form clots and stop bleeding. This is called **disseminated intravascular coagulopathy** (**DIC**).

Blood **lactate** rises due **anaerobic respiration** in the hypo-perfused tissues with inadequate oxygen. A waste product of anaerobic respiration is lactate.

Septic Shock

Septic shock is defined when arterial blood pressure drops resulting in organ hypo-perfusion. This leads to a rise in blood lactate as the organs begin **anaerobic respiration**. This can be measured as either:
- **Systolic blood pressure** less than 90 despite fluid resuscitation
- **Hyperlactaemia** (lactate > 4 mmol/L)

This should be treated aggressively with IV fluids to improve the blood pressure and tissue perfusion. If IV fluid boluses don't improve the blood pressure and lactate level they should be escalated to the high dependency or intensive care unit where they can use medication called **inotropes** (such as **noradrenalin**) that help stimulate the cardiovascular system and improve blood pressure and tissue perfusion.

Severe Sepsis

Severe sepsis is defined when sepsis is present and results in organ dysfunction, for example:
- Hypoxia
- Oliguria
- Acute kidney injury
- Thrombocytopenia
- Coagulation dysfunction
- Hypotension
- Hyperlactaemia (> 2 mmol/L)

Risk Factors

Any condition that impacts the immune system or makes the patient more frail or prone to infection is a risk factor for developing sepsis:
- Very young or old patients (under 1 or over 75 years)
- Chronic conditions such as COPD and diabetes
- Chemotherapy, immunosuppressants or steroids
- Surgery, recent trauma or burns
- Pregnancy or peripartum
- Indwelling medical devices such as catheters or central lines

Presentation

The **national early warning score** (**NEWS**) is used in the UK to pick up the signs of sepsis. This involves checking physical observations and consciousness level:
- Temperature
- Heart rate
- Respiratory rate
- Oxygen saturations
- Blood pressure
- Consciousness level

Other signs on examination:
- Signs of potential sources such as cellulitis, discharge from a wound, cough or dysuria
- Non-blanching rash can indicate **meningococcal septicaemia**
- Reduced urine output
- Mottled skin
- Cyanosis
- Arrhythmias such as new onset **atrial fibrillation**

There are a few key points worth being aware of:
- High respiratory rate (**tachypnoea**) is often the first sign of sepsis
- Elderly patients often present with confusion, drowsiness or simply "off legs"
- **Neutropenic** or **immunosuppressed** patients may have normal observations and temperature despite being life threateningly unwell

Investigations

Arrange blood tests for patients with suspected sepsis:
- **Full blood count** to assess cell count including white cells and neutrophils
- **U&Es** to assess kidney function and for acute kidney injury
- **LFTs** to assess liver function and for possible source of infection
- **CRP** to assess inflammation
- **Clotting** to assess for **disseminated intravascular coagulopathy** (**DIC**)
- **Blood cultures** to assess for **bacteraemia**
- **Blood gas** to assess lactate, pH and glucose

Additional investigations can be helpful in locating the source of the infection:

- Urine dipstick and culture
- Chest xray
- CT scan if intra-abdominal infection or abscess is suspected
- Lumbar puncture for meningitis or encephalitis

Management

Every hospital will have a sepsis protocol and pathway that should be followed for patients with presumed sepsis. Patients should also be escalated to the senior decision maker and the appropriate level of care such as HDU or ICU if needed.

NICE recommend risk stratifying patients into **low**, **medium** and **high risk** based on their presentation. High risk patients need urgent attention and management. Moderate risk patients may be managed in the community where the diagnosis is clear and it is safe to do so. Always remember **safety-netting advice** when managing patients in the community and giving clear instructions about when they need to seek help

Patients should be assessed and have treatment initiated **within 1 hour** of presenting with suspected sepsis. This involves performing the **sepsis six**. This involves three tests and three treatments.

Sepsis Six

Three Tests:
- Blood lactate level
- Blood cultures
- Urine output

Three Treatments:
- Oxygen to maintain oxygen saturations 94-98% (or 88-92% in COPD)
- Empirical broad spectrum antibiotics
- IV fluids

Neutropenic Sepsis

Neutropenic sepsis is a very important medical emergency. It is sepsis in a patient with a low neutrophil count of **less than 1 x 10^9/L**.

A low neutrophil count is usually the consequence of anti-cancer or immunosuppressant treatment. Medication that may cause neutropenia include:
- Anti-cancer **chemotherapy**
- **Clozapine** (schizophrenia)
- **Hydroxychloroquine** (rheumatoid arthritis)
- **Methotrexate** (rheumatoid arthritis)
- **Sulfasalazine** (rheumatoid arthritis)
- **Carbimazole** (hyperthyroidism)
- **Quinine** (malaria)
- **Infliximab** (monoclonal antibody use for immunosuppression)
- **Rituximab** (monoclonal antibody use for immunosuppression)

Have a low threshold for suspecting **neutropenic sepsis** in patients taking immunosuppressants or medications that may cause neutropenia. Treat any temperature above 38°C as neutropenic sepsis in these patients until proven otherwise. They are at high risk of death from sepsis as their immune system cannot adequately fight the infection. They need emergency admission and careful management.

Each local hospital will have a **neutropenic sepsis policy**. Treatment is with immediate broad spectrum antibiotics such as **piperacillin with tazobactam** (**tazocin**). The other aspects of management are essentially the same as for sepsis, however extra precaution needs to be taken. Time is precious so don't delay antibiotics while waiting for investigation results.

Chest Infections

See the **pneumonia** section (page 108) in the respiratory chapter for more on chest infections.

Chest infections typically present with a cough and sputum production, shortness of breath, fever, lethargy and crackles on the chest. Remember that **viral bronchitis** is very common, will also present with a productive cough and does not require antibiotics.

Common causes

- **Streptococcus pneumoniae** (50%)
- **Haemophilus influenzae** (20%)

Other Causes and Associations

- **Moraxella catarrhalis** in immunocompromised patients or those with chronic pulmonary disease
- **Pseudomonas aeruginosa** in patients with cystic fibrosis or bronchiectasis
- **Staphylococcus aureus** in patients with cystic fibrosis

Atypical Bacteria

You can remember the 5 causes of atypical pneumonia with the mnemonic "**legions of psittaci MCQs**":
- Legions - **Legionella pneumophila**
- Psittaci - **Chlamydia psittaci**
- M - **Mycoplasma pneumoniae**
- C - **Chlamydydophila pneumoniae**
- Qs - **Q fever** (**coxiella burnetii**)

Antibiotic Choice

An appropriate initial antibiotic in the community would be:
- Amoxicillin

Alternatives:
- Erythromycin / clarithromycin
- Doxycycline

To treat *atypical bacteria*:
- Macrolides such as clarithromycin
- Quinolones such as levofloxacin
- Tetracyclines such as doxycycline

Urinary Tract Infections

Urinary tract infections involve infection in the bladder causing **cystitis** (inflammation of the bladder). They can spread up to the kidneys and cause **pyelonephritis**. They are far more common in women where the urethra is much shorter, making it easy for bacteria to get into the bladder.

The main source of bacteria for urinary tract infections is from the faeces, where the normal intestinal bacteria such as *E. coli* can easily make the short journey to the urethral opening from the anus. Sexual activity is a key method for spreading bacteria around the *perineum*. They are also very common in women where incontinence or hygiene are a problem.

Urinary catheters are a key source of infection and catheter associated urinary tract infections tend to be more significant and difficult to treat.

Presentation

Lower urinary tract infections present with:
- Dysuria (pain, stinging or burning when passing urine)
- Suprapubic pain or discomfort
- Frequency
- Urgency
- Incontinence
- Confusion is commonly the only symptom in older more frail patients

Pyelonephritis presents with:
- *Fever* is a more prominent feature than lower urinary tract infections
- *Loin*, *suprapubic* or *back pain*. This may be bilateral or unilateral.
- Looking and feeling generally unwell
- Vomiting
- Loss of appetite
- *Haematuria*
- *Renal angle tenderness* on examination

Urine Dipstick

Nitrites – gram negative bacteria (such as *E. coli*) break down **nitrates**, a normal waste product in urine, into **nitrites**. The presence of nitrites suggest bacteria in the urine.

Leukocytes – this means **white blood cells**. There are normally a small number of leukocytes in the urine but a significant rise can be the result of an infection or other cause of inflammation. Urine dipsticks test for **leukocyte esterase**, a product of leukocytes that gives an indication to the number of leukocytes in the urine.

Nitrites are a better indication of infection than **leukocytes**. If both are present the patient should be treated as a UTI. If only nitrites are present it is worth treating as a UTI. If only **leukocytes** are present the patient should not be treated as a UTI unless there is clinical evidence they have one.

If **nitrites** or **leukocytes** are present, the urine should be sent to the microbiology lab. If neither are present the patient is unlikely to have a UTI.

Send a **midstream urine** (**MSU**) sample to the microbiology lab to be cultured and have sensitivity testing.

Causes

Most common cause is **Escherichia coli** (**E. coli**). This is a gram negative, anaerobic, rod shaped bacteria that is part of the normal lower intestinal microbiome. It is found in faeces and can easily spread to the bladder.

Other causes:
- **Klebsiella pneumoniae** (gram negative anaerobic rod)
- **Enterococcus**
- **Pseudomonas aeruginosa**
- **Staphylococcus saprophyticus**
- **Candida albicans** (fungal)

Antibiotics Choice

Follow local guidelines. An appropriate initial antibiotic in the community would be:
- Trimethoprim
- Nitrofurantoin

Alternatives:
- Pivmecillinam
- Amoxicillin
- Cefalexin

Duration of Antibiotics

- **3 days** of antibiotics for a simple lower urinary tract infection in women
- **5-10 days** of antibiotics for women that are immunosuppressed, have abnormal anatomy or impaired kidney function
- **7 days** of antibiotics for men, pregnant women or catheter related UTIs

It is worth noting that NICE recommend changing the catheter when someone is diagnosed with a catheter related urinary tract infection.

Pregnancy

Urinary tract infections in pregnancy increase the risk of **pyelonephritis**, **premature rupture of membranes** and **pre-term labour**.

Management in pregnancy:
- 7 days of antibiotics (even with *asymptomatic bacteriuria*)
- Urine for culture and sensitivities
- First line: nitrofurantoin
- Second line: cefalexin or amoxicillin

Nitrofurantoin is generally avoided in the third trimester as it is linked with *haemolytic anaemia* in the newborn.

Trimethoprim is generally considered safe in pregnancy but avoided in the first trimester or if they are on another medication that affects folic acid (such as anti-epileptics) due to the anti-folate effects.

Management of Pyelonephritis

Referral to hospital if there are features of sepsis

NICE recommend the following first line antibiotics for 7-10 days when treating pyelonephritis in the community:
- Cefalexin
- Co-amoxiclav
- Trimethoprim
- Ciprofloxacin

Skin and Soft Tissue Infections

Cellulitis is an infection of the skin and the soft tissues underneath. The skin normally acts as a very effective physical barrier between the environment and soft tissues. When a patient presents with cellulitis look for a breach in the skin barrier and a point of entry for the bacteria. This may be due to skin trauma, eczematous skin, fungal nail infections or ulcers.

Presentation

The skin will demonstrate changes:
- Erythema (red discolouration)
- Warm or hot to touch
- Tense
- Thickened
- Oedematous
- *Bullae* (fluid filled blisters)
- A *golden-yellow crust* can be present and indicates a *staphylococcus aureus* infection

Causes

The most common causes are:
- *Staphylococcus aureus*
- *Group A streptococcus* (mainly *streptococcus pyogenes*)
- *Group C streptococcus* (mainly *streptococcus dysgalactiae*)

MRSA is another cause that needs to be considered.

Eron Classification

This is the classification system NICE recommends for the assessment of the severity of cellulitis:
- Class 1 - no systemic toxicity or comorbidity
- Class 2 - systemic toxicity or comorbidity
- Class 3 - significant systemic toxicity or significant comorbidity
- Class 4 - sepsis or life threatening infection

Admit the patient for intravenous antibiotics if they are class 3 or 4. Also consider admission for frail, very young or immunocompromised patients.

Antibiotics

Flucloxacillin is very effective against staph infections and also works well against other gram positive cocci. It is usually the first choice in treating cellulitis and can be given oral or intravenous.

Alternatives:
- Clarithromycin
- Clindamycin
- Co-amoxiclav

Ear, Nose and Throat Infections

Tonsillitis, **otitis media** and **rhinosinusitis** are most commonly caused by **viral infections** and do not require antibiotics. These infections will resolve without treatment over 1 to 3 weeks.

Antibiotics should be reserved for immunocompromised patients, those with significant co-morbidities, severe infections or infections that fail to resolve. NICE guidelines are supportive of considering a **delayed prescription** in the community where patients can collect antibiotics if the symptoms don't improve or get worse after 3 days.

Bacteria

Bacterial tonsillitis is most commonly caused by **group A streptococcus** (**GAS**) infections, mainly **streptococcus pyogenes**.

Otitis media, **sinusitis** and **tonsillitis** not caused by **GAS** are most commonly caused by:
- *Streptococcus pneumoniae*

Other causes of *otitis media*, *sinusitis* and *tonsillitis*:
- *Haemophilus influenzae*
- *Morazella catarrhalis*
- *Staphylococcus aureus*

Tonsillitis

Tonsillitis is most commonly viral and does not require antibiotics.

The **Centor criteria** are used to estimate the probability that tonsillitis is due to a bacteria infection and requires antibiotics. A score of less than 3 indicates they are unlikely to benefit from antibiotics. A score of 3 or more gives a 40 to 60% probability of bacterial tonsillitis and it is appropriate to offer antibiotics. One point is given for each of the following:
- Fever ≥ 38°C
- Tonsillar exudates
- Absence of cough
- Tender anterior cervical lymph nodes (lymphadenopathy)

Penicillin V (also called **phenoxymethylpenicillin**) for a **10 day** course is typically first line.

Alternatives antibiotics and for a broader spectrum of activity:
- Co-amoxiclav
- Clarithromycin
- Doxycycline

Otitis Media

It is difficult to distinguish between bacterial and viral *otitis media*. It presents with ear pain. Examination will reveal a bulging red **tympanic membrane**. If the ear drum perforates there can be discharge from the ear.

Otitis media usually resolves within 3 to 7 days without antibiotics. If systemically unwell consider admission.

An appropriate initial antibiotic in the community:
- Amoxicillin

Alternatives in penicillin allergy:
- Clarithromycin
- Erythromycin

Second line if not responding to amoxicillin after 2 days:
- Co-amoxiclav

Sinusitis

Sinusitis can be bacterial or viral. NICE recommend providing an antibiotic if the patient is systemically very unwell, however most patients do not require antibiotics. Sinusitis usually last 2-3 weeks and resolves without treatment.

NICE guidelines suggest the following management:
- Symptoms for less than 10 days: no antibiotics.
- No improvement after 10 days: 2 weeks of high-dose steroid nasal spray
- No improvement after 10 days and likely bacterial cause: consider delayed or immediate prescription of antibiotics

Penicillin V (also called **phenoxymethylpenicillin**) for a 5 day course is typically first line. Co-amoxiclav is used second line if they do not respond after at least 2-3 days.

Alternatives in penicillin allergy:
- Clarithromycin
- Erythromycin (pregnancy)
- Doxycycline

Intra-Abdominal Infections

There is a long list of possible intra-abdominal infections:
- Acute diverticulitis
- Cholecystitis (with secondary infection)
- Ascending cholangitis
- Appendicitis
- Spontaneous bacterial peritonitis
- Intra-abdominal abscess

Common Causes of Intra-Abdominal Infections

- **Anaerobes** (e.g. *bacteroides* and *clostridium*)
- *E. coli*
- *Klebsiella*
- *Enterococcus*
- *Streptococcus*

Treating Intra-Abdominal Infections

When treating intra abdominal infections a broad spectrum of antibiotic cover is required unless culture results are available. It needs to cover gram positive, gram negative and anaerobic bacteria. Always follow the **local guidelines** as these are frequently changed based on local resistance and infection control issues.

Antibiotics for Intra-Abdominal Infections

Co-amoxiclav
This provides good gram positive, gram negative and anaerobic cover. It does not cover pseudomonas or atypical bacteria.

Quinolones
Ciprofloxacin and levofloxacin provide reasonable gram positive and gram negative cover and also cover atypical bacteria, however they don't cover anaerobes so are usually paired with metronidazole when treating intra-abdominal infections.

Metronidazole
This provides exceptional anaerobic cover but does not provide any cover against aerobic bacteria.

Gentamicin
This provides very good gram negative cover with some gram positive cover particularly against staphylococcus. It is **bactericidal**, so works to kill the bacteria rather than just slowing it down.

Vancomycin
This provides very good gram positive cover including MRSA. It is often combined with gentamicin (to cover gram negatives) and metronidazole (to cover anaerobes) in patients with penicillin allergy.

Cephalosporins
These provide good broad spectrum cover against gram positive and gram negative bacteria but are not very effective against anaerobes. They are often avoided due to the risk of developing **C. difficile** infection.

Tazocin and Meropenem

Piperacillin/tazobactam (tazocin) and meropenem are heavy hitting antibiotics that cover gram positive, gram negative and anaerobic bacteria. They don't cover atypical bacteria or MRSA and tazocin doesn't cover ESBLs, but they cover almost everything else. They are usually reserved for very unwell patients or those not responding to other antibiotics.

Common Regimes

Some common regimes for intra abdominal infection are:
- **Co-amoxiclav** alone
- **Amoxicillin** plus **gentamicin** plus **metronidazole**
- **Ciprofloxacin** plus **metronidazole** (penicillin allergy)
- **Vancomycin** plus **gentamicin** plus **metronidazole** (penicillin allergy)

Antibiotics can be given orally where an oral version is available, for example in mild diverticulitis, or intravenous in more serious infections.

A stat dose of **gentamicin** is often added to regimes not including gentamicin if the patient is severely septic to provide initial strong **bactericidal** gram negative action

Spontaneous Bacterial Peritonitis

This is a serious infection that typically occurs in patients with liver failure.
- Pipcracillin and tazobactam (tazocin) is often first line
- Cephalosporins such as cefotaxime are also often used
- Levofloxacin plus metronidazole is an common alternative in penicillin allergy

Septic Arthritis

Septic arthritis is where an infection occurs in a **joint**. This could be a **native** joint, meaning the persons original joint, or in a joint replacement. Infection in a joint is an emergency as the infection can quickly begin to destroy the joint and cause systemic illness. Septic arthritis has a mortality of around 10%.

Septic arthritis is a common and important complication of **joint replacement**. It occurs in around 1% of straight forward hip or knee replacements. This percentage is higher in revision surgery.

Presentation

It usually it only affects a single joint. This is often a knee. It presents with a rapid onset of:
- Hot, red, swollen and painful joint
- Stiffness and reduced range of motion
- Systemic symptoms such as fever, lethargy and sepsis

Common Bacteria

Staphylococcus aureus is the most common causative organism.

Other bacteria:
- **Neisseria gonorrhoea** (**gonococcus**) in sexually active individuals
- **Group A Streptococcus** (most commonly **Streptococcus pyogenes**)
- **Haemophilus influenza**
- **Escherichia coli** (**E. coli**)

TOM TIP: In a young patient presenting with a single acutely swollen joint always consider gonococcus septic arthritis until proven otherwise. Gonorrhoea infection is common and delaying treatment puts the joint in danger. In your exams it might say the gram stain revealed a "gram negative diplococcus". The patient may have urinary or genital symptoms to trick you into thinking of reactive arthritis but remember that it is important to exclude gonococcal septic arthritis first as this is the more serious condition.

Differential Diagnosis

- **Gout** (fluid shows **urate crystals** that are **negatively birefringent** of polarised light)
- **Pseudogout** (fluid shows **calcium pyrophosphate crystals** that are rod shaped intracellular crystals **positively birefringent** of polarised light)
- **Reactive arthritis** typically triggered by **urethritis** or **gastroenteritis** and associated with **conjunctivitis**
- **Haemarthrosis** (bleeding into the joint)

Management

Have a low threshold for treating a patient for septic arthritis until it has been excluded with examination of the joint fluid. Be particularly cautious with immunosuppressed patients.

There will be a local **hot joint policy** at your hospital to guide what team admits the patient (orthopaedics, rheumatology or infectious diseases), what antibiotics to use and for how long.

Aspirate the joint prior to antibiotics and send the sample for **gram staining**, **crystal microscopy**, **culture** and **antibiotic sensitivities**. The joint fluid may be **purulent** (full of pus). The gram stain will come back quite quickly and may give a clue about the organism. The full culture will take longer.

Empirical IV antibiotics should be given until the sensitivities are known. Antibiotics are usually continued for **3 to 6 weeks** in total. Choice of antibiotic depends on the local guidelines. Example regimes are:
- **Flucloxacillin** plus **rifampicin** is often first line
- **Vancomycin** plus **rifampicin** for penicillin allergy, MRSA or prosthetic joint
- **Clindamycin** is an alternative

Influenza

The influenza virus is an **RNA virus**. There are three types: **A**, **B** and **C**, of which A and B are the most common. The A type has different H and N subtypes. Examples of different A type strains are H1N1 (**swine flu**) and H5N1 (**avian flu**). Outbreaks typically occur during the winter.

Vaccination

Every year the vaccine is changed to target multiple strains of influenza that are likely to cause flu that year. It needs to be given yearly to keep the person protected.

It is given free on the NHS to people at higher risk of developing flu or flu related complications:
- Aged 65 and over
- Young children
- Pregnant women
- Chronic health conditions such as asthma, COPD, heart failure and diabetes
- Healthcare workers and carers

Presentation

- Fever
- Coryzal symptoms
- Lethargy and fatigue
- Anorexia (loss of appetite)
- Muscle and joint aches
- Headache
- Dry cough
- Sore throat

Diagnosis

Treatment is usually started based on the history, risk factors and clinical presentation.

Viral nasal or **throat swabs** can be sent to the local virology lab for **polymerase chain reaction** (**PCR**) analysis. This will confirm the diagnosis and also provide data to **public health** so that they can monitor the number of cases of influenza.

Management

Public health monitor the number of cases of flu and provide guidance on when there is enough flu in the area to justify treating patients with suspected flu.

Healthy patients that are not at risk of complications do not need treatment with antiviral medications. The infection will resolve with self care measures such as adequate fluid intake and rest.

There are two options for treatment in someone **at risk** of complications of influenza:
- Oral **oseltamivir** 75mg twice daily for 5 days
- Inhaled **zanamivir** 10mg twice daily for 5 days

Treatment needs to be started **within 48 hours** of the onset of symptoms to be effective.

Post-exposure prophylaxis can be given to **higher risk patients**, such as those with chronic diseases or immunosuppression, **within 48 hours** of close contact with influenza. This aims to minimise the risk of developing flu and complications.

Options for post-exposure prophylaxis are:
- Oral **oseltamivir** 75mg once daily for 10 days
- Inhaled **zanamivir** 10mg once daily for 10 days

Complications

- Otitis media, sinusitis and bronchitis
- Viral pneumonia
- Secondary bacteria pneumonia
- Worsening of chronic health conditions such as COPD and heart failure
- Febrile convulsions (young children)
- Encephalitis

Gastroenteritis

Acute gastritis is inflammation of the stomach and presents with nausea and vomiting. **Enteritis** is inflammation of the intestines and presents with diarrhoea. **Gastroenteritis** is inflammation all the way from the stomach to the intestines and presents with nausea, vomiting and diarrhoea.

The most common cause of gastroenteritis is **viral**. It is very easily spread and patients presenting with gastroenteritis often have an affected family member or contact. It is essential to **isolate** the patient in a healthcare environment such as a hospital ward as they can easily spread it to other patients.

Most people recover well, but beware that it can be potentially fatal, especially in very young or old patients or those with other health conditions.

Viral Gastroenteritis

Viral gastroenteritis is common. It is highly contagious. Causes are:
- **Rotavirus**
- **Norovirus**
- **Adenovirus** is a less common cause and presents with a more **subacute** diarrhoea

E. coli

Escherichia coli (**E. coli**) is a normal intestinal bacteria. Only certain strains cause gastroenteritis. It is spread through contact with infected faeces, unwashed salads or contaminated water.

E. coli 0157 produces the **Shiga toxin**. This causes abdominal cramps, bloody diarrhoea and vomiting. The **Shiga toxin** destroys blood cells and leads to **haemolytic uraemic syndrome** (**HUS**).

The use of antibiotics increases the risk of **haemolytic uraemic syndrome**, therefore antibiotics should be avoided if **E. coli** gastroenteritis is considered.

Campylobacter Jejuni

Campylobacter is a common cause of **travellers diarrhoea**. It is the most common bacterial cause of gastroenteritis worldwide. Campylobacter means "curved bacteria". It is a gram negative bacteria that is curved or spiral shaped. It is spread by:
- Raw or improperly cooked poultry
- Untreated water
- Unpasteurised milk

Incubation is usually 2 to 5 days. Symptoms resolve after 3 to 6 days. Symptoms are:
- Abdominal cramps
- Diarrhoea often with blood
- Vomiting
- Fever

Antibiotics can be considered after isolating the organism where patients have severe symptoms or other risk factors such as HIV or heart failure. Popular antibiotic choices are **azithromycin** or **ciprofloxacin**.

Shigella

Shigella is spread by faeces contaminating drinking water, swimming pools and food. The incubation period is 1 to 2 days and symptoms usually resolve within 1 week without treatment. It causes bloody diarrhoea, abdominal cramps and fever. Shigella can produce the **Shiga toxin** and cause **haemolytic uraemic syndrome**. Treatment of severe cases is with **azithromycin** or **ciprofloxacin**.

Salmonella

Salmonella is spread by eating raw eggs or poultry and food contaminated with the infected faeces of small animals. Incubation is 12 hours to 3 days and symptoms usually resolve within 1 week. Symptoms are watery diarrhoea that can be associated with mucus or blood, abdominal pain and vomiting. Antibiotics are only necessary in severe cases and guided by stool culture and sensitivities.

Bacillus Cereus

Bacillus cereus is a **gram positive rod** that is spread through inadequately cooked food. It grows well on food not immediately refrigerated after cooking. The typical food is fried rice left out at room temperature.

Whilst growing on the food it produces a **toxin** called **cereulide** that causes abdominal cramping and vomiting within 5 hours of ingestion. When it arrives in the intestines it produces different **toxins** that cause a **watery diarrhoea**. This occurs more than 8 hours after ingestion. All of the symptoms usually resolves within 24 hours.

The typical course is vomiting within 5 hours, then diarrhoea after 8 hours, then resolution within 24 hours.

TOM TIP: The typical exam patient with bacillus cereus develops symptoms soon after eating leftover fried rice that has been left at room temperature. It has a short incubation period after eating the rice and they then recover within 24 hours. Examiners like this question because the course of bacillus cereus is easy to distinguish from the other causes of gastroenteritis.

The other place you may come across **bacillus cereus** is in **intravenous drug users** (**IVDU**) that develop **infective endocarditis**. **Staphylococcus** is the most common cause of infective endocarditis in IVDUs, but bacillus cereus is one to keep in mind.

Yersinia Enterocolitica

Yersinia is a **gram negative bacillus**. Pigs are key carriers of Yersinia and eating raw or undercooked pork can cause infection. It is also spread through contamination with the urine or faeces of other mammal such as rat and rabbits.

Yersinia most frequently affects children, causing watery or bloody diarrhoea, abdominal pain, fever and **lymphadenopathy**. Incubation is 4 to 7 days and the illness can last longer than other causes of enteritis with symptoms lasting 3 weeks or more. Older children or adults can present with right sided abdominal pain due **mesenteric lymphadenitis** (inflammation in the intestinal lymph nodes) and fever, which can give the impression of **appendicitis**.

Antibiotics are only necessary in severe cases and guided by stool culture and sensitivities.

Staphylococcus Aureus Toxin

Staphylococcus aureus can produce **enterotoxins** when growing on food such as eggs, dairy and meat. When eaten these toxins cause small intestine inflammation. This causes symptoms of diarrhoea, perfuse vomiting, abdominal cramps and fever. These symptoms start within hours of ingestion and settle within 12 to 24 hours. It is not actually the bacteria causing the enteritis but the staphylococcus **enterotoxin**.

Giardiasis

Giardia lamblia is a type of microscopic **parasite**. It lives in the **small intestines** of mammals. These mammals may be pets, farmyard animals or humans. It releases cysts in the stools of infected mammals. The cysts contaminate food or water and are eaten, infecting a new host. This is called **faecal-oral transmission**.

Infection may not cause any symptoms or it may cause chronic diarrhoea. Diagnosis is made by stool **microscopy**. Treatment is with **metronidazole**.

Principles of Gastroenteritis Management

Good hygiene helps prevent gastroenteritis. When patients develop symptoms they should immediately be isolated to prevent spread. Barrier nursing and rigorous infection control is important for inpatients to prevent spread to other patients.

A sample of the faeces can be tested with **microscopy, culture and sensitivities** to establish the causative organism and antibiotic sensitivities.

Assess patients for dehydration. Attempt a **fluid challenge** and if they are able to tolerate oral fluid and are adequately hydrated consider outpatient management. If not vomiting and tolerated then rehydration solutions (e.g. **dioralyte**) can be used. If dehydrated then intravenous fluids can be used to rehydrate them and prevent dehydration until oral intake is adequate again.

Slowly introduce a light diet in small quantities once oral intake is tolerated again. Advise them to stay off work or school for 48 hours **after** symptoms have **completely** resolved.

Antidiarrhoeal medication such as **loperamide** and **antiemetic** medication such as **metoclopramide** are generally **not** recommended but may be useful for mild to moderate symptoms. Antidiarrhoeals should be avoided in **e. coli 0157** and **shigella** infections and where there is bloody diarrhoea or high fever.

Antibiotics should only be given in patients that are at risk of complications once the causative organism is confirmed.

Post Gastroenteritis Complications

The are possible post-gastroenteritis complications:
- Lactose intolerance
- Irritable bowel syndrome
- Reactive arthritis
- Guillain–Barré syndrome

Meningitis

Meningitis is inflammation of the **meninges**. The **meninges** are the lining of the brain and spinal cord. This inflammation is usually due to a bacterial or viral infection.

Neisseria meningitidis is a **gram negative diploccous** bacteria. They are circular bacteria (**cocci**) that occur in pairs (**diplo-**). It is commonly known as **meningococcus**.

Meningococcal septicaemia is when the meningococcus bacterial infection is in the bloodstream. **Meningococcal** refers to the bacteria and **septicaemia** refers to infection in the blood stream. Meningococcal septicaemia is the cause of the classic "**non-blanching rash**" that everybody worries about. This rash indicates the infection has caused **disseminated intravascular coagulopathy** (**DIC**) and **subcutaneous haemorrhages**.

Meningococcal meningitis is when the bacteria is infecting the **meninges** and the **cerebrospinal fluid** around the brain and spinal cord.

Bacterial Meningitis

Bacterial meningitis is inflammation of the meninges caused by a bacterial infection. The most common causes of bacterial meningitis in children and adults are **Neisseria meningitidis** (**meningococcus**) and **Streptococcus pneumoniae** (**pneumococcus**).

In **neonates** the most common cause is **group B Streptococcus** (**GBS**). GBS is usually contracted during birth from GBS bacteria that often live harmlessly in the mother's vagina.

Presentation

Typical symptoms of meningitis are fever, neck stiffness, vomiting, headache, photophobia, altered consciousness and seizures. Where there is **meningococcal septicaemia** children can present with a **non-blanching rash**. Other causes of bacterial meningitis do not usually cause the non-blanching rash.

Neonates and babies can present with very **non-specific** signs and symptoms such as hypotonia, poor feeding, lethargy, hypothermia and a **bulging fontanelle**. For this reason NICE recommend **lumbar puncture** as part of the investigations for all children:
- Under 1 months presenting with fever
- 1 to 3 months with fever and are unwell
- Under 1 years with unexplained fever and other features of serious illness

There are two **special tests** you can perform to look for meningeal irritation:
- Kernigs test
- Brudzinski's test

Kernig's test involves lying the patient on their back, flexing one hip and knee to 90 degrees and then slowly straightening the knee whilst keeping the hip flexed at 90 degrees. This creates a slight stretch in the meninges and where there is meningitis it will produce spinal pain or resistance to this movement.

Brudzinski's test involves lying the patient flat on their back and gently using your hands to lift their head and neck off the bed and flex their chin to their chest. A positive test is when this causes the patient to involuntarily flex their hips and knees.

Management of Bacteria Meningitis

Meningococcal septicaemia and bacterial meningitis are medical emergencies and should be treated immediately.

Community
Children seen in the primary care setting with suspected meningitis AND a non blanching rash should receive an urgent stat injection (IM or IV) of **benzylpenicillin** prior to transfer to hospital as time is so important:
- Under 1 year: 300mg
- 1-9 years: 600mg
- Above 10 years and adults: 1200mg

This shouldn't delay transfer. Where there is a true penicillin allergy transfer should be the priority rather than other antibiotics.

Hospital
Ideally a blood culture and a **lumbar puncture** for **cerebrospinal fluid** (**CSF**) should be performed prior to starting antibiotics however if the patient is acutely unwell antibiotics should not be delayed.

Send blood tests for **meningococcal PCR** if meningococcal disease is suspected. This tests directly for the **meningococcal DNA**. It can give a result quicker than blood culture depending on local services and will still be positive after the bacteria has been treated with antibiotics.

There should be a low threshold for treating suspected bacterial meningitis, particularly in babies and younger children. Always follow the local guidelines. Typical antibiotics are:
- **Under 3 months** – **cefotaxime** plus **amoxicillin** (the amoxicillin is to cover listeria potentially contracted during pregnancy from the mother)
- **Above 3 months** – **ceftriaxone**

Vancomycin should be added to these if there is a risk of penicillin resistant pneumococcal infection, for example from recent foreign travel or prolonged antibiotic exposure.

Steroids are also used in bacterial meningitis to reduce the frequency and severity of hearing loss and neurological damage. **Dexamethasone** is given 4 times daily for 4 days to children over 3 months if the lumbar puncture is suggestive of bacterial meningitis.

Bacteria meningitis and meningococcal infection are **notifiable diseases**, so **public health** need to be informed of all cases.

Post Exposure Prophylaxis

Significant exposure to a patient with **meningococcal infections** such as meningitis or septicaemia puts people at risk of contracting this illness. This risk of highest for people that have had close prolonged contact within the **7 days** prior to the onset of the illness. The risk of developing this disease decreases 7 days after the exposure, so if no symptoms have developed at this point they are unlikely to develop the illness.

Post exposure prophylaxis is guided by **public health**. The usual antibiotic choice for this is a **single dose** of **ciprofloxacin**. It should be given as soon as possible and ideally within 24 hours of the initial diagnosis.

Viral Meningitis

The most common causes of viral meningitis are **herpes simplex virus** (**HSV**), **enterovirus** and **varicella zoster virus** (**VZV**). A sample of the CSF from the lumbar puncture should be sent for **viral PCR** testing.

Viral meningitis tends to be milder than bacterial and often only requires supportive treatment. **Aciclovir** can be used to treat suspected or confirmed **HSZ meningitis**.

Lumbar Puncture

A lumbar puncture involves inserting a needle into the lower back to collect a sample of **cerebrospinal fluid** (**CSF**). The spinal cord ends at the L1-L2 vertebral level so the needle is usually inserted into the L3-L4 intervertebral space. Samples are sent for bacterial culture, viral PCR, cell count, protein and glucose. A blood glucose sample should be sent at the same time so that it can be compared to the CSF sample. The samples need to be sent immediately.

Cerebrospinal Fluid	Normal	Bacterial	Viral
Appearance	Clear	Cloudy	Clear
Protein	0.2 - 0.4 g/L	> 1.5 g/L	Mildly raised or normal
Glucose	0.6 - 0.8	< 0.5	0.6 - 0.8
White Cell Count	< 5	> 1000 and neutrophils	> 1000 and lymphocytes
Culture	Negative	Bacteria	Negative

TOM TIP: Interpreting lumbar puncture results is a common exam question. It is easier to think about what will happen to the CSF with bacteria or viruses living in it rather than trying to rote learn the results. It makes sense that bacteria swimming in the CSF will release proteins and use up the glucose. Viruses don't use glucose but may release a small amount of protein. The immune system releases neutrophils in response to bacteria and lymphocytes in response to viruses.

Complications

- *Hearing loss* is a key complication
- Seizures and epilepsy
- Cognitive impairment and learning disability
- Memory loss
- Focal neurological deficits such as limb weakness or spasticity

Tuberculosis

Tuberculosis (*TB*) is an infectious disease caused by the *mycobacterium tuberculosis* bacteria. This is a small **rod shaped** bacteria (a *bacillus*). It has a waxy coating that makes gram staining ineffective. They are resistant to the acids used in the staining procedure. This property is called *acid-fastness*. Therefore, the TB bacteria are described as *acid-fast bacilli*. They require a special staining technique using the *Zeihl-Neelsen stain*. This turns TB bacteria **bright red** against a blue background.

TOM TIP: A common exam question involves a patient coughing up sputum that grow acid-fast bacilli that stain red with Zeihl-Neelsen staining. Remember these key words, this is a description of TB in your exams.

TB is more prevalent in non-UK born patients (i.e. from South Asia), those who are immunocompromised (i.e. HIV) and those with close contacts with TB. *Multi-Drug Resistant TB* (*MDR TB*) are strains that are resistant to more than one TB drug, making them very difficult to treat.

Disease Course

The TB bacteria are very slow dividing with high oxygen demands. This makes them difficult to culture and treat. They are mostly spread by inhaling saliva droplets from infected people. It then spreads through the lymphatics and blood. *Granulomas* containing the bacteria form around the body.

Active TB is where there is active infection in various areas in the body. In the majority of cases the immune system is able to kill and clear the infection. The immune system may encapsulate sites of infection and stop the progression of the disease and this is referred to as *latent TB*. When latent TB *reactivates* this is known as *secondary TB*. When the immune system is unable to control the disease this causes a *disseminated*, severe disease and is referred to as *miliary TB*.

The most common site for TB infection is in the lungs, where they get plenty of oxygen. *Extrapulmonary TB* is where it infects other areas:
- **Lymph nodes**. A "*cold abscess*" is a firm painless abscess caused by TB, usually in the neck. They do not have the inflammation, redness and pain you would expect from an acutely infected abscess.
- Pleura
- Central nervous system
- Pericardium
- Gastrointestinal system
- Genitourinary system
- Bones and joints
- *Cutaneous TB* affecting the skin

Risk Factors

- Known contact with active TB
- Immigrants from areas of high TB prevalence
- People with relatives or close contacts from countries with a high rate of TB
- Immunocompromised due to conditions like HIV or immunosuppressant medications
- Homeless people, drug users or alcoholics

BCG Vaccine

The BCG vaccine involves an *intradermal* infection of *live attenuated* (weakened) TB. It offers protection against severe and complicated TB but is less effective at protecting against *pulmonary TB*.

Prior to the vaccine patients are tested with the *Mantoux test* and given the vaccine only if this test is negative. They are also assessed for the possibility of *immunosuppression* and *HIV* due to the risks related to a *live* vaccine.

BCG vaccine is offered to patients that are at higher risk of contact with TB:
- Neonates born in areas of the UK with high rates of TB
- Neonates with relatives from countries with a high rate of TB
- Neonates with a family history of TB
- Unvaccinated older children and young adults (under 35) who have close contact with TB
- Unvaccinated children or young adults that recently arrived from a country with a high rate of TB
- Healthcare workers

Presentation

Tuberculosis usually presents with a history of chronic, gradually worsening symptoms. Most cases are of *pulmonary TB* (around 70%) but they often have systemic symptoms.

Typical signs and symptoms of TB include:
- Lethargy
- Fever or night sweats
- Weight loss
- Cough with or without *haemoptysis*
- Lymphadenopathy
- *Erythema nodosum*
- Spinal pain in *spinal TB* (also known as *Pott's disease of the spine*)

Investigations

Tuberculosis can be very difficult to diagnose. The bacteria grows very slowly in a culture compared with other bacteria. It also can't be stained with traditional gram stains and requires specialist stains like the *Ziehl-Neelsen stain*.

There are two tests for an *immune response to TB* caused by previous, latent or active TB. These are the *Mantoux test* and *interferon-gamma release assay*. In patients where active disease is suspected a *chest xray* and *cultures* are used to support the diagnosis.

Mantoux Test

The Mantoux test is used to look for a previous immune response to TB. This indicates possible **previous vaccination**, *latent* or *active* TB.

This involves injecting **tuberculin** into the **intradermal** space on the forearm. Tuberculin is a collection of **tuberculosis proteins** that have been isolated from the bacteria. It does not contain any live bacteria.

Injecting the tuberculin creates a *bleb* under the skin. After 72 hours the test is "read". This involves measuring the induration of the skin at the site of the injection. NICE suggest considering an **induration of 5mm or more** a positive result. After a positive result they should be assessed for active disease.

Interferon-Gamma Release Assays (IGRAs)

This test involves taking a sample of blood and mixing it with antigens from the TB bacteria. In a person that has had previous contact with TB the **white blood cells** have become sensitised to those antigens and they will release **interferon-gamma** as part of an immune response. If interferon-gamma is released from the white blood cells this is considered a positive result.

The *IGRA test* is to confirm *latent TB* in patients with a positive *Mantoux test* but no active disease.

Chest Xray

- **Primary TB** may show patchy consolidation, pleural effusions and hilar lymphadenopathy
- **Reactivated TB** may show patchy or nodular consolidation with cavitation (gas filled spaces in the lungs) typically in the upper zones
- **Disseminated Miliary TB** give a picture of "*millet seeds*" uniformly distributed throughout the lung fields

TOM TIP: Disseminated miliary TB gives quite a characteristic appearance on a chest xray. This makes it a popular spot diagnosis in exams so it is worth looking at some pictures and remembering this.

Cultures

Performing a **bacterial culture** and collecting a sample of the bacteria is very useful prior to starting treatment. This allows testing of the bacteria for **resistance** to antibiotics. Unfortunately cultures can take several months to grown an organism. Treatment is usually started whilst waiting for the culture results.

There are several ways to collect cultures:
- **Sputum**. 3 samples should be collected and tested. If they are not producing sputum hypertonic saline can be used to **induce** sputum production. They might require **bronchoscopy** with **lavage** to collect sputum samples.
- **Mycobacterium blood cultures**. These require special blood culture bottle.
- **Lymph node aspiration** or **biopsy**

Nucleic Acid Amplification Test

Nucleic acid amplification testing is a way of looking for the **DNA** of the TB bacteria. It is tested on a sample containing the bacteria (i.e. sputum sample). It provides information about the bacteria faster than a traditional culture but is only used where having this information would affect treatment or they are at higher risk of developing complications (i.e. in HIV).

Management of Latent TB

Otherwise healthy patients do not necessarily need treatment for **latent TB**. Patients at risk of **reactivation** of latent TB can be treated with either:
- **Isoniazid** and **rifampicin** for 3 months
- **Isoniazid** for 6 months

Management of Acute Pulmonary TB

Management of active TB is coordinated by a specialist TB service with an **MDT approach**.

RIPE is the mnemonic used to remember the treatment for TB. It involves a combination of 4 drugs used at the same time:
- **R** - **R**ifampicin for 6 months
- **I** - **I**soniazid for 6 months
- **P** - **P**yrazinamide for 2 months
- **E** - **E**thambutol for 2 months

TOM TIP: Remember that Isoniazid causes peripheral neuropathy and pyridoxine (vitamin B6) is usually co-prescribed prophylactically to help prevent this. An exam question might ask "they are started on R, I, P and E, what should also be prescribed?" The answer would be pyridoxine.

Other Management Considerations

- Test for other infectious diseases (**HIV**, **hepatitis B** and **hepatitis C**).
- Test **contacts** for TB.
- Notify **Public Health** of all suspected cases.
- Patients with active TB should be isolated to prevent spread until they are established on treatment (usually 2 weeks). In hospital **negative pressure rooms** are used to prevent airborne spread. Negative pressure rooms have ventilation systems that actively remove air to prevent it spreading on to the ward.
- Management and followup should be guided by a **specialist MDT**.
- Treatment is slightly different for **extrapulmonary disease** and often includes using corticosteroids.
- Individualised drug regimes are required for **multidrug-resistant** TB.

Side Effects of Treatment

Rifampicin can cause red/orange discolouration of secretions like urine and tears. It is a potent inducer of cytochrome P450 enzymes therefore reduces the effect of drugs metabolised by this system. This is important for medications such as the contraceptive pill.

Isoniazid can cause peripheral neuropathy. Pyridoxine (vitamin B6) is usually co-prescribed prophylactically to reduce the risk of peripheral neuropathy.

Pyrazinamide can cause hyperuricaemia (high uric acid levels) resulting in gout.

Ethambutol can cause colour blindness and reduced visual acuity.

Rifampicin, **isoniazid** and **pyrazinamide** are all associated with **hepatotoxicity**.

TOM TIP: A common exam question starts with "a patient has recently started treatment for tuberculosis. They noticed ... Which medication is most likely to be implicated?" It is worth remembering the common side effects to help you answer these questions. They start feeling numbness or unusual sensations in their fingertips or feet: isoniazide ("I'm-so-numb-azid"). They noticed difficulty recognising colours: ethambutol ("eye-thambutol"). They noticed their urine or tears are orange or red: rifampicin ("red-an-orange-pissin'").

HIV

Definitions

- **HIV** – *Human Immunodeficiency Virus*
- **AIDS** – *Acquired Immunodeficiency Syndrome*
- **AIDS** is usually referred to in the UK as *late stage HIV*

Basics

HIV is an **RNA retrovirus**. **HIV-1** is most common type. **HIV-2** is rare outside West Africa. The virus enters and destroys the **CD4 T helper cells**. An initial **seroconversion** flu like illness occurs within a few weeks of infection. The infection is then asymptomatic until it progresses and the patient becomes immunocompromised and develops **AIDS defining illnesses** and opportunistic infections potentially years later.

Transmission

HIV can't spread through normal day to day activities including kissing. It is spread through:
- Unprotected anal, vaginal or oral sexual activity.
- Mother to child at any stage of pregnancy, birth or breastfeeding. This is referred to as **vertical transmission**.
- Mucous membrane, blood or open wound exposure to infected blood or bodily fluids such as through sharing needles, needle-stick injuries or blood splashed in an eye.

AIDS Defining Illnesses

There is a long list of **AIDS defining illnesses** associated with **end stage HIV** infection where the CD4 count has dropped to a level that allows for unusual opportunistic infections and malignancies to appear. Some examples are:
- Kaposi's sarcoma
- Pneumocystis jirovecii pneumonia (PCP)
- Cytomegalovirus infection
- Candidiasis (oesophageal or bronchial)
- Lymphomas
- Tuberculosis

Screening

HIV is a treatable condition and most patients are fit and healthy on treatment. There are many people that have HIV that do not know the diagnosis and these patients are at risk of complications and spreading the disease. Generally the earlier a patient is diagnosed the better the outcome.

We should test practically everyone admitted to hospital with an infectious disease regardless of their risk factors. Patients with any risk factors should be tested. **Antibody tests** can be negative for **3 months** following exposure so repeat testing is necessary if an initial test is negative within 3 months of a potential exposure.

Patients need to give **consent** for a test. **Verbal consent** should be documented prior to a test. Consent only needs to be as simple as "are you happy for us to test you for HIV?" Patients no longer require formal counselling or education prior to a test.

Testing

Antibody blood test. This is the typical test used in hospitals to screen for HIV. There is an option for patients to ***self sample*** by requesting a kit online and posting a sample of their blood to get tested for the antibody.

PCR testing for the ***p24 antigen*** tests directly for this HIV antigen in the blood. It can be positive before the antibody test.

PCR testing for the **HIV RNA** levels tests directly for the quantity of the HIV virus in the blood and gives a ***viral load***.

Monitoring

CD4 count
This is a count of the number of CD4 cells in the blood. These are the cells destroyed by the HIV virus. The lower the count the higher the risk of opportunistic infection:
- 500-1200 cells/mm^3 is the normal range
- Under 200 cells/mm^3 is considered end stage HIV / AIDS and puts the patient at high risk of opportunistic infections

Viral Load (VL)
Viral load is the number of copies of **HIV RNA** per ml of blood. "**Undetectable**" refers to a viral load below the lab's recordable range (usually 50 – 100 copies/ml). The viral load can be in the hundreds of thousands in untreated HIV.

Treatment

Treatment should be coordinated by specialist HIV or GUM centres. It revolves around a combination of ***antiretroviral therapy*** (**ART**) medications. ART is offered to everyone with a diagnosis of HIV irrespective of ***viral load*** or **CD4 count** Some regimes involve only a single combination tablet once per day that has the potential to completely suppress the infection. Specialist blood tests can establish the resistance of each HIV strain to different medications to help tailor treatment. **BHIVA guidelines** (2015) recommend a starting regime of 2 **NRTIs** (e.g. tenofovir and emtricitabine) plus a third agent.

The aim of treatment is to achieve a normal CD4 count and undetectable viral load. As a general rule when a patient has a normal CD4 and undetectable VL on ART treat their physical health problems (e.g. routine chest infections) as you would an HIV -ve patient. When prescribing be aware and check interactions any medication might have with the HIV therapy.

Highly Active Anti-Retrovirus Therapy (HAART) Medication Classes

- Protease inhibitors (PIs)
- Integrase inhibitors (IIs)
- Nucleoside reverse transcriptase inhibitors (NRTIs)
- Non-nucleoside reverse transcriptase inhibitors (NNRTIs)
- Entry inhibitors (EIs)

Additional Management

Prophylactic *co-trimoxazole* (*Septrin*) is given to patients with a CD4 under 200/mm³ to protect against **pneumocystis jirovecii pneumonia** (**PCP**).

HIV infection increases the risk of developing **cardiovascular disease**. Patients with HIV have close monitoring of cardiovascular risk factors and blood lipids and appropriate treatment (such as statins) to reduce their risk of developing cardiovascular disease.

Yearly **cervical smears** are required for women. HIV predisposes to developing cervical **human papillomavirus** (**HPV**) infection and **cervical cancer**, so female patients need close monitoring to ensure early detection of these complications.

Vaccinations should be up to date including annual influenza, pneumococcal (every 5-10 years), hepatitis A and B, tetanus, diphtheria and polio. Patients should avoid **live vaccines**.

Reproductive Health

Advise condoms for vaginal and anal sex and dams for oral sex even with when both partners are positive. If the viral load is undetectable then transmission through unprotected sex is unheard of in large studies but not impossible. Partners should have regular HIV tests.

Where the affected partner has an undetectable viral load, unprotected sex and pregnancy may be considered. It is also possible to conceive safely through techniques like sperm washing and IVF. **Caesarean section** should be used unless the mother has an undetectable viral load. Vaginal birth may be considered where the viral load is undetectable. Newborns to HIV positive mothers should receive ART for 4 weeks after birth to reduce the risk of **vertical transmission**.

Breastfeeding is only considered where the viral load is undetectable. There may still be a risk of contracting HIV through breastfeeding.

Post Exposure Prophylaxis

Post exposure prophylaxis can be used after exposure to HIV to reduce the risk of transmission. It is not 100% effective and must be commenced within a short period (less than 72 hours). The sooner it is started the better. A risk assessment about the probability of developing HIV should be balanced against the side effects of post exposure prophylaxis.

It involves a combination of ART therapy. The current regime is **Truvada** (emtricitabine / tenofovir) and **raltegravir** for 28 days.

HIV tests should be done initially but also a minimum of 3 months after exposure to confirm a negative status. Individuals should abstain from unprotected sexual activity for a minimum of 3 months until confirmed negative.

Malaria

Malaria is an infectious disease caused by members of the *Plasmodium* family of *protozoan parasites*. *Protozoa* are single celled organisms.

The most severe and dangerous member of the family is **Plasmodium falciparum**. This accounts for about 75% of the cases of malaria in the UK.

Malaria is spread through bites from the **female Anopheles mosquitoes** that carry the disease. It commonly occurs in travellers to areas where malaria is known to be present.

Types

- Plasmodium falciparum is the most severe and dangerous form
- Plasmodium vivax
- Plasmodium ovale
- Plasmodium malariae

Life Cycle

Malaria is spread by female **Anopheles** mosquitoes, usually at night time. Infected blood is sucked up by feeding mosquito. The malaria in the blood reproduces in the gut of the mosquito producing thousands of **sporozoites** (malaria spores).

When that mosquito bites another human or animal the **sporozoites** are injected by the mosquito. These sporozoites travel to the **liver** of the newly infected person. They can lie dormant as **hypnozoites** for several years in *P. vivax* and *P. ovale*.

They mature in the liver into **merozoites**, which enter the blood and infect **red blood cells**. In red blood cells the **merozoites** reproduce over **48 hours**, after which the red blood cells **rupture**, releasing loads more **merozoites** into the blood and causing a **haemolytic anaemia**. This is why people infected with malaria have high fever spikes every 48 hours.

Presentation

Suspected malaria in someone who lives or has travelled to an area of malaria. The incubation period is 1 to 4 weeks after infection with malaria although it can lie dormant for years.

Non-Specific Symptoms
- Fever, sweats and rigors
- Malaise
- Myalgia
- Headache
- Vomiting

Signs
- Pallor due to the *anaemia*
- *Hepatosplenomegaly*
- *Jaundice* as bilirubin is released during the rupture of red blood cells

Diagnosis

A diagnosis can be made using a **malaria blood film**. This is sent in an **EDTA bottle** (the red top bottle used for a full blood count). Examining the malaria blood film will show the parasites, the number and what type they are.

Three samples are sent over 3 consecutive days to **exclude** malaria. This is due to the **48 hour cycle** of malaria being released into the blood from red blood cells. The sample may be negative on days where the parasite is not released but becomes positive a day or two later when they are released from the RBCs.

Management

Discuss patients with the local **infectious diseases** unit for advice on management. All patients with **falciparum malaria** should be admitted for treatment as they can deteriorate quite quickly.

Oral options in uncomplicated malaria:
1. Artemether with lumefantrine (**Riamet**)
2. Proguanil and atovaquone (**Malarone**)
3. **Quinine sulphate**
4. **Doxycycline**

Intravenous options in severe or complicated malaria:
1. **Artesunate**. This is the most effective treatment but is not licensed.
2. **Quinine dihydrochloride**

TOM TIP: Remember artesunate and quinine as treatment options for your exams as these are the most likely to be relevant. Remember that Plasmodium falciparum is the most common and severe cause and these patients should be admitted for artesunate treatment and monitoring for complications.

Falciparum Complications

Plasmodium falciparum is the most severe form and has multiple complications. Patients should be carefully monitored for complications and treated appropriately. There is a long list of complications:
- Cerebral malaria
- Seizures
- Reduced consciousness
- Acute kidney injury
- Pulmonary oedema
- Disseminated intravascular coagulopathy (DIC)
- Severe haemolytic anaemia
- Multi-organ failure and death

Malaria prophylaxis

General advice:
- Be aware of locations that are high risk
- No method is 100% effective alone
- Use mosquito spray (e.g. 50% DEET spray) in mosquito exposed areas
- Use mosquito nets and barriers in sleeping areas
- Seek medical advice if symptoms develop
- Take antimalarial medication as recommended

Antimalarials

Antimalarial medications are around 90% effective at preventing infections. There are several options.

Proguanil and atovaquone (*Malarone*)
- Taken *daily* 2 days before, during and 1 week after being in endemic area
- Most expensive (around £1 per tablet)
- Best side effect profile

Mefloquine
- Taken *once weekly* 2 weeks before, during and 4 weeks after being in endemic area
- Can cause bad dreams and rarely psychotic disorders or seizures

Doxycycline
- Taken *daily* 2 days before, during and 4 weeks after being in endemic area
- Broad spectrum antibiotic therefore it causes side effects like diarrhoea and thrush
- Makes patients sensitive to the sun causing a rash and sunburn

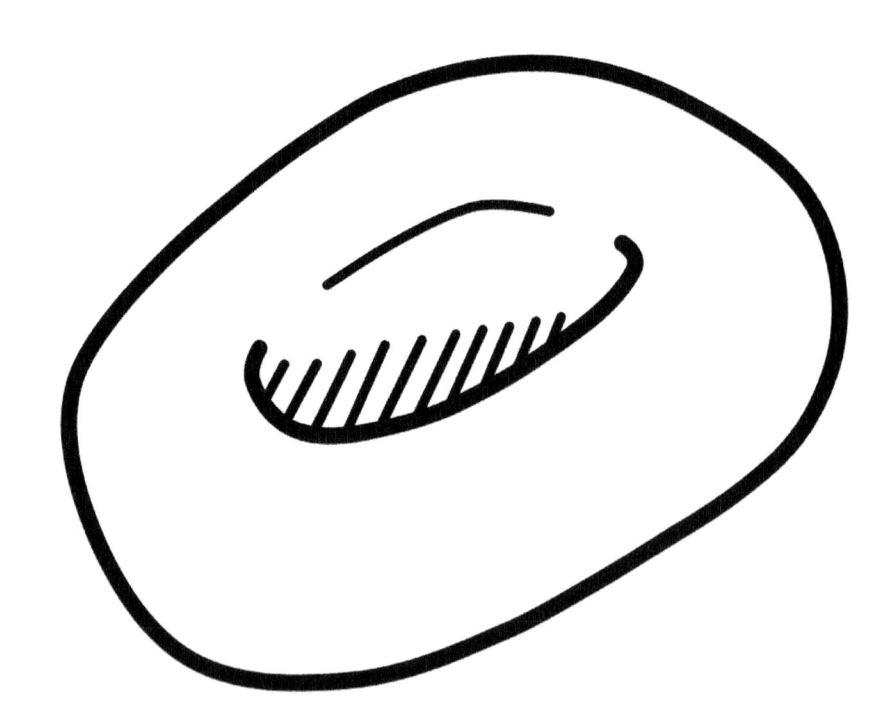

HAEMATOLOGY

6.1	Components of Blood	171
6.2	Anaemia	173
6.3	Iron Deficiency Anaemia	175
6.4	Pernicious Anaemia	177
6.5	Haemolytic Anaemia	178
6.6	Thalassaemia	181
6.7	Sickle Cell Anaemia	183
6.8	Leukaemia	185
6.9	Lymphoma	189
6.10	Myeloma	191
6.11	Myeloproliferative Disorders	195
6.12	Myelodysplasic Syndrome	197
6.13	Thrombocytopenia	198
6.14	Von Willebrand Disease	200
6.15	Haemophilia	201
6.16	Deep Vein Thrombosis and Venous Thromboembolism	202

Components of Blood

Blood is made of *plasma* (the liquid of the blood) that contains **red blood cells**, **white blood cells** and **platelets**. The plasma also contains lots of **clotting factors** such as **fibrinogen**.

Once the clotting factors are removed from the blood what is left is called the **serum**. **Serum** contains:
- **Glucose**
- **Electrolytes** such as **sodium** and **potassium**
- **Proteins** such as **immunoglobulins** and **hormones**

Blood Cells

Blood cells develop in the **bone marrow**. Bone marrow is mostly found in the **pelvis**, **vertebrae**, **ribs** and **sternum**. It is important to understand the different cell lines to understand the conditions where things go wrong with these cells. I strongly suggest watching the Zero to Finals video on "understanding the cells of the immune system" to get your head around the development of blood cells in the bone marrow.

Pluripotent Haematopoietic Stem Cell
These are undifferentiated cells that have the potential to transform into a variety of blood cells. They initially become:
- Myeloid stem cells
- Lymphoid stem cells
- Dendritic cells (via various intermediate stages)

Red Blood Cells
Red blood cells (RBCs) develop from **reticulocytes** that come from the **myeloid stem cells**. Reticulocytes are immature red blood cells. Red blood cells survive up to 3 months.

Platelets
Platelets are made by **megakaryocytes**. Their lifespan is 10 days. The normal count is 150,000 - 450,000 /mm^3. Their role is to clump together (**platelet aggregation**) and plug gaps where blood clots need to form.

White Blood Cells

Myeloid stem cells become **promyelocytes** that can become:
- **Monocytes** then **macrophages**
- **Neutrophils**
- **Eosinophils**
- **Mast Cells**
- **Basophils**

Lymphocytes come from the **lymphoid stem cells** and become **B cells** or **T cells**.

B lymphocytes (B cells) (mature in the **bone marrow**) and differentiate into:
- Plasma Cells
- Memory B Cells

T lymphocytes (T cells) (mature in the ***thymus gland***) and differentiate into:
- CD4 cells (T helper cells)
- CD8 cells (cytotoxic T cells)
- Natural killer cells

Blood Film Findings

A ***blood film*** involves a specialist examining the blood using a microscope to manually check for abnormal shapes, sizes and contents of the cells and note abnormal ***inclusions*** in the blood. Exam questions will often say "… was seen on a blood film" to give you a clue about the diagnosis. There are a lot of possible findings on a blood film but the key ones worth knowing for your exams are included below.

Anisocytosis refers to a variation in size of the red blood cells. These can be seen in ***myelodysplasic syndrome*** as well as some forms of anaemia.

Target cells have a central pigmented area, surrounded by a pale area, surrounded by a ring of thicker cytoplasm on the outside. This makes it look like a bull's eye target. These can be seen in ***iron deficiency anaemia*** and ***post-splenectomy***.

Heinz bodies are individual blobs seen inside red blood cells caused by denatured ***globin***. They can be seen in ***G6PD*** and ***alpha-thalassaemia***.

Howell-Jolly bodies are individual blobs of DNA material seen inside red blood cells. Normally this DNA material is removed by the spleen during circulation of red blood cells. They can be seen ***post-splenectomy*** and in patients with ***severe anaemia*** where the body is regenerating red blood cells quickly.

Reticulocytes are immature red blood cells that are slightly larger than standard erythrocytes (RBCs) and still have ***RNA material*** in them. The RNA has a ***reticular*** ("mesh like") appearance inside the cell. It is normal for about 1% of red blood cells to be reticulocytes. This percentage goes up where there is rapid turnover of red blood cells, such as ***haemolytic anaemia***. They demonstrate that the bone marrow is active in replacing lost cells.

Schistocytes are fragments of red blood cells. They indicate the red blood cells are being physically damaged by trauma during their journey through the blood vessels. They may indicate networks of clots in small blood vessels caused by ***haemolytic uraemic syndrome***, ***disseminated intravascular coagulation*** (DIC) or ***thrombotic thrombocytopenic purpura***. They can also be present in replacement ***metallic heart valves*** and ***haemolytic anaemia***.

Sideroblasts are immature red blood cells that contain blobs of iron. They occur when the bone marrow is unable to incorporate iron into the haemoglobin molecules. They can indicate a ***myelodysplasic syndrome***.

Smudge cells are ruptured white blood cells that occur during the process of preparing the blood film due to aged or fragile white blood cells. They can indicate ***chronic lymphocytic leukaemia***.

Spherocytes are spherical red blood cells without the normal bi-concave disk shape. They can indicated ***autoimmune haemolytic anaemia*** or ***hereditary spherocytosis***.

Anaemia

Anaemia is defined as a low level of **haemoglobin** in the blood. This is the result of an underlying disease and is not a disease itself. The prefix **an-** means without and the suffix **-aemia** refers to blood.

Haemoglobin is a protein found in **red blood cells**. It is responsible for picking up **oxygen** in the lungs and transporting it to the cells of the body. **Iron** is an essential ingredient in creating **haemoglobin** and forms part of the structure of the molecule. When a patient has a low level of **haemoglobin** they have a condition called **anaemia**.

You can diagnose a patient with anaemia when they have a **low haemoglobin**. When you find an anaemic patient you should check the **mean cell volume (MCV)**. This is the size of the red blood cells. The normal ranges are:

	Haemoglobin	Mean Cell Volume (MCV)
Women	120 - 165 grams/litre	80-100 femtolitres
Men	130 -180 grams/litre	80-100 femtolitres

Anaemia is initially subdivided into three main categories based on the size of the red blood cell (the MCV). These have different underlying causes:

- **Microcytic anaemia** (low MCV indicating small RBCs)
- **Normocytic anaemia** (normal MCV indicating normal sized RBCs)
- **Macrocytic anaemia** (large MCV indicating large RBCs)

Microcytic Anaemia Causes

A helpful mnemonic for understanding the causes of **microcytic anaemia** is **TAILS**.
- **T** - **T**halassaemia
- **A** - **A**naemia of chronic disease
- **I** - **I**ron deficiency anaemia
- **L** - **L**ead poisoning
- **S** - **S**ideroblastic anaemia

Normocytic Anaemia Causes

There are **3 As** and **2 Hs** for normocytic anaemia:
- **A** - **A**cute blood loss
- **A** - **A**naemia of Chronic Disease
- **A** - **A**plastic Anaemia
- **H** - **H**aemolytic Anaemia
- **H** - **H**ypothyroidism

Macrocytic Anaemia Causes

Macrocytic anaemia can be **megaloblastic** or **normoblastic**. **Megaloblastic anaemia** is the result of impaired **DNA synthesis** preventing the cell from dividing normally. Rather than dividing it keeps growing into a large, abnormal cell. This is caused by a **vitamin deficiency**.

Megaloblastic anaemia is caused by:
- B12 deficiency
- Folate deficiency

Normoblastic macrocytic anaemia is caused by:
- Alcohol
- **Reticulocytosis** (usually from haemolytic anaemia or blood loss)
- Hypothyroidism
- Liver disease
- Drugs such as *azathioprine*

Symptoms of Anaemia

There are many generic symptoms of anaemia:
- Tiredness
- Shortness of breath
- Headaches
- Dizziness
- Palpitations
- Worsening of other conditions such as angina, heart failure or peripheral vascular disease

There are symptoms specific to **iron deficiency anaemia**:
- **Pica** describes dietary cravings for abnormal things such as dirt and can signify iron deficiency
- **Hair loss** can indicate iron deficiency anaemia

Signs of Anaemia

Generic signs of anaemia:
- Pale skin
- Conjunctival pallor
- Tachycardia
- Raised respiratory rate

Signs of specific causes of anaemia:
- **Koilonychia** is spoon shaped nails and can indicate iron deficiency
- **Angular chelitis** can indicate iron deficiency
- **Atrophic glossitis** is a smooth tongue due to atrophy of the papillae and can indicate iron deficiency
- Brittle hair and nails can indicate iron deficiency
- **Jaundice** occurs in **haemolytic anaemia**
- Bone deformities occur in **thalassaemia**
- Oedema, hypertension and excoriations on the skin can indicate **chronic kidney disease**

Investigating Anaemia

Initial Investigations:
- Haemoglobin
- Mean Cell Volume (MCV)
- B12
- Folate
- Ferritin
- Blood film

Further Investigations:
- **Oesophago-gastroduodenoscopy** (OGD) and **colonoscopy** to investigate for a gastrointestinal cause of unexplained **iron deficiency anaemia**. This is done on an urgent cancer referral for suspected gastrointestinal cancer.
- **Bone marrow biopsy** may be required if the cause is unclear

Iron Deficiency Anaemia

The **bone marrow** requires **iron** to produce **haemoglobin**. There are several scenarios where **iron stores** can be used up and the patient can become **iron deficient**:
- Insufficient dietary iron
- Iron requirements increase (for example in pregnancy)
- Iron is being lost (for example slow bleeding from a colon cancer)
- Inadequate iron absorption

Iron is mainly absorbed in the **duodenum** and **jejunum**. It requires the acid from the stomach to keep the iron in the soluble **ferrous** (Fe^{2+}) form. When the acid drops it changes to the insoluble **ferric** (Fe^{3+}) form. Therefore, medications that reduce the stomach acid such as **proton pump inhibitors** (lansoprazole and omeprazole) can interfere with iron absorption. Conditions that result in inflammation of the **duodenum** or **jejunum** such as **coeliac disease** or **Crohn's disease** can also cause inadequate iron absorption.

Causes

- Blood loss is the most common cause in adults
- Dietary insufficiency is the most common cause in growing children
- Poor iron absorption
- Increased requirements during pregnancy

Whilst growing the dietary requirements of children often exceed their dietary intake, particularly if their diet is low in red meat.

The most common cause in adults in blood loss. In **menstruating women**, particularly in women with heavy periods (**menorrhagia**) there is a clear source of blood loss. In women that are not menstruating or men the most common source of blood loss is the gastrointestinal tract. It is important to be suspicious of a **GI tract cancer**. **Oesophagitis** and **gastritis** are the most common causes of GI tract bleeding. **Inflammatory bowel disease** (**Crohn's** and **ulcerative colitis**) should also be considered.

Understanding Tests for Iron Deficiency

Iron travels around the blood as **ferric ions** (Fe^{3+}) bound to a carrier protein called **transferrin**. **Total iron binding capacity (TIBC)** basically means the total space on the **transferrin** molecules for the iron to bind. Therefore, **total iron binding capacity** is directly related to the amount of **transferrin** in the blood. If you measure **iron** in the blood and then measure the **total iron binding capacity** of that blood, you can calculate the proportion of the **transferrin** molecules that are bound to iron. This is called the transferrin saturation. It is expressed as a percentage. The formula is:

Transferrin Saturation = Serum Iron / Total Iron Binding Capacity

Ferritin is the form that iron takes when it is deposited and stored in cells. Extra ferritin is released from cells in **inflammation**, such as with infection or cancer. If ferritin in the blood is low it is highly suggestive of **iron deficiency**. High ferritin is difficult to interpret and is likely to be related to inflammation rather than iron overload. A patient with a **normal ferritin can still have iron deficiency anaemia**, particularly if they have reasons to have a raised ferritin such as infection.

Serum iron varies significantly throughout the day with higher levels in the morning and after eating iron containing meals. On its own serum iron is not a very useful measure.

Total iron binding capacity can be used as a marker for how much **transferrin** is in the blood. It is an easier test to perform than measuring **transferrin**. Both **TIBC** and **transferrin** levels **increase in iron deficiency** and **decrease in iron overload**.

Transferrin saturation gives a good indication of the **total iron in the body**. In normal adults it is around 30%, however if there is less iron in the body, transferrin will be less saturated, and if iron levels go up, transferrin will be more saturated. It can temporarily increase after eating a meal rich in iron or taking iron supplements so a fasting sample gives the most accurate results.

Blood Test	Normal Range
Serum Ferritin	41 – 400 ug/L
Serum Iron	12 - 30 µmol/L
Total Iron Binding Capacity	45 - 80 µmol/L
Transferrin Saturation	15 - 50%

Two things can increase the values of all of these results giving the impression of iron overload:
- Supplementation with iron
- Acute liver damage (lots of iron is stored in the liver)

Management

New iron deficiency in an adult without a clear underlying cause (for example heavy menstruation or pregnancy) should be investigated with suspicion. This involves doing a **oesophago-gastroduodenoscopy** (**OGD**) and a **colonoscopy** to look for **cancer of the gastrointestinal tract**.

Management involves treating the underlying cause and correcting the anaemia. The anaemia can be treated depending on the severity and symptoms with three methods that range from fastest to slowest and most invasive to least invasive:

1. **Blood transfusion**. This will immediately correct the anaemia but not the underlying iron deficiency and also carries risks.
2. **Iron infusion** e.g. "**cosmofer**". There is a very small risk of anaphylaxis but it quickly corrects the iron deficiency. It should be avoided during sepsis as iron "feeds" bacteria.
3. **Oral iron** e.g. **ferrous sulfate** 200mg three times daily. This slowly corrects the iron deficiency. Oral iron causes constipation and black coloured stools. It is unsuitable where malabsorption is the cause of the anaemia.

When correcting iron deficiency anaemia with iron you can expect the haemoglobin to rise by around 10 grams/litre per week.

Pernicious Anaemia

Pernicious anaemia is a cause of **B12 deficiency anaemia**. B12 deficiency can be caused by **insufficient dietary intake** of vitamin B12 or **pernicious anaemia**.

Pathophysiology

The parietal cells of the stomach produce a protein called **intrinsic factor**. Intrinsic factor is essential for the absorption of **vitamin B12** in the **ileum**. Pernicious anaemia is an **autoimmune condition** where **antibodies** form against the **parietal cells** or **intrinsic factor**. A lack of intrinsic factor prevents the absorption of vitamin B12 and the patient becomes vitamin B12 deficient.

Vitamin B12 deficiency can cause **neurological symptoms**:
- **Peripheral neuropathy** with numbness or **paraesthesia** (pins and needles)
- Loss of **vibration sense** or **proprioception**
- Visual changes
- Mood or cognitive changes

TOM TIP: For your exams remember testing for vitamin B12 deficiency and pernicious anaemia in patients presenting with peripheral neuropathy, particularly with pins and needles.

Antibodies

Testing for auto-antibodies is used to diagnose pernicious anaemia.
- **Intrinsic factor antibody** is the first line investigation
- **Gastric parietal cell antibody** can also be tested but is less helpful

Management

Dietary deficiency can be treated with oral replacement with **cyanocobalamin** unless the deficiency is severe.

In pernicious anaemia, oral replacement is inadequate because the problem is with absorption rather than intake. They can be treated with 1mg of intramuscular **hydroxycobalamin** 3 times weekly for 2 weeks, then every 3 months. More intense regimes are used where there are neurological symptoms (e.g. 1mg every other day until the symptoms improve).

If there is also **folate deficiency** it is important to **treat the B12 deficiency first** before correcting the folate deficiency. Treating patients with folic acid when they have a B12 deficiency can lead to **subacute combined degeneration of the cord**.

Haemolytic Anaemia

Haemolytic anaemia is where there is destruction of red blood cells (**haemolysis**) leading to anaemia. There are a number of **inherited conditions** that cause the red blood cells to be more fragile and break down faster than normal, leading to chronic haemolytic anaemia. There are also a number of **acquired conditions** that lead to increased breakdown of red blood cells and haemolytic anaemia.

Inherited Haemolytic Anaemias

- Hereditary spherocytosis
- Hereditary elliptocytosis
- Thalassaemia
- Sickle cell anaemia
- G6PD deficiency

Acquired Haemolytic Anaemias

- Autoimmune haemolytic anaemia
- Alloimmune haemolytic anaemia (transfusions reactions and haemolytic disease of newborn)
- Paroxysmal nocturnal haemoglobinuria
- Microangiopathic haemolytic anaemia
- Prosthetic valve related haemolysis

Features

The features are a result of the destruction of red blood cells:
- **Anaemia** due to the reduction in circulating red blood cells
- **Splenomegaly** as the spleen becomes filled with destroyed red blood cells
- **Jaundice** as bilirubin is released during the destruction of red blood cells

Investigations

- **Full blood count** shows a **normocytic anaemia**
- **Blood film** shows **schistocytes** (fragments of red blood cells)
- **Direct Coombs test** is positive in **autoimmune haemolytic anaemia**

Hereditary Spherocytosis

Hereditary spherocytosis is the most common inherited haemolytic anaemia in northern Europeans. It is an **autosomal dominant** condition. It causes sphere shaped **red blood cells** that are fragile and easily break down when passing through the spleen.

It presents with jaundice, gallstones, splenomegaly and notably **aplastic crisis** in the presence of the **parvovirus**. It is diagnosed by family history and clinical features with **spherocytes** on the **blood film**. The **mean corpuscular haemoglobin concentration** (**MCHC**) is raised on a full blood count. **Reticulocytes** will be raised due to rapid turnover of red blood cells.

Treatment is with **folate** supplementation and **splenectomy**. Removal of the gallbladder (**cholecystectomy**) may be required if gallstones are a problem.

Hereditary Elliptocytosis

Hereditary elliptocytosis is very similar to hereditary spherocytosis except that the red blood cells are **ellipse** shaped. It is also **autosomal dominant**. Presentation and management are the same.

G6PD Deficiency

G6PD deficiency is a condition where there is a defect in the red blood cell enzyme **G6PD**. It is more common in Mediterranean and African patients and is **X linked recessive**. It causes **crises** that are triggered by **infections**, **medications** or **fava beans** (broad beans).

It presents with jaundice (usually in the neonatal period), gallstones, anaemia, splenomegaly and **Heinz bodies** on blood film. Diagnosis can be made by doing a **G6PD enzyme assay**.

Medications that trigger haemolysis include primaquine (an antimalarial), ciprofloxacin, sulfonylureas, sulfasalazine and other sulphonamide drugs.

TOM TIP: The key piece of knowledge for G6PD deficiency relates to triggers. In your exam look out for a patient that turns jaundice and becomes anaemic after eating broad beans, developing an infection or being treated with antimalarials. The underlying diagnosis might be G6PD deficiency.

Autoimmune Haemolytic Anaemia (AIHA)

Autoimmune haemolytic anaemia occurs when **antibodies** are created against the patient's **red blood cells**. These antibodies lead to destruction of the red blood cells. There are two types based on the temperature at which the auto-antibodies cause destruction of red blood cells.

Warm Type Autoimmune Haemolytic Anaemia
Warm type autoimmune haemolytic anaemia is the more common type. Haemolysis occurs at normal or above normal temperatures. It is usually **idiopathic**, meaning that it arises without a clear cause.

Cold Type Autoimmune Haemolytic Anaemia
This is also called **cold agglutinin disease**. At lower temperatures (e.g. less than 10°C) the **antibodies** against **red blood cells** attach themselves to the red blood cells and cause them to clump together. This is called **agglutination**. This agglutination results in the destruction of the red blood cells as the immune system is activated against them and they get filtered and destroyed in the spleen. Cold type AIHA is often secondary to other conditions such as **lymphoma**, **leukaemia**, **systemic lupus erythematosus** and infections such as **mycoplasma**, **EBV**, **CMV** and **HIV**.

Management of Autoimmune Haemolytic Anaemia
- Blood **transfusions**
- **Prednisolone** (steroids)
- **Rituximab** (a monoclonal antibody against B cells)
- **Splenectomy**

Alloimmune Haemolytic Anaemia

Alloimmune haemolytic anaemia occurs where an there is either foreign red blood cells circulating in the patients blood causing an immune reaction that destroys those red blood cells or there is a foreign antibody circulating in their blood that acts against their own red blood cells and causes haemolysis. The two scenarios where this occurs are **transfusion reactions** and **haemolytic disease of the newborn**.

In **haemolytic transfusion reactions** red blood cells are transfused into the patient. The immune system produces **antibodies** against **antigens** on those foreign red blood cells. This creates an immune response that leads to the destruction of those red blood cells.

In **haemolytic disease of the newborn** there are antibodies that cross the **placenta** from the mother to the fetus. These maternal **antibodies** target **antigens** on the **red blood cells** of the **fetus**. This causes destruction of the red blood cells in the fetus and neonate.

Paroxysmal Nocturnal Haemoglobinuria

Paroxysmal nocturnal haemoglobinuria is a rare condition that occurs when a specific genetic mutation in the **haematopoietic stem cells** in the **bone barrow** occurs **during** the patients lifetime. The specific mutation results in a loss of the **proteins** on the **surface of red blood cells** that **inhibit** the **complement cascade**. The loss of protection against the complement system results in activation of the **complement cascade** on the surface of red blood cells and destruction of the red blood cells.

The characteristic presentation is **red urine** in the morning containing **haemoglobin** and **haemosiderin**. The patient becomes anaemic due to the haemolysis. They are also predisposed to **thrombosis** (e.g. DVT, PE and hepatic vein thrombosis) and **smooth muscle dystonia** (e.g. oesophageal spasm and erectile dysfunction).

Management is with **eculizumab** or **bone marrow transplantation**. **Eculizumab** is a **monoclonal antibody** that targets **complement component 5** (**C5**) causing suppression of the **complement system**. **Bone marrow transplantation** can be curative.

Microangiopathic Haemolytic Anaemia (MAHA)

Microangiopathic haemolytic anaemia (MAHA) is where the small blood vessels have structural abnormalities that cause haemolysis of the blood cells travelling through them. Imagine a mesh inside the small blood vessels shredding the red blood cells. This is usually secondary to an underlying condition:
- Haemolytic uraemic syndrome (HUS)
- Disseminated intravascular coagulation (DIC)
- Thrombotic thrombocytopenia purpura (TTP)

- Systemic lupus erythematosus (SLE)
- Cancer

Prosthetic Valve Haemolysis

Haemolytic anaemia is a key complication of **prosthetic heart valves**. It occurs in both **bioprosthetic** and **metallic** valve replacement. It is caused by turbulence around the valve and collision of red blood cells with the implanted valve. Basically the valve churns up the cells and they break down.

Management involves:
- Monitoring
- Oral iron
- Blood transfusions if severe
- Revision surgery may be required in severe cases

Thalassaemia

Thalassaemia is related to a **genetic defect** in the **protein chains** that make up **haemoglobin**. Normal haemoglobin consists of 2 **alpha** and 2 **beta globin chains**. Defects in **alpha globin chains** lead to **alpha thalassaemia**. Defects in the **beta globin chains** lead to **beta thalassaemia**. Both conditions are **autosomal recessive**. The overall effect is varying degrees of anaemia dependent on the type and mutation.

In thalassaemia the red blood cells are more fragile and break down more easily. The spleen acts as a sieve to filter the blood and remove older blood cells. In thalassaemia the spleen collects all the destroyed red blood cells resulting in **splenomegaly**.

The bone marrow expands to produce extra red blood cells to compensate for the chronic anaemia. This causes a susceptibility to fractures and prominent features such as a **pronounced forehead** and **malar eminences** (cheek bones).

Potential Signs and Symptoms

- Microcytic anaemia (low **mean corpuscular volume**)
- Fatigue
- Pallor
- Jaundice
- Gallstones
- Splenomegaly
- Poor growth and development
- Pronounced forehead and malar eminences

Diagnosis

- **Full blood count** shows a microcytic anaemia.
- **Haemoglobin electrophoresis** is used to diagnose **globin** abnormalities.
- **DNA testing** can be used to look for the genetic abnormality

Pregnant women in the UK are offered a screening test for thalassaemia at booking.

Iron Overload

Iron overload occurs in **thalassaemia** as a result of faulty creation of red blood cells, recurrent transfusions and increased absorption of iron in response to the anaemia.

Patients with thalassaemia have **serum ferritin** levels monitored to check for iron overload. Management involves limiting transfusions and **iron chelation**.

Iron overload in thalassaemia causes effects similar to haemochromatosis:
- Fatigue
- Liver cirrhosis
- Infertility and impotence
- Heart failure
- Arthritis
- Diabetes
- Osteoporosis and joint pain

Alpha-Thalassaemia

Alpha-thalassaemia is caused by defects in **alpha globin chains**. The gene coding for this protein is on **chromosome 16**.

Management:
- Monitoring full blood count
- Monitoring for complications
- Blood transfusions
- Splenectomy may be performed
- **Bone marrow transplant** can be curative

Beta-Thalassaemia

Beta-thalassaemia is caused by defects in **beta globin chains**. The gene coding for this protein is on **chromosome 11**.

The genes defect can either consist of **abnormal copies** that retain some function or **deletion genes** where there is no function in the beta globin protein at all. Based on this, beta-thalassamia can be split into three types:
- *Thalassaemia minor*
- *Thalassaemia intermedia*
- *Thalassaemia major*

Thalassaemia Minor

Patients with beta thalassaemia minor are carriers of an abnormally functioning beta globin gene. They have **one abnormal** and **one normal** gene.

Thalassaemia minor causes a mild *microcytic anaemia* and usually patients only require monitoring and no active treatment.

Thalassaemia Intermedia

Patients with beta thalassaemia intermedia have two abnormal copies of the beta globin gene. This can be either **two defective** genes or **one defective** gene and **one deletion** gene.

Thalassaemia intermedia causes a more significant microcytic anaemia and patients require monitoring and occasional blood transfusions. If they need more transfusions they may require iron chelation to prevent iron overload.

Thalassaemia Major

Patients with beta thalassaemia major are **homozygous** for the **deletion** genes. They have no functioning beta globin genes at all. This is the most severe form and usually presents with severe anaemia and failure to thrive in early childhood.

Thalassaemia major causes:
- Severe microcytic anaemia
- Splenomegaly
- Bone deformities

Management involves regular transfusions, iron chelation and splenectomy. Bone marrow transplant can potentially be curative.

Sickle Cell Anaemia

Sickle cell anaemia is a **genetic** condition that causes **sickle** (crescent) shaped **red blood cells**. This makes the red blood cells fragile and more easily destroyed, leading to a **haemolytic anaemia**. Patients with sickle cell anaemia are prone to various types of **sickle cell crises**.

Pathophysiology

Haemoglobin is the protein in red blood cells that transports oxygen. **Fetal haemoglobin** (**HbF**) is usually replaced by **haemoglobin A** (**HbA**) at around 6 weeks of age. Patients with sickle-cell disease have an abnormal variant called **haemoglobin S** (**HbS**). HbS causes red blood cells to be an abnormal "sickle" shape.

Sickle cell anaemia is an **autosomal recessive** condition where there is an abnormal gene for **beta-globin** on **chromosome 11**. One copy of the gene results in **sickle-cell trait**. Patients with sickle-cell trait are usually asymptomatic. Two abnormal copies are required for **sickle-cell disease**.

Relation to Malaria

Sickle cell disease is more common in patients from areas traditionally affected by malaria such as Africa, India, the Middle East and the Caribbean. Having one copy of the gene (sickle-cell trait) reduces the severity of malaria. As a result, patients with sickle-cell trait are more likely to survive malaria and pass on their genes. Therefore, there is a **selective advantage** to having the sickle cell gene in areas of malaria.

Diagnosis

Pregnant women at risk of being carriers of the sickle cell gene are offered testing during pregnancy. Sickle cell disease is also tested for on the on the **newborn screening heel prick test** at 5 days of age.

Complications

- Anaemia
- Increased risk of infection
- Stroke
- **Avascular necrosis** in large joints such as the hip
- **Pulmonary hypertension**
- Painful and persistent penile erection (**priapism**)
- **Chronic kidney disease**
- **Sickle cell crises**
- **Acute chest syndrome**

General Management

- Avoid dehydration and other triggers of crises
- Ensure vaccines are up to date
- **Antibiotic prophylaxis** to protect against infection with **penicillin V** (**phenoxymethypenicillin**)
- **Hydroxycarbamide** can be used to stimulate production of **fetal haemoglobin** (**HbF**). Fetal haemoglobin does not lead to sickling of red blood cells. This has a protective effect against sickle cell crises and acute chest syndrome.
- **Blood transfusion** for severe anaemia
- **Bone marrow transplant** can be curative

Sickle Cell Crisis

Sickle cell crisis is an umbrella term for a spectrum of acute crises related to the condition. These range from mild to life threatening. They can occur spontaneously or be triggered by stresses such as infection, dehydration, cold or significant life events.

There is no specific treatment for sickle cell crises and they are managed **supportively**:
- Have a low threshold for admission to hospital
- Treat any infection
- Keep warm
- Keep well hydrated (IV fluids may be required)
- Simple analgesia such as paracetamol and ibuprofen (NSAIDs should be avoided where there is renal impairment)
- Penile aspiration in **priapism**

Vaso-occlusive Crisis (AKA painful crisis)

Vaso-occlusive crisis is caused by the sickle shaped blood cells clogging **capillaries** causing **distal ischaemia**. It is associated with dehydration and raised **haematocrit**. Symptoms are typically pain, fever and those of the triggering infection. It can cause **priapism** in men by trapping blood in the penis, causing a painful and persistent erection. This is a urological emergency and is treated with aspiration of blood from the penis.

Splenic Sequestration Crisis

Splenic sequestration crisis is caused by red blood cells blocking blood flow within the **spleen**. This causes an acutely enlarged and painful spleen. The pooling of blood in the spleen can lead to **severe anaemia** and **circulatory collapse** (hypovolaemic shock).
Splenic sequestration crisis is considered an emergency. Management is supportive with blood transfusions and fluid resuscitation to treat anaemia and shock.

Splenectomy prevents sequestration crisis and is often used in cases of recurrent crises. Recurrent crises can lead to splenic infarction and therefore susceptibility to infections.

Aplastic Crisis

Aplastic crisis describes a situation where there is temporary loss of the creation of new blood cells. This is most commonly triggered by infection with **parvovirus B19**.

It leads to significant anaemia. Management is supportive with blood transfusions if necessary. It usually resolves spontaneously within a week.

Acute Chest Syndrome

A diagnosis of acute chest syndrome requires:
- Fever or respiratory symptoms with
- New infiltrates seen on a chest xray

This can be due to infection (e.g. pneumonia or bronchiolitis) or non-infective causes (e.g. pulmonary vaso-occlusion or fat emboli).

It is a medical emergency with a high mortality and requires prompt supportive management and treatment of the underlying cause:
- **Antibiotics** or **antivirals** for infections
- **Blood transfusions** for anaemia
- **Incentive spirometry** using a machine that encourages effective and deep breathing
- **Artificial ventilation** with NIV or intubation may be required

Leukaemia

Leukaemia is the name for **cancer** of a particular line of the **stem cells** in the **bone marrow**. This causes unregulated production of certain types of blood cells. They can be classified depending on how rapidly they progress (**chronic** is slow and **acute** is fast) and the cell line that is affected (**myeloid** or **lymphoid**) to make four main types:

- *Acute myeloid leukaemia*
- *Acute lymphoblastic leukaemia*

- *Chronic myeloid leukaemia*
- *Chronic lymphocytic leukaemia*

There are other rarer and more specialist leukaemias such as *acute promyelocytic leukaemia*. You are unlikely to come across these in your exams.

Pathophysiology

Leukaemia is a form of cancer of the cells in the bone marrow. A genetic mutation in one of the precursor cells in the bone marrow leads to excessive production of a single type of abnormal white blood cell.

The excessive production of a single type of cell can lead to suppression of the other cell lines causing underproduction of other cell types. This results in a *pancytopenia*, which is a combination of low red blood cells (*anaemia*), white blood cells (*leukopenia*) and platelets (*thrombocytopenia*).

Ages

You can use the mnemonic "**ALL CeLL**mates have **CoM**mon **AM**bitions" to remember the progressive ages of the different leukaemia from 45-75 in steps of 10 years. Remember that **ALL** (the first in the mnemonic) most commonly affects children under 5 years.

- Under 5 and over 45 - **a**cute **l**ymphoblastic **l**eukaemia (**ALL**)
- Over 55 - **c**hronic **l**ymphocytic **l**eukaemia (**CeLL**mates)
- Over 65 - **c**hronic **m**yeloid leukaemia (**CoM**mon)
- Over 75 - **a**cute **m**yeloid leukaemia (**AM**bitions)

Presentation

The presentation of leukaemia is quite *non-specific*. If leukaemia appears on your list of differentials then get an urgent *full blood count*. Some typical features are:
- Fatigue
- Fever
- Failure to thrive (children)
- Pallor due to anaemia
- Petechiae and abnormal bruising due to thrombocytopenia
- Abnormal bleeding
- Lymphadenopathy
- Hepatosplenomegaly

Differential Diagnosis of Petechiae

One of the key presenting features of leukaemia is bleeding under the skin leading to bruising and petechiae. This is caused by *thrombocytopenia* (low platelets). It is important to be aware of the differential diagnoses for this type of non-blanching rash:
- Leukaemia
- Meningococcal septicaemia
- Vasculitis
- Henoch-Schonlein Purpura (HSP)

- Idiopathic Thrombocytopenia Purpura (ITP)
- Non-accidental injury

Don't ever forget **non-accidental injury** (abuse) as a differential, particularly in children and vulnerable adults.

Diagnosis

Full blood count is the initial investigation. NICE recommend a **full blood count** within 48 hours for patients with suspected leukaemia. Children or young adults with **ptechiae** or **hepatosplenomegaly** should be referred immediately to hospital.

Blood film can be used to look for **abnormal cells** and **inclusions**.

Lactate dehydrogenase (**LDH**) is a blood test that is often raised in leukaemia but is not specific to leukaemia. It can be raised in other cancers and many non-cancerous diseases.

Bone marrow biopsy can be used to analyse the cells in the bone marrow. This is the main investigation for establishing a definitive diagnosis of leukaemia.

Chest xray may show infection or mediastinal lymphadenopathy.

Lymph node biopsy can be used to assess lymph node involvement or investigate for lymphoma.

Lumbar puncture may be used if there is central nervous system involvement.

CT, **MRI** and **PET** scans can be used for staging and assessing for lymphoma and other tumours.

Bone Marrow Biopsy

Bone marrow aspiration involves taking a liquid sample full of cells from within the bone marrow.

Bone marrow trephine involves taking a solid core sample of the bone marrow and provides a better assessment of the cells and structure.

Bone marrow biopsy is usually taken from the iliac crest. It involves a local anaesthetic and a specialist needle. Samples from bone marrow aspiration can be examined straight away however a trephine sample requires a few days of preparation.

Acute Lymphoblastic Leukaemia

Acute lymphocytic leukaemia is where there is malignant change in one of the lymphocyte precursor cells. It causes **acute** proliferation of a single type of lymphocyte, usually **B-lymphocytes**. Excessive proliferation of these cells cause them to replace the other cell types in the bone marrow, leading to a pancytopenia.

This is the most common cancer in children and peaks around 2-4 years. It can also affect adults over 45. It is often associated with **Downs syndrome**.

Blood film shows **blast cells**.

It is associated with the the **t(15:17) translocation** in 30% of children with ALL and the **Philadelphia chromosome** (**t(9:22) translocation**) in 30% of adults with ALL.

Chronic Lymphocytic Leukaemia

Chronic lymphocytic leukaemia is where there is **chronic** proliferation of a single type of well differentiated lymphocyte, usually **B-lymphocytes**. This usually affects adults over 55 years of age. Often it is asymptomatic but it can present with infections, anaemia, bleeding and weight loss. It can cause **warm autoimmune haemolytic anaemia**.

CLL can transform into **high-grade lymphoma**. This is called **Richter's transformation**.

Blood film shows "**smear**" or "**smudge**" cells. These occur during the process of preparing the blood film where aged or fragile white blood cells rupture and leave a smudge on the film.

Chronic Myeloid Leukaemia

Chronic myeloid leukaemia has three phases: the **chronic phase**, the **accelerated phase** and the **blast phase**. The **chronic phase** can last around 5 years, is often asymptomatic and patients are diagnosed incidentally with a raised white cell count.

The **accelerated phase** occurs where the abnormal blast cells take up a high proportion of the cells in the bone marrow and blood (10-20%). In the accelerated phase patients become more symptomatic, develop anaemia and thrombocytopenia and become immunocompromised.

The **blast phase** follows the accelerated phase and involves an even higher proportion of blast cells in the blood (> 30%). This phase has severe symptoms and pancytopenia. It is often fatal.

The cytogenetic change that is characteristic of CML is the **Philadelphia chromosome,** which is a translocation of genes between chromosome 9 and 22: it is a **t(9:22) translocation**.

Acute Myeloid Leukaemia

Acute myeloid leukaemia is the most common acute leukaemia in adults. There are many different types of acute myeloid leukaemia, all with slightly different cytogenetic differences and differences in presentation.

It can present at any age but normally presents from middle age onwards. It can be the result of a **transformation** from a **myeloproliferative disorder** such as **polycythaemia ruby vera** or **myelofibrosis.**

A blood film will show a high proportion of **blast cells**. These blast cells can have **rods** inside their **cytoplasm** that are named **auer rods**.

TOM TIP: There are some key bits of information that you should learn to be able to spot which leukaemia is in the exam:
- *Acute lymphoblastic leukaemia: Most common leukaemia in children. Associated with Down syndrome.*
- *Chronic lymphocytic leukaemia: Most common leukaemia in adults overall. Associated with warm haemolytic anaemia, Richter's transformation into lymphoma and smudge / smear cells.*

- *Chronic myeloid leukaemia: Has three phases including a 5 year "asymptomatic chronic phase". Associated with the Philadelphia chromosome.*
- *Acute myeloid leukaemia: Most common acute adult leukaemia. It can be the result of a transformation from a myeloproliferative disorder. Associated with auer rods.*

Management

Treatment will be coordinated by an oncology **multi-disciplinary team**. Leukaemia is primarily treated with **chemotherapy** and **steroids**.

Other therapies include:
- Radiotherapy
- Bone marrow transplant
- Surgery

Complications of Chemotherapy

- Failure
- Stunted growth and development in children
- Infections due to immunodeficiency
- Neurotoxicity
- Infertility
- Secondary malignancy
- Cardiotoxicity
- Tumour lysis syndrome

Tumour lysis syndrome is caused by the release of **uric acid** from cells that are being destroyed by chemotherapy. The uric acid can form crystals in the **interstitial space** and **tubules** of the **kidneys** and causes **acute kidney injury**. **Allopurinol** or **rasburicase** are used to reduce the high **uric acid** levels. Other chemicals such as **potassium** and **phosphate** are also released so these need to be monitored and treated appropriately. High phosphate can lead to low calcium, which can have adverse effects, so calcium is also monitored.

Lymphoma

Lymphomas are a group of cancers that affect the lymphocytes inside the **lymphatic system**. These cancerous cells proliferate within the **lymph nodes** and cause the lymph nodes to become abnormally large (**lymphadenopathy**).

There are two main categories of lymphoma: **Hodgkin's lymphoma** and **non-Hodgkin's lymphoma**. Hodgkin's lymphoma is a specific disease and non-Hodgkins lymphoma encompasses all the other lymphomas. Hodgkin's lymphoma is the most likely specific lymphoma to appear in your exams.

Hodgkin's Lymphoma

Overall 1 in 5 lymphomas are Hodgkin's lymphoma. It is caused by proliferation of **lymphocytes**. There is a **bimodal age distribution** with peaks around aged 20 and 75 years.

Risk factors

- HIV
- Epstein-Barr Virus
- Autoimmune conditions such as rheumatoid arthritis and sarcoidosis
- Family history

Presentation

Lymphadenopathy is the key presenting symptom. The enlarged lymph node or nodes might be in the neck, axilla or inguinal (armpit) region. They are characteristically **non-tender** and feel "**rubbery**". Some patients will experience pain in the lymph nodes when they drink with **alcohol**.

B symptoms are the systemic symptoms of lymphoma:
- Fever
- Weight loss
- Night sweats

Other symptoms can include:
- Fatigue
- Itching
- Cough
- Shortness of breath
- Abdominal pain
- Recurrent infections

Investigations

Lactate dehydrogenase (**LDH**) is a blood test that is often raised in Hodgkin's lymphoma but is not specific and can be raised in other cancers and many non-cancerous diseases.

Lymph node biopsy is the key diagnostic test.

The **Reed-Sternberg** cell is the key finding from lymph node biopsy in patients with Hodgkin's lymphoma. They are **abnormally large B cells** that have **multiple nuclei** that have **nucleoli** inside them. They look like the face of an owl with large eyes. The Reed-Sternberg cell is a popular feature in medical exams.

CT, **MRI** and **PET** scans can be used for diagnosing and staging lymphoma and other tumours.

Ann Arbor Staging

The Ann Arbor staging system is used for both **Hodgkins** and **non-Hodgkins lymphoma**. The system puts importance on whether the affected nodes are above or below the **diaphragm**. A simplified version is:
- Stage 1: Confined to one region of lymph nodes.
- Stage 2: In more than one region but on the same side of the diaphragm (either above or below).
- Stage 3: Affects lymph nodes both above and below the diaphragm.
- Stage 4: Widespread involvement including non-lymphatic organs such as the lungs or liver.

Management

The key treatments are **chemotherapy** and **radiotherapy**. The aim of treatment is to cure the condition. This is usually successful however there is a risk of relapse, other haematological cancers and side effects of medications. **Chemotherapy** creates a risk of **leukaemia** and **infertility**.

Radiotherapy creates a risk of **cancer**, damage to tissues and hypothyroidism.

Non-Hodgkin Lymphoma

Non-Hodgkins lymphoma is a group of lymphomas. There are almost endless types of lymphoma. A few notable ones are:
- **Burkitt lymphoma** is associated with Epstein-Barr virus, malaria and HIV.
- **MALT lymphoma** affects the **mucosa-associated lymphoid tissue**, usually around the **stomach**. It is associated with **H. pylori** infection.
- **Diffuse large B cell lymphoma** often presents as a rapidly growing painless mass in patients over 65 years.

Risk factors for non-Hodgkin's lymphoma include:
- HIV
- Epstein-Barr Virus
- H. pylori (MALT lymphoma)
- Hepatitis B or C infection
- Exposure to pesticides and a specific chemical called **trichloroethylene** used in several industrial processes
- Family history

The presentation is similar to Hodgkin's lymphoma and often they can only be differentiated when the lymph node is biopsied.

Management involves a combination of treatments depending on the type and staging of the lymphoma:
- Watchful waiting
- Chemotherapy
- Monoclonal antibodies such as **rituximab**
- Radiotherapy
- Stem cell transplantation

Myeloma

Myeloma is a cancer of the **plasma cells**. These are a type of **B lymphocyte** that produce **antibodies**. Cancer in a specific type of plasma cell results in large quantities of a single type of **antibody** being produced. Myeloma accounts for around 1% of all cancers.

Multiple myeloma is where the myeloma affects multiple areas of the body.

Monoclonal gammopathy of undetermined significance (**MGUS**) is where there is an excess of a single type of antibody or antibody components without other features of myeloma or cancer. This is often an incidental finding in an otherwise healthy person and as the name suggests the significance is unclear. It may progress to myeloma and patients are often followed up routinely to monitor for progression.

Smouldering myeloma is where there is progression of **MGUS** with higher levels of antibodies or antibody components. It is premalignant and more likely to progress to myeloma than MGUS. **Waldenstrom's macroglobulinemia** is a type of smouldering myeloma where there is excessive **IgM** specifically.

Pathophysiology

Plasma cells are **B cells** (**B lymphocytes**) of the immune system that have become activated to produce a certain antibody. They are called B cells because they are found in the bone marrow. **Myeloma** is a cancer of a specific type of plasma cell where there is a **genetic mutation** causing it to rapidly and uncontrollably multiply.

These plasma cells produce one type of **antibody**. **Antibodies** are also called **immunoglobulins**. They are complex molecules made up of two **heavy chains** and two **light chains** arranged in a Y shape. They help the immune system recognise and fight infections by targeting specific proteins on the pathogen. They come in 5 main types: A, G, M, D and E. When you measure the **immunoglobulins** in a patient with **myeloma**, one of those types will be significantly abundant. More than 50% of the time this is immunoglobulin type G (**IgG**). This single type of antibody that is produced by all the identical cancerous plasma cells is called a **monoclonal paraprotein**. This means a single type of abnormal protein.

The "**Bence Jones protein**" that can be found in the urine of patients with **myeloma** is actually a part (**subunit**) of the **antibodies**, called the **light chains**.

Anaemia

The cancerous plasma cells invade the bone marrow. This is described as **bone marrow infiltration**. This causes suppression of the development of other blood cell lines leading to **anaemia** (low red cells), **neutropenia** (low neutrophils) and **thrombocytopenia** (low platelets).

Myeloma Bone Disease

Myeloma bone disease is a result of increased **osteoclast** activity and suppressed **osteoblast** activity. **Osteoclasts** absorb bone and **osteoblasts** deposit bone. This results in the metabolism of bone becoming imbalanced as more bone is being reabsorbed than constructed. This is caused by **cytokines** released from the **plasma cells** and the **stromal cells** (other bone cells) when they are in contact with the plasma cells.

Common places for myeloma bone disease to happen are the skull, spine, long bones and ribs. The abnormal bone metabolism is patchy, meaning that in some areas the bone becomes very thin whereas others remain relatively normal. These patches of thin bone can be described as **osteolytic** lesions. These weak points in bone lead to **pathological fractures**. For example, a **vertebral body** in the spine may collapse (**vertebral fracture**) or a long bone such as the **femur** may break under minimal force.

All the **osteoclast** activity causes a lot of calcium to be reabsorbed from the bone into the blood. This results in **hypercalcaemia** (high blood calcium).

People with myeloma can also develop **plasmacytomas**. These are individual **tumours** formed by **cancerous plasma cells**. They can occur in the bones, replacing normal bone tissue or can occur outside bones in the soft tissues of the body.

Myeloma Renal Disease

Patients with myeloma often develop renal impairment. This is due to a number of factors:

- High levels of **immunoglobulins** (antibodies) can block the flow through the tubules
- Hypercalcaemia impairs renal function
- Dehydration
- Medications used to treat the conditions such as bisphosphonates can be harmful to the kidneys

Hyperviscocity

The normal **plasma viscosity**, or internal friction in the flow of blood, is between 1.3 and 1.7 times that of water. To oversimplify it: blood is 1.3 to 1.7 times thicker than water. **Plasma viscosity** increases when there are more **proteins** in the blood. These are proteins like **immunoglobulins** and **fibrinogen**, both of which increase with **inflammation**. In myeloma there are large amounts of immunoglobulins in the blood causing the plasma viscosity to be significantly higher.

Raised **plasma viscosity** can cause many issues:
- Easy bruising
- Easy bleeding
- Reduced or loss of sight due to vascular disease in the eye
- Purple discolouration to the extremities (purplish palmar erythema)
- Heart failure

Four Features to Remember for Exams

You can use the mnemonic **CRAB** to remember four key features of myeloma:
- **C** - **C**alcium (elevated)
- **R** - **R**enal failure
- **A** - **A**naemia (normocytic, normochromic) from replacement of bone marrow.
- **B** - **B**one lesions and bone pain

Risk Factors

- Older age
- Male
- Black African ethnicity
- Family history
- Obesity

Suspecting Myeloma

This is a simplified version of the 2016 **NICE guidelines** on suspected myeloma. They suggest considering myeloma in anyone over 60 with persistent bone pain, particularly back pain, or an unexplained fractures. Perform initial investigations:
- **FBC** (low white blood cell count in myeloma)
- **Calcium** (raised in myeloma)
- **ESR** (raised in myeloma)
- **Plasma viscosity** (raised in myeloma)

If any of these are positive or myeloma is still suspected do an urgent **serum protein electrophoresis** and a **urine Bence-Jones protein** test.

Testing for Myeloma

NICE guidelines from 2016 provide guidance on investigating and managing myeloma. They recommend the following **initial investigations** when myeloma is suspected. You can remember these with the mnemonic "**BLIP**". You cannot exclude myeloma with just one investigation.

- **B** - **B**ence–Jones protein (request **urine electrophoresis**)
- **L** - Serum-free **L**ight-chain assay
- **I** - Serum **I**mmunoglobulins
- **P** - Serum **P**rotein electrophoresis

Bone marrow biopsy is necessary to confirm the diagnosis of myeloma and get more information on the disease.

Imaging is required to assess for bone lesions. The order of preference to establish this is:
1. Whole body **MRI**
2. Whole body **CT**
3. **Skeletal survey** (xray images of the full skeleton)

Patients only require one investigation but may not tolerate or be suitable for MRI or CT.

Xray Signs

- Punched out lesions
- Lytic lesions
- "**Pepperpot skull**" caused by many punched out lesions throughout the skull

Management

The aim of treatment is to control disease. It usually takes a relapsing-remitting course and treatment aims to improve quality and quantity of life. Management will be undertaken by the haematology and oncology specialist **multidisciplinary team**.

First line treatment usually involves a combination of **chemotherapy** with:
- Bortezomid
- Thalidomide
- Dexamethasone

Stem cell transplantation can be used as part of a clinical trial where patients are suitable.

Patients require **venous thromboembolism prophylaxis** with aspirin or low molecular weight heparin whilst on certain chemotherapy regimes (e.g. thialidomide) as there is a higher risk of developing a thrombus.

Management of Myeloma Bone Disease

- **Myeloma bone disease** can be improved using **bisphosphonates**. These suppress osteoclast activity.
- **Radiotherapy** to bone lesions can improve bone pain.
- **Orthopaedic surgery** can stabilise bones (e.g. by inserting a prophylactic intramedullary rod) or treat fractures.
- **Cement augmentation** involves injecting cement into **vertebral fractures** or **lesions** and can improve spine stability and pain

Complications

There are a number of complications of myeloma itself and the treatments:
- Infection
- Pain
- Renal failure
- Anaemia
- Hypercalcaemia
- Peripheral neuropathy
- Spinal cord compression
- Hyperviscocity

Myeloproliferative Disorders

These conditions occur due to uncontrolled **proliferation** of a single type of stem cell. They are considered a type of bone marrow cancer.

The three myeloproliferative disorders to remember are:
- *Primary myelofibrosis*
- *Polycythaemia vera*
- *Essential thrombocythaemia*

Primary myelofibrosis is the result of proliferation of the **haematopoietic stem cells**. **Polycythaemia vera** is the result of proliferation of the **erythroid cell line**. **Essential thrombocythaemia** is the result of proliferation of the **megakaryocytic cell line**.

Proliferating Cell Line	Disease
Haematopoietic Stem Cell	Primary Myelofibrosis
Erythroid Cells	Polycythaemia Vera
Megakaryocyte	Essential Thrombocythaemia

Myeloproliferative disorders have the potential to progress and transform into **acute myeloid leukaemia**.

These conditions are associated with mutations in certain genes:
- JAK2
- MPL
- CALR

TOM TIP: Remember the JAK2 mutation for your exams. This can be the target of JAK2 inhibitors such as ruxolitinib as part of a treatment regime.

Myelofibrosis

Myelofibrosis can be the result of **primary myelofibrosis**, **polycythaemia vera** or **essential thrombocythaemia**.

Myelofibrosis is where the proliferation of the cell line leads to **bone marrow fibrosis**. The bone marrow is replaced by scar tissue. This is in response to **cytokines** that are released from the proliferating cells. One particular cytokine is **fibroblast growth factor**. This fibrosis affects the production of blood cells and can lead to **anaemia** and low white blood cells (**leukopenia**).

When the bone marrow is replaced with scar tissue the production of blood cells (**haematopoiesis**) starts to happen in other areas such as the **liver** and **spleen**. This is known as **extramedullary haematopoiesis** and can lead to **hepatomegaly** and **splenomegaly**. This can lead to **portal hypertension**. If it occurs around the spine it can lead to **spinal cord compression**.

Presentation

Initially myeloproliferative disorders can be asymptomatic.

They can present with **systemic symptoms**:
- Fatigue
- Weight loss
- Night sweats
- Fever

There may be signs and symptoms of underlying complications:
- Anaemia (except in polycythaemia)
- Splenomegaly (abdominal pain)
- Portal hypertension (ascites, varices and abdominal pain)
- Low platelets (bleeding and petechiae)
- **Thrombosis** is common in polycythaemia and thrombocythaemia
- Raised red blood cells (thrombosis and red face)
- Low white blood cells (infections)

Full Blood Count Findings

Polycythaemia Vera:
Raised haemoglobin (more than 185g/l in men or 165g/l in women).

Primary Thrombocythaemia:
Raised platelet count (more than 600×10^9/l).

Myelofibrosis (due to **primary MF** or secondary to **PV** or **ET**) can give variable findings:
- Anaemia

- Leukocytosis or leukopenia (high or low white cell counts)
- Thrombocytosis or thrombocytopenia (high or low platelet counts)

A **blood film** in **myelofibrosis** can show **teardrop-shaped RBCs**, varying sizes of red blood cells (**anisocytosis**) and immature red and white cells (**blasts**).

Diagnosis

Bone marrow biopsy is the test of choice to establish a diagnosis. **Bone marrow aspiration** is usually "**dry**" as the bone marrow has turned to scar tissue.

Testing for the **JAK2**, **MPL** and **CALR** genes can help guide management.

Management of Primary Myelofibrosis

- Patients with mild disease with minimal symptoms might be monitored and not actively treated.
- **Allogeneic stem cell transplantation** is potentially curative but carries risks.
- **Chemotherapy** can help control the disease, improve symptoms and slow progression but is not curative on its own.
- **Supportive management** of the anaemia, splenomegaly and portal hypertension.

Management of Polycythaemia Vera

- **Venesection** can be used to keep the haemoglobin in the normal range. This is the first line treatment.
- **Aspirin** can be used to reduce the risk of developing blood clots (**thrombus formation**).
- **Chemotherapy** can be used to control the disease.

Management of Essential Thrombocythaemia

- **Aspirin** can be used to reduce the risk of developing blood clots (**thrombus formation**).
- **Chemotherapy** can be used to control the disease.

Myelodysplastic Syndrome

Myelodysplastic syndrome is caused by the **myeloid bone marrow cells** not maturing properly and therefore not producing healthy blood cells. There are a number of specific types of myelodysplastic syndrome.

It causes low levels of blood components that originate from the myeloid cell line:
- *Anaemia*
- *Neutropenia* (low neutrophil count)
- *Thrombocytopenia* (low platelets)

It is more common in patients above 60 years of age and in patients that have previously had treatment with **chemotherapy** or **radiotherapy**.

There is an increased risk of transforming into **acute myeloid leukaemia**.

Presentation

Patients may be asymptomatic and incidentally diagnosed based on a full blood count.

They may present with symptoms of *anaemia* (fatigue, pallor or shortness of breath), *neutropenia* (frequent or severe infections) or *thrombocytopenia* (purpura or bleeding).

Diagnosis

Full blood count will be abnormal. There may be *blasts* on the *blood film*.

The diagnosis is confirmed by *bone marrow aspiration* and *biopsy*.

Management

Depending on the symptoms, risk of progression and overall prognosis the treatment options are:
- Watchful waiting
- Supportive treatment with blood transfusions if severely anaemic
- Chemotherapy
- Stem cell transplantation

Thrombocytopenia

Thrombocytopenia describes a low platelet count. The normal platelet count is between 150 to 450 x 10^9/L. There are a long list of causes of a low platelet count. They can be split into problems with *production* or *destruction*.

Problems with Production

- Sepsis
- B12 or folic acid deficiency
- Liver failure causing reduced *thrombopoietin* production in the liver
- Leukaemia
- Myelodysplastic syndrome

Problems with Destruction

- Medications (sodium valproate, methotrexate, isotretinoin, antihistamines and proton pump inhibitors)
- Alcohol
- Immune thrombocytopenic purpura
- Thrombotic thrombocytopenic purpura
- Heparin induced thrombocytopenia
- Haemolytic-uraemic syndrome

Presentation

A mild thrombocytopenia may be asymptomatic and found incidentally on a full blood count.

Platelet counts below 50 x 10⁹/L will result in easy or spontaneous bruising and prolonged bleeding times. They may present with nosebleeds, bleeding gums, heavy periods, easy bruising or blood in the urine or stools.

Patients with platelet counts below 10 x 10⁹/L are high risk for spontaneous bleeding. Spontaneous intracranial haemorrhage or GI bleeds are particularly concerning.

Differential Diagnosis of Abnormal or Prolonged Bleeding

The blood contains a clotting system that allow it to make blood clots to stop bleeding. This system can break down in a number of ways. A few key differentials to remember for your exams are:
- **Thrombocytopenia** (low platelets)
- **Haemophilia A** and **haemophilia B**
- **Von Willebrand disease**
- **Disseminated intravascular coagulation** (usually secondary to sepsis)

Immune Thrombocytopenic Purpura (ITP)

Confusing this is also called **autoimmune thrombocytopenic purpura**, **idiopathic thrombocytopenic purpura** and **primary thrombocytopenic purpura**. They all refer to the same condition.

ITP is a condition where **antibodies** are created against **platelets**. This causes an immune response against platelets, resulting in the destruction of platelets and a low platelet count.

Management options include:
- **Prednisolone** (steroids)
- IV **immunoglobulins**
- **Rituximab** (a monoclonal antibody against B cells)
- **Splenectomy**

The platelet count needs to be monitored and the patient needs education about concerning signs of bleeding such as **persistent headaches** and **melaena** and when to seek help. Additional measures such as carefully controlling **blood pressure** and suppressing **menstrual periods** are also important.

Thrombotic Thrombocytopenic Purpura

This is a condition where tiny blood clots develop throughout the **small vessels** of the body using up platelets and causing thrombocytopenia, bleeding under the skin and other systemic issues. It affect the small vessels so it is described as a **microangiopathy**.

The blood clots develop due to a problem with a specific protein called **ADAMTS13**. This protein normally *inactivates von Willebrand factor* and reduces **platelet adhesion** to vessel walls and **clot formation**. A shortage in this protein leads to von Willebrand factor overactivity and the formation of blood clots in small vessels. This causes platelets to be used up, leading to thrombocytopenia. The blood clots in the small vessels break up red blood cells, leading to **haemolytic anaemia**.

Deficiency in the **ADAMTS13** protein can be due to an inherited **genetic mutation** or **autoimmune disease** where **antibodies** are created against the protein.

Treatment is guided by a haematologist and may involve **plasma exchange**, **steroids** and **rituximab** (a monoclonal antibody against B cells).

Heparin Induced Thrombocytopenia

Heparin induced thrombocytopenia (**HIT**) involves the development of **antibodies** against platelets in response to exposure to **heparin.** These **heparin induced antibodies** specifically target a protein on the platelets called **platelet factor 4** (**PF4**). These are **anti-PF4/heparin antibodies**.

The HIT antibodies bind to platelets and **activate clotting mechanisms**. This causes a **hypercoagulable state** and leads to **thrombosis**. They also break down platelets and cause **thrombocytopenia**. Therefore there is an unintuitive situation where a patient on heparin with low platelets forms unexpected blood clots.

Diagnosis is by testing for the **HIT antibodies** in the patients blood. Management is by stopping heparin and using an alternative anticoagulant guided by a specialist.

Von Willebrand Disease

Von Willebrand disease (VWD) is the most common **inherited** cause of **abnormal bleeding** (**haemophilia**). There are many different underlying genetic causes, most of which are **autosomal dominant**. The causes involve a deficiency, absence or malfunctioning of a **glycoprotein** called **von Willebrand factor** (**VWF**). There are three types based on the underlying cause ranging from type 1 to type 3. Type 3 is the most severe.

Presentation

Patients present with a history of unusually easy, prolonged or heavy bleeding:
- Bleeding gums with brushing
- Nose bleeds (**epistaxis**)
- Heavy menstrual bleeding (**menorrhagia**)
- Heavy bleeding during surgical operations

Family history of heavy bleeding or von Willebrand disease is very relevant.

Diagnosis

Diagnosis is based on a history of abnormal bleeding, family history, **bleeding assessment tools** and laboratory investigations. Due to all the underlying causes there is no easy von Willebrand disease test. This can make diagnosis challenging and beyond the scope of most medical exams.

Management

Von Willebrand disease does not require day to day treatment. Management is required either in response to major bleeding or trauma (to stop bleeding) or in preparation for operations (to prevent bleeding):

- **Desmopressin** can be used to stimulates the release of vWF
- **VWF** can be infused
- **Factor VIII** is often infused along with plasma derived vWF

Women with vWD that suffer with heavy periods can be managed by a combination of:
- Tranexamic acid
- Mefanamic acid
- Norethisterone
- Combined oral contraceptive pill
- Mirena coil

Hysterectomy may be required in severe cases.

Haemophilia

Haemophilia A and **haemophilia B** are **inherited severe bleeding disorders**. Haemophilia A is caused by a deficiency in **factor VIII**. Haemophilia B (also known as **Christmas disease**) is caused by a deficiency in **factor IX**.

X Linked Recessive

Both haemophilia A and B are **X linked recessive**. This means in order to have the condition all of the **X chromosomes** need to have the **abnormal gene**. Men only require one abnormal copy as they only have one X chromosome. Women require abnormal copies on both their X chromosomes, and if only one copy is affected they are a **carrier** of the condition.

Therefore haemophilia A and B almost **exclusively affect males**. For a female to be affected they would require an affected father and a mother that is either a carrier or also affected.

Signs and Symptoms

Both haemophilia A and B are severe bleeding disorders. Patients can bleed excessively in response to minor trauma and are also at risk of **spontaneous haemorrhage** without any trauma.

Most cases present in neonates or early childhood. It can present with **intracranial haemorrhage**, **haematomas** and **cord bleeding** in neonates.

Spontaneous bleeding into **joints** (**haemoathrosis**) and **muscles** are a classic feature of severe haemophilia and worth remembering for your exams. If untreated this can lead to joint damage and deformity.

Abnormal bleeding can occur in other areas:
- Gums
- Gastrointestinal tract
- Urinary tract causing haematuria
- Retroperitoneal space
- Intracranial
- Following procedures

Diagnosis

Diagnosis is based on **bleeding scores**, **coagulation factor assays** and **genetic testing**.

Management

Management should be coordinated by a specialist.

The affected **clotting factors** (**VIII** or **IX**) can be replaced by **intravenous infusions**. This can be either prophylactically or in response to bleeding. A complication of this treatment is formation of **antibodies** against the **clotting factor**, resulting in the treatment becoming ineffective.

Treating acute episodes of bleeding or prevention of excessive bleeding during surgical procedures involve:
- **Infusions** of the affected factor (VIII or IX)
- **Desmopressin** to stimulate the release of **von Willebrand Factor**
- **Antifibrinolytics** such as **tranexamic acid**

Deep Vein Thrombosis and Venous Thromboembolism

Venous thromboembolism (**VTE**) is a common and potentially fatal condition. It involves blood clots (**thrombosis**) developing in the circulation. This usually occurs secondary to stagnation of blood and **hyper-coagulable** states. When a **thrombosis** develops in the venous circulation it is called a **deep vein thrombosis** (**DVT**). Once a thrombosis has developed, it can mobilise (**embolise**) from the deep veins and travel through the right side of the heart and into the lungs, where it becomes lodged in the **pulmonary arteries**. This blocks blood flow to areas of the lungs and is called a **pulmonary embolism** (**PE**).

If the patient has a hole in their heart (for example, an **atrial septal defect**) the blood clot can pass through to the left side of the heart to the systemic circulation. If it travels to the brain it can cause a large **stroke**.

Risk Factors

There are a number of factors that can put patients at higher risk of developing a DVT or PE. In many of these situations (e.g. surgery) we give patients **prophylactic treatment** to prevent VTE.
- Immobility
- Recent surgery
- Long haul flights
- Pregnancy
- Hormone therapy with **oestrogen** (combined oral contraceptive pill and hormone replacement therapy)
- Malignancy
- Polycythaemia
- Systemic lupus erythematosus
- Thrombophilia

TOM TIP: In your exams when a patient is presenting with possible features of a DVT or PE, ask about risk factors such as periods of immobility, surgery and long haul flights to score extra points.

Thrombophilias

Thrombophilias are conditions that predispose patients to developing blood clots. There are large number of these:
- **Antiphospholipid syndrome** (this is the one to remember for your exams)
- Antithrombin deficiency
- Protein C or S deficiency
- Factor V Leiden
- Hyperhomocysteinaemia
- Prothombin gene variant
- Activated protein C resistance

VTE Prophylaxis

Every patient admitted to hospital should be assessed for their risk of **venous thromboembolism** (**VTE**). If they are at increased risk of VTE they should receive prophylaxis with a **low molecular weight heparin** such as **enoxaparin** unless contraindicated. Contraindications include active bleeding or existing anticoagulation with **warfarin** or a **NOAC**. **Anti-embolic compression stockings** are also used unless contraindicated. The main contraindication for compression stockings is significant **peripheral arterial disease**.

DVT Presentation

DVTs are almost always **unilateral**. Bilateral DVT is rare and bilateral symptoms are more likely due to an alternative diagnosis such as **chronic venous insufficiency** or **heart failure**. DVTs can present with:
- Calf or leg swelling
- Dilated superficial veins
- Tenderness to the calf (particularly over the site of the deep veins)
- Oedema
- Colour changes to the leg

To examine for leg swelling measure the circumference of the calf 10cm below the **tibial tuberosity**. **More than 3cm** difference between calves is significant.

Always ask questions and examine with the suspicion of a potential **pulmonary embolism** as well.

Wells Score

The **Wells score** predicts the risk of a patient presenting with symptoms actually having a **DVT** or **PE**. It takes into account risk factors such as recent surgery and clinical findings such as unilateral calf swelling 3cm greater than the other leg.

Diagnosis

D-dimer is a **sensitive** (95%) but **not specific** blood test for VTE. This makes it useful for **excluding VTE** where there is a low suspicion. It is almost always raised if there is a DVT, however other conditions can also cause a raised d-dimer:

- Pneumonia
- Malignancy
- Heart failure
- Surgery
- Pregnancy

Ultrasound doppler of the leg is required to diagnose deep vein thrombosis. NICE recommend repeating negative ultrasound scans after 6-8 days if there is a positive D-dimer and the **Wells score** suggest a DVT is **likely**.

Pulmonary embolism can be diagnosed with a **CT pulmonary angiogram** or **ventilation–perfusion** (**VQ**) **scan**.

Management

Initial Management

The initial management is with treatment dose **low molecular weight heparin** (**LMWH**). It should be started immediately before confirming the diagnosis in patients where DVT or PE is suspected and there is a delay in getting the scan. Examples are **enoxaparin** and **dalteparin**.

Switching to Long Term Anticoagulation

The options for long term anticoagulation in VTE are **warfarin**, a **NOAC** or **LMWH**.

Warfarin is a vitamin K antagonist. The target INR for warfarin is between 2 and 3. When switching to warfarin continue LMWH for 5 days or the INR is between 2 and 3 for 24 hours on warfarin (whichever is longer).

NOACs (or **DOACs**) are essentially oral anticoagulants that are not warfarin. They are an alternative option for anticoagulation that does not require monitoring. Originally they were called "**novel oral anticoagulants**" but this has been changed to "**non-vitamin K oral anticoagulants**" because they are no longer novel. This is changing to DOACs, standing for "**direct-acting oral anticoagulants**". The main three options are **apixaban**, **dabigatran** and **rivaroxaban**.

LMWH long term is first line treatment in pregnancy or cancer.

Continue anticoagulation for:
- **3 months** if there is an obvious reversible cause (then review)
- **Beyond 3 months** if the cause is unclear, there is recurrent VTE or there is an irreversible underlying cause such as thrombophilia. This is often 6 months in practice.
- **6 months** in active cancer (then review)

Inferior Vena Cava Filter

Inferior vena cava filters are devices inserted into the **inferior vena cava** designed to filter the blood and catch any blood clots traveling from the venous system towards the heart and lungs. They act like a sieve, allowing blood to flow through whilst stopping larger blood clots. They are used in unusual cases of patients with **recurrent PEs** or those that are unsuitable for anticoagulation.

Investigating Unprovoked DVT

When patients have their first VTE without a clear cause, NICE recommend investigating them for possible **cancer**. To screen for **cancer** they recommend:
- History and examination
- Chest X-ray

- Bloods (FBC, calcium and LFTs)
- Urine dipstick
- **CT abdomen and pelvis** in patients over 40
- **Mammogram** in women over 40

They also recommend testing for **antiphospholipid syndrome** by checking for **antiphospholipid antibodies**.

In patients with an unprovoked VTE **with** a family history of VTE they recommend testing for **hereditary thrombophilias**:
- Factor V Leiden (most common hereditary thrombophilia)
- Prothrombin G20210A
- Protein C
- Protein S
- Antithrombin

Budd-Chiari Syndrome

Budd-Chiari syndrome is where a blood clot (thrombosis) develops in the **hepatic vein**, blocking the outflow of blood. It is associated with hyper-coagulable states. It causes an acute hepatitis

It presents with a classic **triad** of:
- Abdominal pain
- Hepatomegaly
- Ascites

Management involves anticoagulation (heparin or warfarin), investigating for the underlying cause of hyper-coagulation and treating the hepatitis.

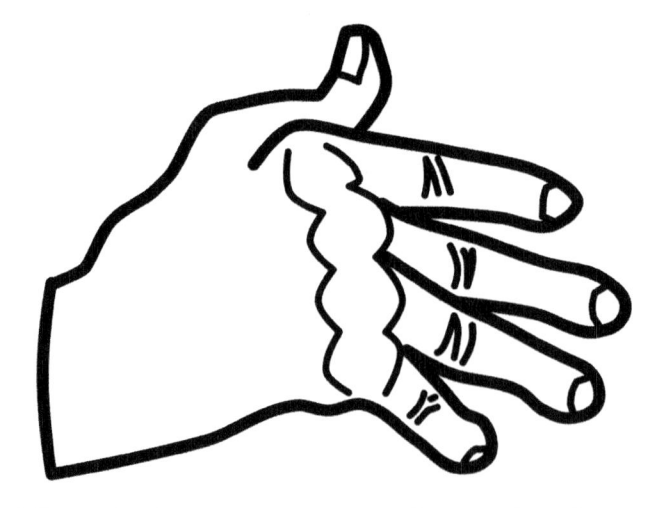

RHEUMATOLOGY

7.1	Osteoarthritis	207
7.2	Rheumatoid Arthritis	208
7.3	Psoriatic Arthritis	214
7.4	Reactive Arthritis	216
7.5	Ankylosing Spondylitis	217
7.6	Systemic Lupus Erythematosus	219
7.7	Discoid Lupus Erythematosus	221
7.8	Systemic Sclerosis	222
7.9	Polymyalgia Rheumatica	225
7.10	Giant Cell Arteritis	227
7.11	Polymyositis and Dermatomyositis	229
7.12	Antiphosphlipid Syndrome	230
7.13	Sjogren's Syndrome	231
7.14	Vasculitis	232
7.15	Behçet's Disease	236
7.16	Gout	238
7.17	Pseudogout	239
7.18	Osteoporosis	240
7.19	Osteomalacia	243
7.20	Paget's Disease	244

Osteoarthritis

Osteoarthritis is often described as "wear and tear" in the joints. It is not an inflammatory condition like rheumatoid arthritis. It occurs in the synovial joints and is a result of a combination of genetic factors, overuse and injury.

Risk factors include obesity, age, occupation, trauma, being female and family history.

It is thought to be the result of an imbalance between the cartilage being worn down and the chondrocytes repairing it, leading to structural issues in the joint. These abnormalities can be seen on an xray:

Four Key Xray Changes (LOSS)

- **L - L**oss of joint space
- **O - O**steophytes
- **S - S**ubarticular sclerosis (increased density of the bone along the joint line)
- **S - S**ubchondral cysts (fluid filled holes in the bone)

Xray changes do not necessarily correlate with symptoms. Significant xray changes might be found incidentally in someone without symptoms. Equally, someone with severe symptoms of osteoarthritis may have only mild changes on an xray.

Presentation

Osteoarthritis presents with joint pain and stiffness. This pain and stiffness tends to be worsened by activity in contrast to inflammatory arthritis where activity improves symptoms. It also leads to deformity, instability and reduced function in the joint.

Commonly Affected Joints

- Hips
- Knees
- Sacro-iliac joints
- Distal-interphalangeal joints in the hands (DIPs)
- The MCP joint at the base of the thumb
- Wrist
- Cervical spine

Signs in the Hands

- **Haberdens nodes** (in the DIP joints)
- **Bouchards nodes** (in the PIP joints)
- Squaring at the base of the thumb at the carpo-metacarpal joint
- Weak grip
- Reduced range of motion

The **carpo-metacarpal joint** at the base of the thumb is a saddle joint with the metacarpal bone of the thumb sat on the trapezius bone, using it like a saddle. It gets a lot of use from everyday activities. This makes it very prone to wear when used for complex movements.

Diagnosis

NICE (2014) suggest that a diagnosis can be made without any investigations if the patient is over 45, has typical activity related pain and has no morning stiffness or stiffness lasting less than 30 minutes.

Management

Start with **patient education** about the condition and advise on lifestyle changes such as **weight loss** if overweight to reduce the load on the joint, **physiotherapy** to improve strength to support the joint and **occupational therapy** and **orthotics** to support activities and function.

Stepwise use of **analgesia** to control symptoms:
1. Oral **paracetamol** and topical **NSAIDs** or topical **capsaicin** (chilli pepper extract).
2. Add oral **NSAIDs** and consider also prescribing a **proton pump inhibitor** (PPI) to protect their stomach such as **omeprazole**. They are better used intermittently rather than continuously.
3. Consider **opiates** such as **codeine** and **morphine**. These should be used cautiously as they can have significant side effects and patients can develop dependence and withdrawal. They also don't work for chronic pain and result in patients becoming depending without benefitting from pain relief.

Intra-articular steroid injections provide a temporary reduction in inflammation and improve symptoms.

Joint replacement can be used in severe cases. The hip and knee are the most commonly replaced joints.

Rheumatoid Arthritis

Rheumatoid arthritis is an autoimmune condition that causes **chronic inflammation** of the **synovial lining** of the **joints**, **tendon sheaths** and **bursa**. It is an **inflammatory arthritis**. Synovial inflammation is called **synovitis**. Rheumatoid arthritis tends to be **symmetrical** and affects **multiple joints**. It is a "**symmetrical polyarthritis**". Inflammation of the tendons increases the risk of tendon rupture.

It is three times more common in women than men. It most often develops in middle age but can present at any age. Family history is relevant and increases the risk of rheumatoid arthritis.

Genetic Associations

- **HLA DR4** (a gene often present in RF positive patients)
- **HLA DR1** (a gene occasionally present in RA patients)

Antibodies

Rheumatoid factor (**RF**) is an **autoantibody** presenting in around 70% of RA patients. It is an autoantibody that targets the **Fc portion** of the **IgG antibody**. All antibodies have an **Fc portion** on them that is used to bind to cells of the immune system. Rheumatoid factor targets this Fc portion on **immunoglobin G** (IgG). This causes activation of the immune system against the patients own IgG resulting in systemic inflammation. Rheumatoid factor is most often **IgM**, however they can be any class of immunoglobulin.

Anti-citrullinated cyclic peptide antibodies (anti-CCP antibodies) are autoantibodies that are more sensitive and specific to rheumatoid arthritis than rheumatoid factor. Anti-CCP antibodies often pre-date the development of rheumatoid arthritis and give an indication that a patient will go on to develop rheumatoid arthritis at some point.

Presentation

It typically presents with a **symmetrical distal polyarthropathy**. The key symptoms are joint:
- Pain
- Swelling
- Stiffness

Patients usually attend complaining of pain and stiffness in the small joints of the hands and feet, typically the wrist, ankle, MCP and PIP joints in the hands. They can also present with larger joints affected such as the knees, shoulders and elbows. The onset can be very rapid (i.e. overnight) or over months to years.

There are also associated systemic symptoms:
- Fatigue
- Weight loss
- Flu like illness
- Muscles aches and weakness

TOM TIP: Pain from an inflammatory arthritis is worse after rest but improves with activity. Pain from a mechanical problem such as osteoarthritis is worse with activity and improves with rest.

Palindromic Rheumatism

This involves self limiting short episodes of **inflammatory arthritis** with joint pain, stiffness and swelling typically affecting only a few joints. The episodes typically only last 1-2 days and then completely resolve. Having positive antibodies (**RF** and **anti-CCP**) may indicate that it will progress to full rheumatoid arthritis.

Common Joints Affected

- Proximal interphalangeal (PIP) joints
- Metacarpophalangeal (MCP) joints
- Wrist and ankle
- Metatarsophalangeal (MTP) joints
- Cervical spine
- Large joints can also be affected such as the knee, hips and shoulders

TOM TIP: The distal interphalangeal joints are almost never affected by rheumatoid arthritis. If you come across enlarged painful distal interphalangeal joints this is most likely to be Heberden's nodes due to osteoarthritis.

Atlantoaxial Subluxation

Atlantoaxial subluxation occurs in the cervical spine. The **axis** (C2) and the **odontoid peg** shift within the **atlas** (C1). This is caused by local synovitis and damage to the ligaments and bursa around the odontoid peg of the axis. Subluxation can cause **spinal cord compression** and is an emergency. This is particularly important if the patient is having a general anaesthetic and requiring intubation. MRI scans can visualise changes in these areas as part of pre-operative assessment.

Signs in the Hands

Palpation of the **synovium** around joints when the disease is active will give a "boggy" feeling related to the inflammation and swelling.

Key changes to look for and mention when examining someone with rheumatoid arthritis are:
- **Z shaped deformity** to the thumb
- **Swan neck deformity** (hyperextended PIP with flexed DIP)
- **Boutonnieres deformity** (hyperextended DIP with flexed PIP)
- **Ulnar deviation** of the fingers at the MCP joints

Boutonnieres Deformity
Boutonnieres deformity is due to a tear in the central slip of the extensor components of the fingers. This means that when the patient tries to straighten their finger, the lateral tendons that go around the PIP (called the **flexor digitorum superficialis** tendons) pull on the **distal phalynx** without any other supporting structure. The DIPs extend and the PIPs flex.

Extra-articular Manifestations

- **Pulmonary fibrosis** with pulmonary nodules (Caplan's syndrome)
- **Bronchiolitis obliterans** (inflammation causing small airway destruction)
- **Felty's syndrome** (RA, neutropenia and splenomegaly)
- Secondary **Sjogren's Syndrome** (AKA **sicca syndrome**)
- Anaemia of chronic disease
- Cardiovascular disease
- Eye manifestations
- Rheumatoid nodules
- Lymphadenopathy
- Carpel tunnel syndrome
- Amyloidosis

Eye Manifestations

There are a number of different eye related complications of rheumatoid arthritis:
- Scleritis
- Epislceritis
- Keratitis
- Keratoconjunctivitis sicca
- Cararacts (secondary to steroids)
- Retinopathy (secondary to chloroquine)

Investigations

The diagnosis of rheumatoid arthritis is clinical in patients with features of rheumatoid arthritis (i.e. **symmetrical polyarthropathy** affecting **small joints**). A few extra investigations are required at diagnosis:
- Check rheumatoid factor
- If RF negative, check anti-CCP antibodies
- Inflammatory markers such as CRP and ESR
- X-ray of hands and feet

Ultrasound scan of the joints can be used to evaluate and confirm **synovitis**. It is particularly useful where the findings of the clinical examination are unclear.

Xray Changes

- Joint destruction and deformity
- Soft tissue swelling
- Periarticular osteopenia
- Boney erosions

Referral

NICE recommend referral for any adult with persistent synovitis, even if they have negative rheumatoid factor, anti-CCP antibodies and inflammatory markers. The referral should be urgent if it involves the small joints of the hands or feet, multiple joints or symptoms have been present for more than 3 months.

Diagnosis

Diagnostic criteria come from the **American College of Rheumatology** (**ACR**) / **European League Against Rheumatism** (**ELAR**) from 2010. Patients are scored based on:
- The joints that are involved (more and smaller joints score higher)
- Serology (rheumatoid factor and anti-CCP)
- Inflammatory markers (ESR and CRP)
- Duration of symptoms (more or less than 6 weeks)

Scores are added up and a score greater than or equal to 6 indicates a diagnosis of rheumatoid arthritis.

DAS28 Score

The DAS28 is the **disease activity score**. It is based on the assessment of 28 joints and points are given for:
- Swollen joints
- Tender joints
- ESR / CRP result

It is useful in monitoring disease activity and response to treatment.

Health Assessment Questionnaire (HAQ)

This questionnaire measures functional ability. NICE recommend using this at diagnosis to check the response to treatment.

Prognosis

Prognosis varies between patients from mild and remitting to severe and progressive. There is a worse prognosis with:
- Younger onset
- Male
- More joints and organs affected
- Presence of RF and anti-CCP antibodies
- Erosions seen on xray

Management

Starting treatment early is associated with better outcomes. It is important to have fully involvement of **multidisciplinary team** including specialist nurses, physiotherapy, occupational therapy, psychology and podiatry.

A short course of steroids can be used at first presentation and during flare ups to quickly settle the disease. **NSAIDs** are often effective but risk upper GI bleeding so are often avoided or co-prescribed with **proton pump inhibitors** (**PPIs**).

The aim is to induce remission or get as close to remission as possible. CRP and DAS28 is used to monitor the success of treatment. Aim to reduce the dose to the "**minimal effective dose**" that controls the disease.

NICE guidelines for Disease Modifying Anti-Rheumatic Drugs (DMARDs):
- First line is monotherapy with **methotrexate**, **leflunomide** or **sulfasalazine**. **Hydroxychloroquine** can be considered in mild disease and is considered the "mildest" anti rheumatic drug.
- Second line is 2 of these used in combination.
- Third line is methotrexate plus a **biological therapy**, usually a **TNF inhibitor**.
- Fourth line is methotrexate plus **rituximab.**

Pregnant women tend to have an improvement in symptoms during pregnancy, probably due to the higher natural production of steroid hormones. Sulfasalazine and hydroxychloroquine are considered as DMARDs in pregnancy.

Biological Therapies
- Anti-TNF (adalimumab, infliximab, etanercept, golimumab and certolizumab pegol)
- Anti-CD20 (rituximab)
- Anti-IL6 (sarilumab)
- Anti-IL6 receptor (tocilizumab)
- JAK inhibitors (tofacitinib and baricitinib)

TOM TIP: The most important biologics to remember are the TNF inhibitors adalimumab, infliximab and etanercept and it is also worth remembering rituximab. The others are very unlikely to come up in your exams but are worth being aware of. Just remember they all lead to immunosuppression so patients are prone to serious infections. They can also lead to reactivation of dormant infections such as TB and hepatitis B.

Surgery
Orthopaedic surgery used to be an important part of management where joint deformities caused significant problems with function, however the DMARDS and biologics mean that now patients are less likely to progress to that stage.

Methotrexate

Methotrexate works by interfering with the metabolism of folate and suppressing certain components of the immune system. It is taken by injection or tablet once a week. **Folic acid** 5mg is also prescribed once a week to be **taken on a different day** to the methotrexate.

Notable Side Effects
- Mouth ulcers and mucositis
- Liver toxicity
- **Pulmonary fibrosis**
- Bone marrow suppression and leukopenia (low white blood cells)
- It is **teratogenic** (harmful to pregnancy) and needs to be avoided prior to conception in mothers and fathers

Leflunomide

Leflunomide is an immunosuppressant medication that works by interfering with the production of **pyrimidine**. Pyrimidine is an important component of RNA and DNA.

Notable Side Effects
- Mouth ulcers and mucositis
- Increased blood pressure
- Rashes
- *Peripheral neuropathy*
- Liver toxicity
- Bone marrow suppression and leukopenia (low white blood cells)
- It is **teratogenic** (harmful to pregnancy) and needs to be avoided prior to conception in mothers and fathers

Sulfasalzine

Sulfasalazine works as an immunosuppressive and anti-inflammatory medication. The mechanism is not clear but may be related to folate metabolism. It appears to be safe in pregnancy however women need adequate folic acid supplementation

Notable Side Effects
- Temporary male infertility (reduced sperm count)
- Bone marrow suppression

Hydroxychloroquine

Hydroxychloroquine is traditionally an anti-malarial medication. It acts as an immunosuppressive medication by interfering with **Toll-like receptors**, disrupting antigen presentation and increasing the pH in the lysosomes of immune cells. It is thought to be safe in pregnancy.

Notable Side Effects
- Nightmares
- Reduced visual acuity (macular toxicity)
- Liver toxicity
- Skin pigmentation

Anti-TNF drugs

Tumour necrosis factor is a cytokine involved in stimulating inflammation. Blocking TNF reduces inflammation. Some examples of anti-TNF drugs are:
- Adalimumab
- Infliximab
- Golimumab
- Certolizumab pegol
- Etanercept

Adalimumab, infliximab, golimumab and certolizumab pegol are **monoclonal antibodies** to tumour necrosis factor. **Etanercept** is a protein that binds TNF to the **Fc portion** of **IgG** and thereby reduces its activity.

Notable Side Effects
- Vulnerability to severe infections and sepsis
- Reactivation of TB and hepatitis B

Rituximab

Rituximab is a **monoclonal antibody** that targets the **CD20 protein** on the surface of **B cells**. This causes destruction of B cells. It is used for immunosuppression in autoimmune conditions such as rheumatoid arthritis and cancers relating to B cells.

Notable Side Effects
- Vulnerability to severe infections and sepsis
- Night sweats
- Thrombocytopenia (low platelets)
- Peripheral neuropathy
- Liver and lung toxicity

TOM TIP: There are a lot of side effects to remember for your exams. Many of them are shared between medications. Try to remember the unique ones as these are more likely to be tested:
- *Methotrexate: pulmonary fibrosis*
- *Leflunomide: Hypertension and peripheral neuropathy*
- *Sulfasalazine: Male infertility (reduces sperm count)*
- *Hydroxychloroquine: Nightmares and reduced visual acuity*
- *Anti-TNF medications: Reactivation of TB or hepatitis B*
- *Rituximab: Night sweats and thrombocytopenia*

Psoriatic Arthritis

Psoriatic arthritis is an **inflammatory arthritis** associated with **psoriasis**. This can vary in severity. Patients may have a mild stiffening and soreness in the joint or the joint can be completely destroyed in a condition called **arthritis mutilans**.

It occurs in 10-20% of patients with psoriasis and usually occurs within 10 years of developing the skin changes. It typically affects people in middle age but can occur at any age.

It is part of the "**seronegative spondyloarthropathy**" group of conditions.

Patterns

The condition does not have a single pattern of affected joints in the same way as osteoarthritis or rheumatoid. There are several recognised patterns:

Symmetrical polyarthritis presents similarly to rheumatoid arthritis and is more common in women. The hands, wrists, ankles and DIP joints are affected. The MCP joints are less commonly affected (unlike rheumatoid).

Asymmetrical pauciarthritis affecting mainly the digits (fingers and toes) and feet. Pauciarthritis describes when the arthritis only affects a few joints.

Spondylitic pattern is more common in men. It presents with:
- Back stiffness
- Sacroiliitis
- Atlanto-axial joint involvement

Other areas can be affected:
- Spine
- Achilles tendon
- Plantar fascia

Signs

- Plaques of psoriasis on the skin
- **Pitting** of the nails (nail pitting)
- **Onycholysis** (separation of the nail from the nail bed)
- **Dactylitis** (inflammation of the full finger)
- **Enthesitis** (inflammation of the entheses, which are the points of insertion of tendons into bone)

Other Associations

- Eye disease (**conjunctivitis** and **anterior uveitis**)
- Aortitis (inflammation of the aorta)
- Amyloidosis

Psoriasis Epidemiological Screening Tool (PEST)

NICE recommend patients with psoriasis complete the **PEST tool** to screen for psoriatic arthritis. This involves several questions asking about joint pain, swelling, a history of arthritis and nail pitting. A high score triggers a referral to a rheumatologist.

Xray Changes

- **Periostitis** is inflammation of the **periosteum** causing a thickened and irregular outline of the bone
- **Ankylosis** is where bones joining together causing joint stiffening
- **Osteolysis** is destruction of bone
- **Dactylitis** is inflammation of the whole digit and appears on the xray as soft tissue swelling
- **Pencil-in-cup** appearance

The classic xray change to the digits is the "**pencil-in-cup appearance**". This is where there are **central erosions** of the bone beside the joints. This causes the appearance of one bone in the joint being hollow and looking like a cup whilst the other is narrow and sits in the cup.

Arthritis Mutilans

This is the most severe form of psoriatic arthritis. This occurs in the **phalanxes**. There is **osteolysis** (destruction) of the bones around the joints in the digits. This leads to progressive shortening of the digit. The skin then folds as the digit shortens giving an appearance that is often called a "**telescopic finger**".

Management

Management is similar to rheumatoid arthritis. There is a crossover between the systemic treatments of psoriasis and treatment of psoriatic arthritis. Treatment is often coordinated between dermatologists and rheumatologists.

Depending on the severity the patient might require:
- NSAIDs for pain
- DMARDS (methotrexate, leflunomide or sulfasalazine)
- Anti-TNF medications (etanercept, infliximab or adalimumab)
- **Ustekinumab** is last line (after anti-TNF medications) and is a monoclonal antibody that targets *interleukin 12 and 23*

Reactive Arthritis

Reactive arthritis is where **synovitis** occurs in the joints as a reaction to a recent infective trigger. It used to be known as **Reiter syndrome**. Typically it causes an **acute monoarthritis**, affecting a single joint in the lower limb (most often the knee) presenting with a warm, swollen and painful joint.

The obvious differential diagnosis is **septic arthritis** (infection in the joint). In reactive arthritis there is no joint infection.

The most common infections that trigger reactive arthritis are **gastroenteritis** or **sexually transmitted infection**. **Chlamydia** is the most common sexually transmitted cause of reactive arthritis. **Gonorrhoea** commonly causes a **gonococcal septic arthritis**.

There is a link with the **HLA B27 gene**. It is considered part of the **seronegative spondyloarthropathy** group of conditions.

Associations

- **Bilateral conjunctivitis** (non-infective)
- **Anterior uveitis**
- **Circinate balanitis** is dermatitis of the head of the penis

TOM TIP: These features of reactive arthritis (eye problems, balanitis and arthritis) lead to the saying "can't see, pee or climb a tree".

Management

Patients presenting with an acute warm, swollen, painful joint need to be treated according to the local "**hot joint**" policy. This will involve giving antibiotics until the possibility of septic arthritis is excluded. **Aspirate** the joint and send a sample for **gram staining**, **culture and sensitivity** testing to exclude septic arthritis.

The aspirated fluid can also be sent for **crystal examination** to look for **gout** and **pseudogout**.

Management of reactive arthritis when septic arthritis is excluded:
- NSAIDs
- Steroid injections into the affected joints
- Systemic steroids may be required, particularly where multiple joints are affected

Most cases resolve within 6 months and don't recur. Recurrent cases may require DMARDs or anti-TNF medications.

Ankylosing Spondylitis

Ankylosing spondylitis (AS) is an *inflammatory* condition mainly affecting the spine that causes progressive stiffness and pain. It is part of the *seronegative spondyloarthropathy* group of conditions relating to the HLA B27 gene. Other conditions in this group are *reactive arthritis* and *psoriatic arthritis*.

The key joints that are affected in AS are the *sacroiliac joints* and the joints of the *vertebral column*. The inflammation causes pain and stiffness in these joints. It can progress to *fusion* of the spine and sacroiliac joints. Fusion of the spine leads to the classical "*bamboo spine*" finding on a spinal xray. This often appears in exams.

There is a strong link with the *HLA B27 gene*. Around 90% of patients with AS have the *HLA B27 gene* however around 2% of people with the gene will get AS. This number is higher (around 20%) if they have a first degree relative that is affected.

Presentation

The typical presentation is a young adult male in their late teens or 20s. It affects males three times more often than females. Symptoms develop gradually over **more than 3 months**.

The main presenting features are **lower back pain and stiffness** and **sacroiliac pain** in the buttock region. The pain and stiffness is worse with rest and improves with movement. The pain is worse at night and in the morning and may wake them from sleep. It takes **at least 30 minutes** for the stiffness to improve in the morning and it gets progressively better with activity throughout the day.

Symptoms can fluctuate with "*flares*" of worsening symptoms and other periods where symptoms improve.

Vertebral fractures are a key complication of AS.

Associations

Ankylosing spondylitis does not only affect the spine. It can affect other organ systems causing:
- *Systemic symptoms* such as weight loss and fatigue
- *Chest pain* related to *costovertebral* and *costosternal* joints
- *Enthesitis* is inflammation of the *entheses*. This is where tendons or ligaments insert in to bone. This can cause problems such as *plantar fasciitis* and *achilles tendonitis*.
- *Dactylitis* is inflammation in a finger or toe.
- *Anaemia*
- *Anterior uveitis*
- *Aortitis* is inflammation of the aorta
- *Heart block* can be caused by fibrosis of the heart's conductive system
- *Restrictive lung disease* can be caused by restricted chest wall movement
- *Pulmonary fibrosis* at the upper lobes of the lungs occurs in around 1% of AS patients
- *Inflammatory bowel disease* is a condition associated with AS

Schober's Test

This is a test used as part of a general examination of the spine to assess how much mobility there is in the spine. You might be asked to do it in your OSCE examinations.

Have the patient stand straight. Find the **L5 vertebrae**. Mark a point 10cm above and 5cm below this point (15cm apart from each other). Then ask the patient to bend forward as far as they can and measure the distance between the points. If the distance with them bending forwards is **less than 20cm**, this indicates a restriction in lumbar movement and will help support a diagnosis of ankylosing spondylitis.

Investigations

- Inflammatory markers (CRP and ESR) may rise with disease activity
- HLA B27 genetic test
- Xray of the spine and sacrum
- MRI of the spine can show **bone marrow oedema** early in the disease before there are any xray changes

Xray Changes

"**Bamboo spine**" is the typical exam description of the xray appearance of the spine in later stage ankylosing spondylitis.

Xray images in ankylosing spondylitis can show:
- **Squaring** of the vertebral bodies
- **Subchondral sclerosis** and **erosions**
- **Syndesmophytes** are areas of bone growth where the ligaments insert into the bone. They occur related to the ligaments supporting the intervertebral joints.
- **Ossification** of the ligaments, discs and joints. This is where these structures turn to bone.
- **Fusion** of the **facet**, **sacroiliac** and **costovertebral** joints

Management

Medication:
- **NSAIDs** can be used to help with pain. If the improvement is not adequate after 2 to 4 weeks of a maximum dose consider switching to another NSAID.
- **Steroids** can be use during flares to control symptoms. This could be oral, intramuscular slow release injections or joint injections.
- **Anti-TNF** medications such as **etanercept** or a **monoclonal antibody** against **TNF** such as **infliximab**, **adalimumab** or **certolizumab pegol** are known to be effective in treating the disease activity in AS.
- **Secukinumab** is a **monoclonal antibody** against **interleukin-17**. It is recommended by NICE if the response to NSAIDS and TNF inhibitors is inadequate.

Additional management:
- Physiotherapy
- Exercise and mobilisation
- Avoid smoking
- Bisphosphonates to treat osteoporosis
- Treatment of complications
- Surgery is occasionally required for deformities to the spine or other joints

Systemic Lupus Erythematosus

Systemic lupus erythematosus ("**lupus**") is an **inflammatory autoimmune connective tissue disease**. It is "**systemic**" because it affects multiple organs and systems, and "**erythematosus**" refers to the typical red **malar rash** that occurs across the face. It presents with varying and non-specific symptoms. It is more common in women and Asians and usually presents in young to middle aged adults, but can present later in life.

It often takes a **relapsing-remitting** course, with flares and periods where symptoms are improved. The result of **chronic inflammation** means patients with lupus often have shortened life expectancy. **Cardiovascular disease** and **infection** are the leading causes of death.

Pathophysiology

SLE is characterised by **anti-nuclear antibodies**. These are **antibodies** to proteins within the persons own **cell nucleus**. This causes the immune system to target theses proteins. When the immune system is activated by these antibodies targeting proteins in the cell nucleus it generates an **inflammatory response**. **Inflammation** in the body leads to the symptoms of the condition. Usually inflammation is a helpful response when fighting off an infection, however it creates numerous problems when it occurs chronically and against the tissues of the body.

Presentation

SLE presents with non-specific symptoms:
- Fatigue
- Weight loss
- Arthralgia (joint pain) and non-erosive arthritis
- Myalgia (muscle pain)
- Fever
- **Photosensitive malar rash**. This is a "butterfly" shaped rash across the nose and cheek bones that gets **worse with sunlight**.
- Lymphadenopathy and splenomegaly
- Shortness of breath
- Pleuritic chest pain
- Mouth ulcers
- Hair loss
- Raynaud's phenomenon

Investigations

- **Autoantibodies** (see below)
- **Full blood count** (normocytic anaemia of chronic disease)
- **C3** and **C4** levels (decreased in active disease)
- **CRP** and **ESR** (raised with active inflammation)
- **Immunoglobulins** (raised due to activation of B cells with inflammation)
- Urinalysis and **urine protein:creatinine ratio** for proteinuria found in **lupus nephritis**
- **Renal biopsy** can be used to investigate for **lupus nephritis**

Autoantibodies

SLE is associated with **anti-nuclear antibodies** (**ANA**). These are antibodies against normal proteins in the cell nucleus. Around 85% of patients with SLE will be positive for ANA. Performing an **ANA blood test** is the initial step in testing for SLE in someone with symptoms of the condition. Antinuclear antibodies can be positive in healthy patients and those with other autoimmune conditions (e.g. autoimmune hepatitis). Therefore, a positive result needs to be interpreted in the context of their symptoms.

Anti-double stranded DNA (**anti-dsDNA**) is specific to SLE, meaning patients without the condition are very unlikely to have these antibodies. Around 70% of patients with SLE will have anti-dsDNA antibodies. The levels vary with disease activity, so they are useful in monitoring disease activity and response to treatment.

If you send a test for **antibodies** to **extractable nuclear antigens** (**anti-ENA antibodies**) the lab will check for antibodies to specific proteins in the cell nucleus. These are all types of antinuclear antibody:
- **Anti-Smith** (highly specific to **SLE** but not very sensitive)
- **Anti-centromere antibodies** (most associated with **limited cutaneous systemic sclerosis**)
- **Anti-Ro** and **anti-La** (most associated with **Sjogren's syndrome**)
- **Anti-Scl-70** (most associated with **systemic sclerosis**)
- **Anti-Jo-1** (most associated with **dermatomyositis**)

Antiphospholipid antibodies and **antiphospholipid syndrome** can occur secondary to SLE. They can occur in up to 40% of patients with SLE and are associated with an increased risk of venous thromboembolism.

Diagnosis

You can use the **SLICC criteria** or the **ACR criteria** for establishing a diagnosis. This involves confirming the presence of **antinuclear antibodies** and establishing a certain number of clinical features suggestive of SLE.

Complications

Systemic lupus erythematosus affects many of the organs in the body. These effects are related to chronic inflammation.

Cardiovascular disease is a leading cause of death. Chronic inflammation in blood vessels leads to hypertension and coronary artery disease.

Infection is more common in patients with SLE as part of the disease process and secondary to immunosuppressants.

Anaemia of chronic disease is common in SLE. It affects the bone marrow causing a chronic normocytic anaemia. Patients can also get **leucopenia** (low white cells), **neutropenia** (low neutrophils) and **thrombocytopenia** (low platelets).

Pericarditis is inflammation in the fluid filled sac around the heart. It causes sharp chest pain worse on lying flat.

Pleuritis is inflammation of the pleural lining of the lungs. This is also called **pleurisy**. It causes typical symptoms of sharp chest pain on inspiration.

Interstitial lung disease can be caused by inflammation in the lung tissue. This leads to **pulmonary fibrosis**.

Lupus nephritis occurs due to inflammation in the kidney. It can progress to end-stage renal failure. It is assessed with a **urine protein:creatinine ratio** and **renal biopsy**. The renal biopsy is often repeated to assess response to treatment.

Neuropsychiatric SLE is caused by inflammation in the central nervous system. It can present with **optic neuritis** (inflammation of the optic nerve), **transverse myelitis** (inflammation of the spinal cord) or **psychosis**.

Recurrent miscarriage is common in systemic lupus erythematosus. It is associated with other pregnancy complications such as intrauterine growth restriction, pre-eclampsia and pre-term labour.

Venous thromboembolism is particularly associated with **antiphospholipid syndrome** occurring secondary to SLE.

Treatment

As with most autoimmune conditions **anti-inflammatory** medication and **immunosuppression** is the mainstay of treatment. There is no cure and the aim is to reduce symptoms and complications. It will be guided by a rheumatology specialist. Treatment is usually titrated upwards to find the minimal medication with the least side effects required to control the symptoms.

First line treatments are:
- NSAIDs
- Steroids (prednisolone)
- **Hydroxychloroquine** (first line for mild SLE)
- Suncream and sun avoidance for the photosensitive malar rash

Other commonly used immunosuppressants in resistant or more severe lupus:
- Methotrexate
- Mycophenolate mofetil
- Azathioprine
- Tacrolimus
- Leflunomide
- Ciclosporin

Biological therapies are considered for patients with severe disease or where patients have not responded to other treatments. The main options in SLE:
- **Rituximab** is a **monoclonal antibody** that targets the **CD20 protein** on the surface of **B cells**
- **Belimumab** is a monoclonal antibody that targets **B-cell activating factor**

Discoid Lupus Erythematosus

Discoid lupus erythematosus is a non-cancerous chronic skin condition. It is more common in women and usually presents in young adulthood between ages 20 and 40. It is more common in darker skinned patients and smokers.

It is associated with an increased risk of developing **systemic lupus erythematosus**, however this risk is still below 5%. Rarely the lesions can progress to **squamous cell carcinoma** (SCC) of the skin.

Presentation

The lesions typically occur on the face, ears and scalp. They are **photosensitive**, meaning that they are made worse by exposure to sunlight. They are associated with **scarring alopecia** (hair loss in affected areas that does not grow back) and **hyper-pigmented** or **hypo-pigmented** scars.

The appearance of the lesions are:
- Inflamed
- Dry
- Erythematous
- Patchy
- Crusty and scaling

Management

Skin biopsy can be used to confirm the diagnosis.

Treatment is with
- Sun protection
- Topical steroids
- Intralesional steroid injections
- Hydroxychloroquine

Systemic Sclerosis

The terms **systemic sclerosis** and **scleroderma** are often used interchangeably. Most patients with **scleroderma** have **systemic sclerosis**, however there is a localised version of scleroderma that only affects the skin. Scleroderma translates directly to **hardening** of the **skin**.

Systemic sclerosis is an **autoimmune inflammatory and fibrotic connective tissue disease**. The cause of the condition is unclear. It most notably affects the skin in all areas but it also affects the internal organs.

There are two main patterns of disease in systemic sclerosis:
- *Limited cutaneous systemic sclerosis*
- *Diffuse cutaneous systemic sclerosis*

Limited Cutaneous Systemic Sclerosis

Limited cutaneous systemic sclerosis is the more limited version of systemic sclerosis. It used to be called **CREST syndrome**. This forms a helpful mnemonic for remembering the features of limited cutaneous systemic sclerosis:
- **C** - **C**alcinosis
- **R** - **R**aynaud's phenomenon
- **E** - o**E**sophageal dysmotility
- **S** - **S**clerodactyly
- **T** - **T**elangiectasia

Diffuse Cutaneous Systemic Sclerosis

Diffuse cutaneous systemic sclerosis includes the features of CREST syndrome plus it affects internal organs causing:
- **Cardiovascular problems**, particularly hypertension and coronary artery disease.
- **Lung problems**, particularly pulmonary hypertension and pulmonary fibrosis.
- **Kidney problems**, particularly glomerulonephritis and a condition called scleroderma renal crisis.

Features

Scleroderma refers to hardening of the skin. This gives a the appearance of shiny, tight skin without the normal folds in the skin. These changes are most notable on the hands and face.

Sclerodactyly describes the skin changes in the hands. As the skin tightens around joints it restricts the range of motion in the joint and reduces the function. As the skin hardens and tightens further the fat pads on the fingers are lost. The skin can break and ulcerate.

Telangiectasia are dilated small blood vessels in the skin. They are tiny veins that have dilated. They have a fine, thready appearance.

Calcinosis is where calcium deposits build up under the skin. This is most commonly found on the fingertips.

Raynaud's phenomenon is where the fingertips go completely white and then blue in response to even mild cold. It is caused by **vasoconstriction** of the vessels supplying the fingers. This commonly occurs without any associated systemic disease, however it is a classical feature of systemic sclerosis.

Oesophageal dysmotility is caused by connective tissue dysfunction in the oesophagus. This is commonly associated with swallowing difficulties, acid reflux and oesophagitis.

Systemic and **pulmonary hypertension** is caused by connective tissue dysfunction in the systemic and pulmonary arterial systems. Systemic hypertension can be worsened by renal impairment.

Pulmonary fibrosis can occur in severe systemic sclerosis. This presents with gradual onset dry cough and shortness of breath.

Scleroderma renal crisis is an acute condition where there is a combination of severe hypertension and renal failure.

Autoantibodies

There are many autoantibodies involved in systemic sclerosis and they are helpful in predicting the extent of the disease and which organs will be affected. It is not worth memorising all of them unless you want to be a rheumatologist. The ones to remember are below.

Antinuclear antibodies (**ANA**) are positive in most patients with systemic sclerosis. They are not specific to systemic sclerosis.

Anti-centromere antibodies are most associated with **limited cutaneous systemic sclerosis**.

Anti-Scl-70 antibodies are most associated with **diffuse cutaneous systemic sclerosis**. They are associated with more severe disease.

Nailfold Capillaroscopy

This is a technique to magnify and examine the area where the skin meets the base of the fingernail (the **nailfold**). This allows us to examine the health of the **peripheral capillaries**. Abnormal capillaries, avascular areas and microhaemorrhages indicate systemic sclerosis. It is useful to support a diagnosis of systemic sclerosis and to investigate patients with Raynaud's phenomenon to exclude systemic sclerosis. Patients with primary Raynaud's without systemic sclerosis will have normal nailfold capillaries.

Diagnosis

Diagnosis is based on classification criteria from the **American College of Rheumatology** (**ACR**) and **European League Against Rheumatism** (**EULAR**) published in 2013. This involves meeting a number of criteria for **clinical features**, **antibodies** and **nailfold capillaroscopy**.

Management

Patients with systemic sclerosis should be managed and followed up by a **specialist multidisciplinary team**.

Steroids and **immunosuppressants** are usually started with diffuse disease and complications such as pulmonary fibrosis. There is no standardised and proven treatment for systemic sclerosis. There is ongoing research trying to find effective ways of treating the condition.

Non-medical management involves:
- Avoid smoking
- Gentle skin stretching to maintain the range of motion
- Regular emollients
- Avoiding cold triggers for Raynaud's
- Physiotherapy to maintain healthy joints
- Occupational therapy for adaptations to daily living to cope with limitations

Medical management focuses on treating symptoms and complications:
- Nifedipine can be used to treat symptoms of Raynaud's phenomenon
- Anti acid medications (e.g. PPIs) and pro-motility medications (e.g. metoclopramide) for gastrointestinal symptoms
- Analgesia for joint pain
- Antibiotics for skin infections
- Antihypertensives can be used to treat hypertension (usually ACE inhibitors)
- Treatment of pulmonary artery hypertension
- Supportive management of pulmonary fibrosis

Polymyalgia Rheumatica

Polymyalgia rheumatica is an *inflammatory* condition that causes pain and stiffness in the shoulders, pelvic girdle and neck. There is a strong association with *giant cell arteritis* and the two conditions often occur together. Both conditions respond well to treatment with steroids.

There are very good **NICE clinical knowledge summaries** on polymyalgia rheumatica. I suggest reading them before treating patients. This is a summary to help with your learning and revision.

Demographics

- It usually affects old adults (above 50 years)
- More common in women
- More common in caucasians

Core Features

The **NICE Clinical Knowledge Summary** gives some core features that can be used to determine which patients may have PMR. These should be present for at least 2 weeks:
- Bilateral shoulder pain that may radiate to the elbow
- Bilateral pelvic girdle pain
- Worse with movement
- Interferes with sleep
- Stiffness for at least 45 minutes in the morning

Other features:
- Systemic symptoms such as weight loss, fatigue, low grade fever and low mood
- Upper arm tenderness
- Carpel tunnel syndrome
- Pitting oedema

Differential Diagnosis

One of the key challenges is to exclude other conditions that can cause similar symptoms and not miss other diagnoses. The list of differentials is very long however some examples are:
- Osteoarthritis
- Rheumatoid arhtirits
- Systemic lupus erythematosus
- Myositis (due to conditions like polymyositis or medications like statins)
- Cervical spondylosis
- Adhesive capsulitis of both shoulders
- Hyper or hypothyroidism
- Osteomalacia
- Fibromyalgia

Diagnosis

Diagnosis is mainly based on the **clinical presentation** and the **response to steroids**. Other conditions need to be excluded in order to make a diagnosis of PMR.

Inflammatory markers (**ESR**, **plasma viscosity** and **CRP**) are usually raised however normal inflammatory markers do not exclude PMR.

The NICE clinical knowledge summaries advise a number of investigations prior to starting steroids to exclude other conditions:
- Full blood count
- Urea and electrolytes
- Liver function tests
- **Calcium** can be raised in hyperparathyroidism or cancer or low in osteomalacia
- **Serum protein electrophoresis** for myeloma and other protein disorders
- **Thyroid stimulating hormone** for thyroid function
- **Creatine kinase** for myositis
- **Rheumatoid factor** for rheumatoid arthritis
- Urine dipstick

Additional investigations to consider:
- **Anti-nuclear antibodies** (**ANA**) for systemic lupus erythematosus
- **Anti-cyclic citrullinated peptide** (**anti-CCP**) for rheumatoid arthritis
- **Urine Bence Jones protein** for myeloma
- **Chest xray** for lung and mediastinal abnormalities

Treatment

Treatment of PMR is with steroids. The NICE CKS have clear guidelines on the steroid regime you should follow if treating patients. This is a summary to help your understanding.

Initially patients are started on **15mg of prednisolone** per day.

Assess 1 week after starting steroids. If there is a poor response in symptoms it is probably not PMR and an alternative diagnosis needs to be considered. Stop the steroids.

Assess 3-4 weeks after starting steroids. You would expect a 70% improvement in symptoms and inflammatory markers to return to normal to make a working diagnosis of PMR.

If 3-4 weeks of treatment with steroids has given a good response then start a **reducing regime** with the aim of getting the patient off steroids:
- 15mg until symptoms are fully controlled, then
- 12.5mg for 3 weeks, then
- 10mg for 4-6 weeks, then
- Reduce by 1mg every 4-8 weeks

If symptoms reoccur whilst on the reducing regime they may need to increase the dose or stay on the dose longer before reducing again. It can take 1 to 2 years to fully wean off. If there is doubt about the diagnosis, difficulty controlling symptoms, difficult weaning steroids or steroids are required for more than 2 years refer to a rheumatologist.

Additional measures for patients on long term steroids. You can use the mnemonic "**Don't STOP**":
- **DON'T** - Make them aware that they will become **steroid dependent** after 3 weeks of treatment and should not stop taking the steroids due to the risk of **adrenal crisis** if steroids are abruptly withdrawn
- **S** - **S**ick day rules: Discuss increasing the steroid dose if they become unwell ("**sick day rules**")
- **T** - **T**reatment card: Provide a **steroid treatment card** to alert others that they are steroid dependent in case they become unresponsive
- **O** - **O**steoporosis prevention: Consider **osteoporosis** prophylaxis whilst on steroids with **bisphosphonates** and **calcium and vitamin D** supplements
- **P** - **P**roton pump inhibitor: Consider **gastric protection** with a **proton pump inhibitor** (e.g. omeprazole)

Giant Cell Arteritis

Giant cell arteritis is a **systemic vasculitis** of the **medium** and **large arteries**. It typically presents with symptoms affecting the **temporal arteries** and is also known as **temporal arteritis**.

There is a strong link with **polymyalgia rheumatica**. The patients at higher risk are female caucasians over 50.

The key complication of **giant cell arteritis** is **vision loss**. This is often irreversible. High dose steroids are used immediately once a diagnosis is suspected to prevent the development or progression of vision loss.

Symptoms

The main presenting feature is a headache:
- Severe unilateral headache typically around temple and forehead
- Scalp tenderness may be noticed when brushing hair
- Jaw claudication
- Blurred or double vision
- Irreversible painless complete sight loss can occur rapidly

There may be associated systemic symptoms such as:
- Fever
- Muscle aches
- Fatigue
- Loss of appetite and weight loss
- Peripheral oedema

Diagnosis

A definitive diagnosis is based on:
- Clinical presentation
- Raised ESR: usually 50 mm/hour or more
- Temporal artery biopsy findings

TOM TIP: Multinucleated giant cells are found on the temporal artery biopsy. This is what gives rise to the giant cell arteritis name. This is worth remembering for your exams as it is a popular question.

Additional Investigations

- **Full blood count** may show a **normocytic anaemia** and **thrombocytosis** (raised platelets)
- **Liver function tests** can show a raised **alkaline phosphatase**
- **C reactive protein** is usually raised
- **Duplex ultrasound** of the temporal artery shows the **hypoechoic halo** sign

Initial Management

Steroids:
Start steroids immediately before confirming the diagnosis to reduce the risk of permanent sight loss. Start 40-60mg prednisolone per day. 60mg is given depending where there are jaw claudication or visual symptoms. Review the response to steroids within 48 hours. There is usually a rapid and significant response to treatment.

Other medications:
- **Aspirin** 75mg daily decreases vision loss and strokes
- **Proton pump inhibitor** (e.g. omeprazole) for gastric prevention while on steroids

Referrals:
- **Vascular surgeons** for a temporal artery biopsy in all patients with suspected GCA
- **Rheumatology** for specialist diagnosis and management
- **Ophthalmology** review as an emergency same day appointment if they develop visual symptoms

Ongoing Management

Once the diagnosis is confirmed they will need to continue high dose steroids (40-60mg) until the symptoms have resolved. They then need to slowly wean off the steroids. This can take several years. This is a similar process to managing polymyalgia rheumatica.

There are additional measures for patients on steroids that can be remembered by the mnemonic "**Don't STOP**":
- **DON'T** - Don't stop taking steroids abruptly. There is a risk of **adrenal crisis**.
- **S** - **S**ick day rules.
- **T** - **T**reatment card.
- **O** - **O**steoporosis prevention with **bisphosphonates** and supplemental **calcium and vitamin D**.
- **P** - **P**roton pump inhibitors for gastric protection.

Complications

Early neuro-ophthalmic complications:
- Vision loss
- Cerebrovascular accident (stroke)

Late:
- Relapses of the condition are common
- Steroid related side effects and complications
- Cerebrovascular accident (stroke)
- **Aortitis** leading to **aortic aneurysm** and **aortic dissection**

Polymyositis and Dermatomyositis

Polymyositis and dermatomyositis are autoimmune disorders where there is inflammation in the muscles (*myositis*). **Polymyositis** is a condition of chronic inflammation of muscles. **Dermatomyositis** is a connective tissue disorder where there is chronic inflammation of the skin and muscles.

Creatine Kinase

The key investigation for diagnosing myositis is a **creatine kinase** blood test. Creatine kinase is an enzyme found inside muscle cells. Inflammation in the muscle cells (*myositis*) leads to the release of creatine kinase. Creatine kinase is usually less than 300 U/L. In **polymyositis** and **dermatomyositis** the result is usually over 1000, often in the multiples of thousands.

Other causes of a raised creatine kinase include:
- Rhabdomyolysis
- Acute kidney injury
- Myocardial infarction
- Statins
- Strenuous exercise

Malignancy

Polymyositis or dermatomyositis can be caused by an underlying malignancy. This makes them *paraneoplastic syndromes*. The most common associated cancers are:
- Lung
- Breast
- Ovarian
- Gastric

Presentation

- Muscle pain, fatigue and weakness
- Occurs bilaterally and typically affects the proximal muscles
- Mostly affects the shoulder and pelvic girdle
- Develops over weeks

Polymyositis occurs without any skin features whereas dermatomyositis is associated with involvement of the skin.

Dermatomyositis Skin Features

- **Gottron lesions** (scaly erythematous patches) on the knuckles, elbows and knees
- **Photosensitive erythematous rash** on the back, shoulders and neck
- Purple rash on the face and eyelids
- Periorbital oedema (swelling around the eyes)
- Subcutaneous calcinosis (calcium deposits in the subcutaneous tissue)

Autoantibodies

- *Anti-Jo-1 antibodies*: polymyositis (but often present in dermatomyositis)
- *Anti-Mi-2 antibodies*: dermatomyositis
- *Anti-nuclear antibodies*: dermatomyositis

Diagnosis

Diagnosis is based on:
- Clinical presentation
- Elevated creatine kinase
- Autoantibodies
- Electromyography (EMG)

Muscle biopsy can be used to establish a definitive diagnosis.

Management

Management is guided by a rheumatologist. New cases should be assessed for possible underling cancer. They may require physiotherapy and occupational therapy to help with muscle strength and function.

Corticosteroids are the first line treatment of both conditions.

Other medical options where the response to steroids is inadequate:
- Immunosuppressants (such as azathioprine)
- IV immunoglobulins
- Biological therapy (such as infliximab or etanercept)

Antiphospholipid Syndrome

Antiphospholipid syndrome is a disorder associated with **antiphospholipid antibodies** where the blood becomes prone to clotting. The patient is in a **hyper-coagulable state**. The main associations are with **thrombosis** and complications in **pregnancy**, particularly **recurrent miscarriage**.

Antiphospholipid syndrome can occur on its own or secondary to an autoimmune condition, particularly **systemic lupus erythematosus**.

It is associated with antiphospholipid antibodies:
- *Lupus anticoagulant*
- *Anticardiolipin antibodies*
- *Anti-beta-2 glycoprotein I antibodies*

These antibodies interfere with coagulation and create a **hypercoagulable state** where the blood is more prone to clotting.

Associations

Venous thromboembolism
- Deep vein thrombosis
- Pulmonary embolism

Arterial thrombosis
- Stroke
- Myocardial infarction
- Renal thrombosis

Pregnancy complications
- Recurrent miscarriage
- Stillbirth
- Preeclampsia

Livedo reticularis is a purple lace like rash that gives a mottled appearance to the skin.

Libmann-Sacks endocarditis is a type of non-bacterial endocarditis where there are growths (**vegetations**) on the valves of the heart. The mitral valve is most commonly affected. It is associated with SLE and antiphospholipid syndrome.

Thrombocytopenia (low platelets) is common in antiphospholipid syndrome.

Diagnosis

Diagnosis is made when there is a history of thrombosis or pregnancy complication plus persistent antibodies:
- Lupus anticoagulant
- Anticardiolipin antibodies
- Anti-beta 2 glycoprotein I antibodies

Management

Patients are usually managed jointly between rheumatology, haematology and obstetrics (if pregnant)

Long term **warfarin** with an INR range of 2 to 3 is used to prevent thrombosis.

Pregnant women are started on **low molecular weight heparin** (e.g. enoxaparin) plus **aspirin** to reduce the risk of pregnancy complications. Warfarin is contraindicated in pregnancy.

Sjogren's Syndrome

This is an **autoimmune condition** that affects the **exocrine glands**. It leads to symptoms of dry **mucous membranes**, such as dry mouth, dry eyes and dry vagina.

Primary Sjogren's is where the condition occurs in isolation.

Secondary Sjogren's is where it occurs related to SLE or rheumatoid arthritis.

It is associated with **anti-Ro** and **anti-La** antibodies.

Schirmer Test

The Schirmer test involves inserting a folded piece of filter paper under the lower eyelid with a strip hanging out over the eyelid. This is left in for 5 minutes and the distance along the strip that becomes moist is measured. The tears should travel 15mm in a healthy young adult. A result of less than 10mm is significant.

Management

- Artificial tears
- Artificial saliva
- Vaginal lubricants
- Hydroxychloroquine is used to halt the progression of the disease.

Complications

- Eye problems such as conjunctivitis and corneal ulcers
- Oral problems such as dental cavities and candida infections
- Vaginal problems such as candidiasis and sexual dysfunction

Sjogrens can rarely affect other organs causing complications such as:
- Pneumonia and bronchiectasis
- Non-Hodgkins lymphoma
- Peripheral neuropathy
- Vasculitis
- Renal impairment

Vasculitis

Vasculitis is the name for **inflammation** of the **blood vessels**. There are many different types of vasculitis that affect different sizes of blood vessel. They are categorised based on whether they affect **small vessels**, **medium sized vessels** or **large vessels**. They each have some unique features that will help you spot them in exams.

Types of Vasculitis Affecting The Small Vessels

- Henoch-Schonlein purpura
- Eosinophilic granulomatosis with polyangiitis (Churg-Strauss syndrome)
- Microscopic polyangiitis
- Granulomatosis with polyangiitis (Wegener's granulomatosis)

Types of Vasculitis Affecting The Medium Sized Vessels

- Polyarteritis nodosa
- Eosinophilic granulomatosis with polyangiitis (Churg-Strauss syndrome)
- Kawasaki disease

Types of Vasculitis Affecting The Large Vessels

- Giant cell arteritis
- Takayasu's arteritis

Presentation

There are some generic features that apply to most types of vasculitis. There are some features that are more specific to individual types and these are discussed separately. Things that should make you think about a possible vasculitis are:
- **Purpura**. These are purple-coloured non-blanching spots caused by blood leaking from the vessels under the skin.
- Joint and muscle pain
- Peripheral neuropathy
- Renal impairment
- Gastrointestinal disturbance (diarrhoea, abdominal pain and bleeding)
- Anterior uveitis and scleritis
- Hypertension

They are also associated with systemic manifestations of:
- Fatigue
- Fever
- Weight loss
- Anorexia (loss of appetite)
- Anaemia

Tests

Inflammatory markers (CRP and ESR) are usually raised in vasculitis.

Anti neutrophil cytoplasmic antibodies (**ANCA**) is the blood test to remember for vasculitis. If you remember this alone you will be able to answer many questions on vasculitis.

There are two type of ANCA blood tests: **p-ANCA** and **c-ANCA**. P-ANCA are also called **anti-PR3** antibodies. C-ANCA are also called **anti-MPO** antibodies. These different ANCA tests are associated with different types of vasculitis:
- **p-ANCA** (PR3 antibodies): **Microscopic polyangiitis** and **Churg-Strauss syndrome**
- **c-ANCA** (MPO antibodies): **Wegener's granulomatosis**

Management

The management of vasculitis depends on the type. Suspected cases should be referred to a specialist, usually a rheumatologist, to guide diagnosis and management. Treatment usually involves a combination of steroids and immunosuppressants.

Steroids can be administered to target the affected area:
- **Oral** (i.e. prednisolone)
- **Intravenous** (i.e. hydrocortisone)
- **Nasal** sprays for nasal symptoms
- **Inhaled** for lung involves (e.g. Churg-Strauss syndrome)

Immunosuppressants that are used include:
- Cyclophosphamide
- Methotrexate
- Azathioprine
- Rituximab and other monoclonal antibodies

The management of HSP and Kawasaki disease (the types mainly affecting children) is different.

Henoch-Schonlein purpura

Henoch-Schonlein -urpura (HSP) is an **IgA vasculitis** that commonly presents with a purpuric rash affecting the lower limbs and buttocks in children. Inflammation occurs due to **immunoglobulin A** deposits in the blood vessels of affected organs such as the skin, kidneys and gastro-intestinal tract. The condition is often triggered by an upper airway infection (e.g. tonsillitis) or a gastroenteritis. It is most common in children under the age of 10 years. The rash is caused by inflammation and leaking of blood from small blood vessels under the skin, forming purpura.

The four classic features are **purpura** (100%), **joint pain** (75%), **abdominal pain** (50%) and **renal involvement** (50%). HSP affects the kidneys in about 50% of patients, causing an **IgA nephritis**.

Management is typically **supportive**, with simple analgesia, rest and proper hydration. The benefits of steroids are unclear.

The abdominal pain usually settles within a few days. Patients without kidney involvement can expect to fully recover within 4 to 6 weeks. A third of patients have a recurrence of the disease within 6 months. 1% of patients will go on to develop end stage renal failure.

Eosinophilic Granulomatosis with Polyangiitis (Churg-Strauss syndrome)

Eosinophilic granulomatosis with polyangiitis used to be called **Churg-Strauss syndrome** and is still often referred to by this name. It is a **small and medium vessel vasculitis**.

It is most associated with **lung** and **skin** problems, but can affect other organs such as the kidneys. It often presents with **severe asthma** in late teenage years or adulthood. A characteristic finding is **elevated eosinophil levels** on the full blood count.

Microscopic Polyangiitis

Microscopic polyangiitis is a **small vessel vasculitis**. The main feature of microscopic polyangiitis is **renal failure**. It can also affect the lungs causing shortness of breath and haemoptysis.

Granulomatosis with Polyangiitis (Wegener's granulomatosis)

Wegener's granulomatosis is a small vessel vasculitis. It affects the respiratory tract and kidneys.

In the upper respiratory tract it commonly affects the nose causing nose bleeds (epistaxis) and **crusty** nasal secretions, ears causing hearing loss and sinuses causing sinusitis. A classic sign in exams is the saddle shaped nose due to a perforated nasal septum. This causes a dip halfway down the nose.

In the lungs it causes a cough, wheeze and haemoptysis. A chest xray may show consolidation and it may be misdiagnosed as pneumonia. In the kidneys it can cause a rapidly progressing **glomerulonephritis**.

Polyarteritis Nodosa

Polyarteritis nodosa (PAN) is a **medium vessel vasculitis**. It is most associated with **hepatitis B** but can also occur without a clear cause or with **hepatitis C** and **HIV**.

It affects the medium sized vessels in locations such as the skin, gastrointestinal tract, kidneys and heart. This can cause renal impairment, strokes and myocardial infarction.

It is associated with a rash called **livedo reticularis**. This is a mottled, purplish, lace like rash.

Kawasaki Disease

Kawasaki disease is a **medium vessel vasculitis**. It affects young children, typically under 5 years of age. There is no clear cause.

Clinical features are:
- Persistent high fever for **more than 5 days**
- Erythematous rash
- Bilateral conjunctivitis
- Erythema and desquamation (skin peeling) of palms and soles
- "**Strawberry tongue**" (red tongue with prominent papillae)

A key complication is **coronary artery aneurysms**. Treatment is with aspirin and IV immunoglobulins.

Takayasu's Arteritis

Takayasu's arteritis is a form of **large vessel vasculitis**. It mainly affects the **aorta** and its branches. It also affect the pulmonary arteries. These large vessels and their branches can swell and form aneurysms or become narrowed and blocked. This leads to its other name of "**pulseless disease**".

It usually presents before the age of 40 years with non-specific systemic symptoms, such as fever, malaise and muscle aches, or with more specific symptoms of arm claudication or syncope. It is diagnosed using **CT** or **MRI angiography**. **Doppler ultrasound** of the carotids can be useful in detecting carotid disease.

Behçet's Disease

Behçet's disease is a **complex inflammatory** condition. It characteristically presents with recurrent **oral** and **genital ulcers**. It can also cause inflammation in a number of other areas such as the skin, gastrointestinal tract, lungs, blood vessels, musculoskeletal system and central nervous system. The presentation can vary a lot between patients, with some patients mildly affected and others affected dramatically.

There is a link with the **HLA B51 gene**. This is a prognostic indicator of severe disease.

Differential Diagnosis

Mouth ulcers are very common. There is a long list of differentials to mouth ulcers:
- **Simple aphthous ulcers** are very common
- **Squamous cell carcinoma**
- **Herpes simplex** ulcers
- **Hand, foot and mouth** disease (coxsackie A virus)
- **Inflammatory bowel disease** (particularly Crohn's disease)
- Inflammatory conditions such as **rheumatoid arthritis**
- **Folate deficiency**

Features

Mouth Ulcers
Patients with Behçet's disease are expected to get at least 3 episodes of oral ulcers per year. They are painful, sharply circumscribed erosions with a **red halo**. They occur on the oral mucosa and heal over 2 to 4 weeks.

Genital Ulcers
Genital ulcers are similar in appearance to the oral ulcers. "**Kissing ulcers**" are where an ulcer develops on two opposing surfaces so that they are facing each other.

Skin
The skin is very easily inflamed in Behçet's disease. Particular skin findings in Behçet's disease are:
- Erythema nodosum
- Papules and pustules (similar to acne)
- Vasculitic type rashes

Eyes
Eye manifestations need emergency review by ophthalmology as they can be sight treating.
- Anterior or posterior uveitis
- Retinal vasculitis
- Retinal haemorrhage

Musculoskeletal System
- Morning stiffness
- Arthralgia
- Oligoarthritis often affecting the knee or ankle. This causes swelling without joint destruction.

Gastrointestinal System
Inflammation and ulceration can occur in the gastrointestinal tract. This tends to affect the:
- Ileum
- Caecum
- Ascending colon

Central Nervous System
- Memory impairment
- Headaches and migraines
- Aseptic meningitis
- Meningoencephalitis

Veins
In Behçet's disease the veins can become inflamed and this can lead to vein thrombosis. These thrombosis tend to stay in place and don't embolism as they are related to inflammation in the vessel wall. Examples are:
- Budd Chiari syndrome
- Deep vein thrombosis
- Thrombus in pulmonary veins
- Cerebral venous sinus thrombosis

Lungs
Pulmonary artery aneurysms can develop. If they rupture they can be fatal.

Investigations

Behçet's disease is a clinical diagnosis based on the features of the condition. One key investigation is the *pathergy test*.

The *pathergy test* involves using a sterile needle to create a subcutaneous abrasion on the forearm. This is then reviewed 24 to 48 hours later to look for a weal 5mm or more in size. It tests for non-specific **hypersensitivity** in the skin. It is positive in **Behçet's disease**, **Sweet's syndrome** and **pyoderma gangrenosum**.

Management

Management is coordinated by a specialist, usually a rheumatologist. Other specialities may be involved depending on the affected areas, for example dermatology, ophthalmology and neurology.

Management involves a combination of:
- Topical steroids to mouth ulcers (e.g. **soluble betamethasone** tablets)
- Systemic steroids (i.e. oral **prednisolone**)
- **Colchicine** is usually effective in treating symptoms (as an anti-inflammatory)
- Topical anaesthetics for genital ulcers (e.g. **lidocaine** ointment)
- Immunosuppressants such as **azathioprine**
- Biologic therapy such as **infliximab**

Prognosis

Behçet's disease is a **relapsing remitting** condition. Patients generally have a normal life expectancy and the condition may go into complete remission. There is an increased mortality with haemoptysis, neurological involvement and other major complications.

Gout

Gout is a type of **crystal arthropathy** associated with chronically high blood **uric acid** levels. **Urate crystals** are deposited in the joint causing it to become hot, swollen and painful. **Gouty tophi** are **subcutaneous** deposits of **uric acid**, typically affect the small joints and connective tissues of the hands, elbows and ears. The **DIP joints** are the most affected joints in the hands.

It typically presents with a single acute hot, swollen and painful joint. The obvious and extremely important differential diagnosis is **septic arthritis**.

Risk Factors

- Male
- Obesity
- High purine diet (e.g. meat and seafood)
- Alcohol
- Diuretics
- Existing cardiovascular or kidney disease
- Family history

Typical Joints

- Base of the big toe (metatarso-phalangeal joint)
- Wrists
- Base of the thumb (carpometacarpal joint)

Gout can also affects big joints like the knee and ankle.

Diagnosis

Gout is diagnosed clinically or by aspiration of fluid from the joint. **Excluding septic arthritis** is essential as this is a potentially joint and life threatening diagnosis.

Aspirated fluid will show:
- No bacterial growth
- **Needle shaped crystals**
- **Negative birefringent of polarised light**
- **Monosodium urate crystals**

Joint xray:
- Typically the joint space is maintained
- **Lytic lesions** in the bone
- **Punched out erosions**
- Erosions can have **sclerotic boarders** with **overhanding edges**

Management

During the acute flare:
- NSAIDs (e.g. ibuprofen) are first line
- Colchicine is second line
- Steroids can be considered third line

Colchicine is used in patients that are inappropriate for NSAIDs, such as those with renal impairment or significant heart disease. A notable side effect is gastrointestinal upset. **Diarrhoea** is a very common side effect. This is dose dependent, meaning lower doses cause less upset than higher doses.

Prophylaxis

Allopurinol is an *xanthine oxidate inhibitor* use for the prophylaxis of gout. It reduces uric acid level.

Lifestyle changes can reduce the risk of developing gout. This involves loosing weight, staying hydrated and minimising the consumption of alcohol and purine-based food (such as meat and seafood).

TOM TIP. Do not initiate allopurinol prophylaxis until after the acute attack is settled. Once treatment of allopurinol has been started then it can be continued during an acute attack.

Pseudogout

Pseudogout is a **crystal arthropathy** caused by **calcium pyrophosphate crystals**. Calcium pyrophosphate crystals are deposited in the joint causing joint problems. It is also known as **chondrocalcinosis**.

Presentation

A typically presentation of pseudogout is an older adult with a hot, swollen, stiff, painful knee. Other joints that are commonly affected are the shoulders, wrists and hips.

It can be a chronic condition and affect multiple joints. It can also be asymptomatic and picked up incidentally on an xray of the joint.

Diagnosis

In any patient presenting with a hot, painful and swollen joint, **septic arthritis** needs to be excluded as it is a **medical emergency** that is joint and life threatening. It tends the be milder in presentation compared with gout and septic arthritis.

To establish a definitive diagnosis the joint needs to be **aspirated** for **synovial fluid**. Aspirated fluid will show:
- No bacterial growth
- **Calcium pyrophosphate crystals**
- **Rhomboid** shaped crystals
- **Positive birefringent of polarised light**

Chondrocalcinosis is the classic xray change in pseudogout. It appears as a thin white line in the middle of the joint space caused by the calcium deposition. This is **pathognomonic** (diagnostic) of pseudogout.

Other joint xray changes are similar to osteoarthritis. Remember the mnemonic **LOSS**:
- **L** - **L**oss of joint space
- **O** - **O**steophytes
- **S** - **S**ubarticular sclerosis
- **S** - **S**ubchondral cysts

Management

Chronic asymptomatic changes found on an xray do not require any action.

Symptoms usually resolve spontaneously over several weeks. Symptomatic management involves:
- NSAIDs
- Colchicine
- Joint aspiration
- Steroid injections
- Oral steroids

Joint washout (**arthrocentesis**) is an option in severe cases.

Osteoporosis

Osteoporosis is a condition where there is a reduction in the density of the bones. **Osteopenia** refers to a less severe reduction in bone density than osteoporosis. Reduced bone density makes bone less strong and more prone to fractures.

Risk Factors for Osteoporosis

- Older age
- Female
- Reduced mobility and activity
- Low BMI (under 18.5 kg/m^2)
- Rheumatoid arthritis
- Alcohol and smoking
- **Long term corticosteroids**. NICE suggest the risk increases significantly with the equivalent of more than 7.5mg of prednisolone per day for more than 3 months)
- **Other medications** such as SSRIs, PPIs, anti-epileptics and anti-oestrogens.

Post-menopausal women are a key group where osteoporosis should be considered. **Oestrogen** is protective against osteoporosis. Unless they are on hormone replacement therapy, postmenopausal women have less oestrogen. They also tend to be are older and often have other risk factors for osteoporosis.

FRAX Tool

The FRAX tool gives a prediction of the risk of a **fragility fracture** over the next **10 years**. This is usually the first step in assessing someones risk of osteoporosis.

It involves inputting information such as their age, BMI, co-morbidities, smoking, alcohol and family history. You can enter a result for **bone mineral density** (from a DEXA scan) for a more accurate result but it can also be performed without the bone mineral density.

It gives results as a percentage 10 year probability of a:
- Major osteoporotic fracture
- Hip fracture

Bone Mineral Density

Bone mineral density (**BMD**) is measured using a **DEXA scan**, which stands for **dual-energy xray absorptiometry**. DEXA scans are brief xray scans that measure how much radiation is absorbed by the bones, indicating how dense the bone is. The **bone mineral density** (**BMD**) can be measured at any location on the skeleton, but the reading at the hip is key for classification and management of osteoporosis.

Bone density can be represented as a **Z score** or **T score**. **Z scores** represent the number of standard deviations the patient's bone density falls below the mean for their age. **T scores** represent the number of standard deviations below the mean for a healthy young adult their bone density is.

The most clinically important outcome is the **T score** at the persons hip. This forms the basis for the **WHO classification** of osteoporosis. DEXA scans can be used to confirm osteoporosis and monitor treatment.

WHO Classification

T Score at the Hip	Bone Mineral Density
More than -1	Normal
-1 to -2.5	Osteopenia
Less than -2.5	Osteoporosis
Less than -2.5 plus a fracture	Severe Osteoporosis

Assessing For Osteoporosis

The first step is to perform a FRAX assessment on patients at risk of osteoporosis:
- Women over 65
- Men over 75
- Younger patients with risk factors such as a previous fragility fracture, history of falls, low BMI, long term steroids, endocrine disorders and rheumatoid arthritis.

The **NOGG Guidelines** from 2017 suggest the next step in management based on the probability of a major osteoporotic fracture from the FRAX score:

FRAX outcome **without** a **BMD** result will suggest one of three outcomes:
- Low risk - reassure
- Intermediate risk - offer DEXA scan and recalculate the risk with the results
- High risk - offer treatment

FRAX outcome **with** a **BMD** result will suggest one of two outcomes:
- Treat
- Lifestyle advice and reassure

Management

Lifestyle Changes:
- Activity and exercise
- Maintain a health weight
- Adequate calcium intake
- Adequate vitamin D
- Avoiding falls
- Stop smoking
- Reduce alcohol consumption

Vitamin D and Calcium:
NICE recommend **calcium** supplementation **with vitamin D** in patients at risk of fragility fractures with an inadequate intake of calcium. An example of this would be **Calcichew-D$_3$**, which contains 1000mg of calcium and 800 units of vitamin D (*colecalciferol*).

Patients with an adequate calcium intake but lacking sun exposure should have vitamin D supplementation.

Bisphosphonates:
Bisphosphonates are the first line treatment for osteoporosis. They work by interfering with **osteoclasts** and reducing their activity, preventing the reabsorption of bone. There are a few key side effects to remember:
- **Reflux** and **oesophageal erosions**. Oral bisphosphonates are taken on an empty stomach sitting upright for 30 minutes before moving or eating to prevent this.
- Atypical fractures (e.g. atypical femoral fractures)
- Osteonecrosis of the jaw
- Osteonecrosis of the external auditory canal

Examples of bisphosphonates are:
- Alendronate 70 mg once weekly (oral)
- Risedronate 35 mg once weekly (oral)
- Zolendronic acid 5 mg once yearly (intravenous)

Other Medical Options:
Other options if bisphosphonates are contraindicated, not tolerated or not effective:
- **Denosumab** is a monoclonal antibody that works by blocking the activity of osteoclasts.
- **Strontium ranelate** is a similar element to calcium that stimulates osteoblasts and blocks osteoclasts but increases the risk of DVT, PE and myocardial infarction.
- **Raloxifene** is used as secondary prevention only. It is a selective oestrogen receptor modulator that stimulates oestrogen receptors on bone but blocks them in the breasts and uterus.
- **Hormone replacement therapy** should be considered in women that go through the menopause early.

Follow Up:
Low risk patients not being put on treatment should be given lifestyle advice and followed up within 5 years for a repeat assessment. Patients on bisphosphonates should have a repeat FRAX and DEXA scan after 3 to 5 years. A **treatment holiday** should be considered if their BMD has improved and they have not suffered any fragility fractures. This involves a break from treatment of 18 months to 3 years before repeating the assessment.

Osteomalacia

Osteomalacia is a condition where there is defective **bone mineralisation** causing "**soft**" bones. **Osteo-** means bone and -**malacia** means soft. This results from insufficient **vitamin D**. It presents with weak bones, bone pain, muscle weakness and fractures. When this occurs in children prior to their growth plates closing this leads to a condition called **rickets**.

Simplified Pathophysiology

Vitamin D is a **hormone** (not technically a vitamin) created from **cholesterol** by the **skin** in response to **UV radiation**. Patients with darker skin require a longer period of sun exposure to generate the same quantity of vitamin D. A standard diet contains inadequate levels of vitamin D to compensate for a lack of sun exposure. Reduced sun exposure without vitamin D supplementation leads to vitamin D deficiency.

Patients with **malabsorption disorders** (such as **inflammatory bowel disease**) are more likely to have vitamin D deficiency. The kidneys are essential in metabolising vitamin D to its active form, therefore vitamin D deficiency is common in **chronic kidney disease**.

Vitamin D is essential in **calcium** and **phosphate** absorption from the **intestines** and **kidneys**. Vitamin D is also responsible for regulating bone turnover and promoting bone reabsorption to boost the serum calcium level.

Inadequate vitamin D leads to a lack of **calcium** and **phosphate** in the blood. Since calcium and phosphate are required for the construction of bone, low levels result in defective bone mineralisation. **Low calcium** causes a **secondary hyperparathyroidism** as the **parathyroid gland** tries to raise the calcium level by secreting parathyroid hormone. Parathyroid hormone stimulates increased reabsorption from the bones. This causes further problems with bone mineralisation.

Presentation

Patients with vitamin D deficiency and osteomalacia may not have any symptoms. Potential symptoms are:
- Fatigue
- Bone pain
- Muscle weakness
- Muscle aches
- Pathological or abnormal fractures

TOM TIP: Think about the risk factors for vitamin D deficiency in your exams and clinical practice. Patients with osteomalacia are likely to have risk factors such as darker skin, low exposure to sunlight, live in colder climates and spend the majority of their time indoors.

Investigations

Serum 25-hydroxyvitamin D is the laboratory investigation for vitamin D. The interpretation of the results is as follows:
- Less than 25 nmol/L - **vitamin D deficiency**
- 25 to 50 nmol/L - **vitamin D insufficiency**
- 75 nmol/L or above is **optimal**

Other investigation results include:
- Serum calcium is low
- Serum phosphate is low
- Serum alkaline phosphatase may be high
- Parathyroid hormone may be high (secondary hyperparathyroidism)
- Xrays may show **osteopenia** (more **radiolucent** bones)
- DEXA scan shows low bone mineral density

Treatment

Treatment is with supplementary vitamin D (**colecalciferol**). There are various regimes suggested by the **NICE CKS** on vitamin D deficiency. They involve correcting the initial **vitamin D deficiency** with one of the following:
- 50,000 IU once weekly for 6 weeks
- 20,000 IU twice weekly for 7 weeks
- 4000 IU daily for 10 weeks

A **maintenance** supplementary dose of 800 IU or more per day should be continued for life after the initial treatment.

Patients with **vitamin D insufficiency** can be started on the maintenance dose without the initial treatment regime.

Paget's Disease of Bone

Paget's disease of bone refers to a disorder of bone turnover. There is excessive bone turnover (formation and reabsorption) due to excessive **osteoblast** and **osteoclast** activity. This excessive turnover is not coordinated, leading to patchy areas of high density (**sclerosis**) and low density (**lysis**). This results in enlarged and misshapen bones with structural problems that increase the risk of **pathological fractures**. It particularly affects the **axial skeleton** (the bones of the head and spine).

Presentation

Paget's disease typically affects older adults. It presents with:
- Bone pain
- Bone deformity
- Fractures
- Hearing loss can occur if it affects the bones of the ear

Key Investigations

Xray Findings
- Bone enlargement and deformity
- **Osteoporosis circumscripta** describes well defined osteolytic lesions that appear less dense compared with normal bone
- **Cotton wool appearance** of the **skull** describes poorly defined patchy areas of increased density (**sclerosis**) and decreased density (**lysis**)
- **V-shaped defects** in the **long bones** are V shaped osteolytic bone lesions surrounded by healthy bone

Biochemistry
- Raised *alkaline phosphatase* (and other LFTs are normal)
- Normal calcium
- Normal phosphate

Management

Bisphosphonates are the main treatment. They are generally very effective. They interfere with osteoclast activity and seem to restore normal bone metabolism. They improve symptoms and prevent further abnormal bone changes.

Other measures include:
- NSAIDs for bone pain
- Calcium and vitamin D supplementation, particularly whilst on bisphosphonates
- Surgery is rarely required to treat fractures, severe deformity and arthritis

Monitoring involves check the serum **alkaline phosphatase** (**ALP**) and reviewing symptoms. Effective treatment should normalise the ALP and eliminate symptoms.

Complications

Two key complications to remember are:
- *Osteogenic sarcoma* (*osteosarcoma*)
- *Spinal stenosis* and *spinal cord compression*

Osteosarcoma is a type of bone cancer with a very poor prognosis. It presents with increased focal bone pain, bone swelling or pathological fractures. The risk is increased in Paget's disease and patients need to be followed up to detect it early. They can usually be seen on a plain xray.

Spinal stenosis may occur where deformity in the spine leads to spinal canal narrowing. If this presses on the spinal nerves it causes neurological signs and symptoms. This is diagnosed with an MRI scan and is often treated effectively with bisphosphonates. Surgical intervention may be considered.

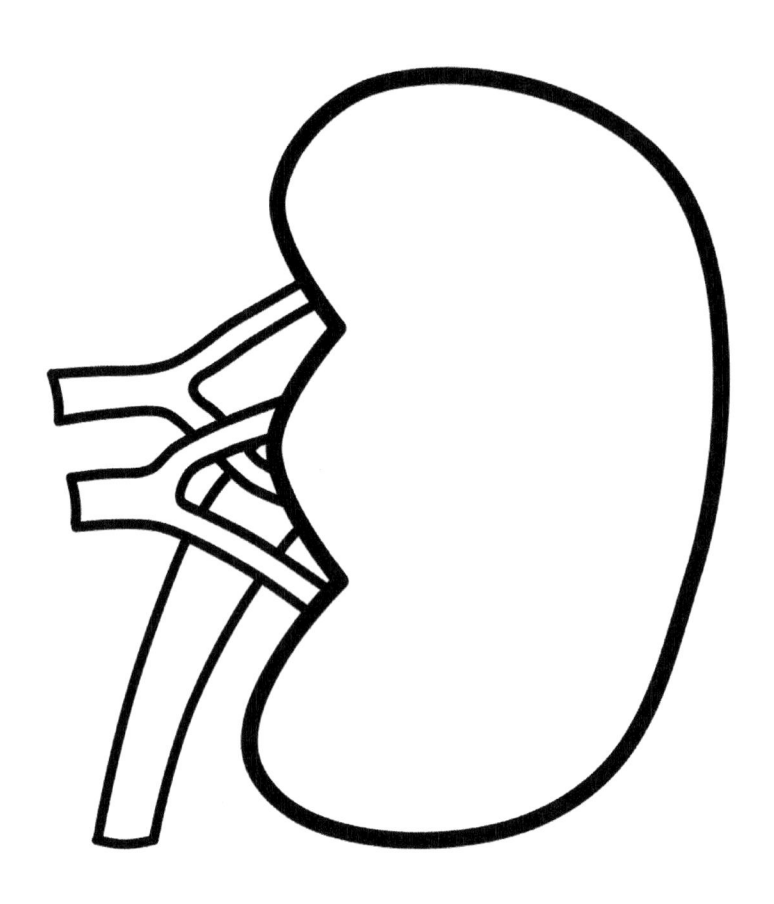

RENAL

8.1	Acute Kidney Injury	247
8.2	Chronic Kidney Disease	249
8.3	Dialysis	252
8.4	Renal Transplant	255
8.5	Glomerulonephritis	256
8.6	Diabetic Nephropathy	258
8.7	Interstitial Kidney Disease	258
8.8	Acute Tubular Necrosis	259
8.9	Renal Tubular Acidosis	260
8.10	Haemolytic Uraemic Syndrome	261
8.11	Rhabdomyolysis	262
8.12	Hyperkalaemia	264
8.13	Polycystic Kidney Disease	265

Acute Kidney Injury

Acute kidney injury (AKI) is defined as an acute drop in kidney function. It is diagnosed by measuring the serum **creatinine**.

NICE Criteria For AKI

- Rise in creatinine of ≥ 25 micromol/L in 48 hours
- Rise in creatinine of ≥ 50% in 7 days
- Urine output of < 0.5ml/kg/hour for more than 6 hours

Risk Factors for Acute Kidney Injury

Consider the possibility of an **acute kidney injury** in patients that are suffering with an acute illness, such as infection or having a surgical operation. Risk factors that would predispose to developing acute kidney injury include:
- Chronic kidney disease
- Heart failure
- Diabetes
- Liver disease
- Older age (above 65 years)
- Cognitive impairment
- Nephrotoxic medications such as NSAIDS and ACE Inhibitors
- Use of a **contrast medium** such as during CT scans

Causes

TOM TIP: Whenever someone asks you the causes of renal impairment always answer "the causes are pre-renal, renal or post-renal". This will impress them and allow you to think through the causes more logically.

Pre-Renal Causes

Pre-renal pathology is the most common cause of acute kidney injury. It is due to **inadequate blood supply** to kidneys reducing the filtration of blood. Inadequate blood supply may be due to:
- Dehydration
- Hypotension (shock)
- Heart failure

Renal Causes

This is where **intrinsic disease** in the kidney is leading to reduced filtration of blood. It may be due to:
- Glomerulonephritis
- Interstitial nephritis
- Acute tubular necrosis

Post-renal Causes

Post renal acute kidney injury is caused by **obstruction to outflow** of urine from the kidney, causing back-pressure into the kidney and reduced kidney function. This is called an **obstructive uropathy**. Obstruction may be caused by:
- Kidney stones
- Masses such as cancer in the abdomen or pelvis
- Ureter or uretral strictures
- Enlarged prostate or prostate cancer

Investigations

Urinalysis for protein, blood, leucocytes, nitrites and glucose.
- **Leucocytes** and **nitrites** suggest infection
- **Protein** and **blood** suggest **acute nephritis** (but can be positive in infection)
- **Glucose** suggests diabetes

Ultrasound of the urinary tract is used to look for obstruction. It is not necessary if an alternative cause is found for the AKI.

Management

Prevention of acute kidney injury is important. This is achieved by avoiding nephrotoxic medications where possible and ensuring adequate fluid input in unwell patients, including IV fluids if they are not taking enough orally.

The first step to treating an acute kidney injury is to correct the underlying cause:
- **Fluid rehydration** with IV fluids in pre-renal AKI
- **Stop nephrotoxic medications** such as NSAIDS and antihypertensives that reduce the filtration pressure (i.e. ACE inhibitors)
- **Relieve obstruction** in a post-renal AKI, for example insert a catheter for a patient in retention from an enlarged prostate

In a severe acute kidney injury, where there is doubt about the cause or where complications develop, input from a renal specialist is required. They may need dialysis.

Complications

- Hyperkalaemia
- Fluid overload, heart failure and pulmonary oedema
- Metabolic acidosis
- Uraemia (high urea) can lead to **encephalopathy** or **pericarditis**

Chronic Kidney Disease

Chronic kidney disease describes a chronic reduction in kidney function. This reduction in kidney function tends to be permanent and progressive.

Causes

- Diabetes
- Hypertension
- Age related decline
- Glomerulonephritis
- Polycystic kidney disease
- Medications such as NSAIDS, proton pump inhibitors and lithium

Risk Factors

- Older age
- Hypertension
- Diabetes
- Smoking
- Use of medications that affect the kidneys

Presentation

Usually chronic kidney disease is **asymptomatic** and diagnosed on routine testing. A number of signs and symptoms might suggest chronic kidney disease:

- Pruritus (itching)
- Loss of appetite
- Nausea
- Oedema
- Muscle cramps
- Peripheral neuropathy
- Pallor
- Hypertension

Investigations

Estimated glomerular filtration rate (**eGFR**) can be checked using a U&E blood test. Two tests are required 3 months apart to confirm a diagnosis of chronic kidney disease.

Proteinuria can be checked using a **urine albumin:creatinine ratio** (ACR). A result of ≥ 3 mg/mmol is significant.

Haematuria can be checked using a **urine dipstick**. A significant result is 1+ of blood. Haematuria should prompt investigation for malignancy (i.e. bladder cancer).

Renal ultrasound can be used to investigate patients with accelerated CKD, haematuria, family history of polycystic kidney disease or evidence of obstruction.

Stages

The **G** score is based on the e**G**FR:
- G1 = eGFR >90
- G2 = eGFR 60-89
- G3a = eGFR 45-59
- G3b = eGFR 30-44
- G4 = eGFR 15-29
- G5 = eGFR <15 (known as "end-stage renal failure")

The **A** score is based on the **a**lbumin:creatinine ratio:
- A1 = < 3mg/mmol
- A2 = 3 - 30mg/mmol
- A3 = > 30mg/mmol

The patient **does not** have CKD if they have a score of A1 combined with G1 or G2. They need at least an **eGFR of less than 60** or **proteinuria** for a diagnosis of CKD.

Complications

- Anaemia
- Renal bone disease
- Cardiovascular disease
- Peripheral neuropathy
- Dialysis related problems

Referral to a Specialist

NICE suggest referral to a specialist when there is:
- eGFR < 30
- ACR ≥ 70 mg/mmol
- Accelerated progression defined as a decrease in eGFR of 15 **or** 25% **or** 15 ml/min **in 1 year**
- Uncontrolled hypertension despite 4 or more antihypertensives

Management

Aims of Management
- Slow the progression of the disease
- Reduce the risk of cardiovascular disease
- Reduce the risk of complications
- Treating complications

Slowing the Progression of the Disease
- Optimise diabetic control
- Optimise hypertensive control
- Treat glomerulonephritis

Reducing the Risk of Complications
- Exercise, maintain a healthy weight and stop smoking
- Special dietary advice about phosphate, sodium, potassium and water intake
- Offer atorvastatin 20mg for primary prevention of cardiovascular disease

Treating Complications
- Oral **sodium bicarbonate** to treat metabolic acidosis
- **Iron** supplementation and **erythropoietin** to treat anaemia
- **Vitamin D** to treat renal bone disease
- **Dialysis** in end stage renal failure
- **Renal transplant** in end stage renal failure

Treating Hypertension

ACE inhibitors are the first line in patients with chronic kidney disease. These are offered to all patients with:
- Diabetes plus ACR > 3mg/mmol
- Hypertension plus ACR > 30mg/mmol
- All patients with ACR > 70mg/mmol

Aim to keep blood pressure < 140/90 (or < 130/80 if the ACR > 70mg/mmol).

Serum potassium needs to be monitored as chronic kidney disease and ACE inhibitors both cause **hyperkalaemia**.

Anaemia of Chronic Kidney Disease

Healthy kidney cells produced **erythropoietin**. Erythropoietin is the hormone that stimulates production of red blood cells. Damaged kidney cells in CKD cause a drop in erythropoietin. Therefore, there is a drop in red blood cells and a subsequent anaemia.

Anaemia can be treated with **erythropoiesis** stimulating agents, such as exogenous **erythropoeitin**. Blood transfusions should be limited as they can sensitise the immune system ("**allosensitisation**") so that transplanted organs are more likely to be rejected.

Iron deficiency should be treated before offering erythropoetin. Intravenous iron is usually given, particularly in dialysis patients. Oral iron is an alternative.

Renal Bone Disease

Renal bone disease is also known as **chronic kidney disease-mineral and bone disorder** (**CKD-MBD**).

Features
- Osteomalacia (softening of bones)
- Osteoporosis (brittle bones)
- Osteosclerosis (hardening of bones)

Xray Changes
Spine xray shows **sclerosis** of both ends of the vertebra (denser white) and **osteomalacia** in the centre of the vertebra (less white). This is classically known as "**rugger jersey**" spine after the stripes found on a rugby shirt.

Pathophysiology

High serum phosphate occurs due to reduced phosphate excretion. **Low active vitamin D** occurs because the kidney is essential in metabolising vitamin D to its active form. **Active vitamin D** is essential in calcium absorption from the intestines and kidneys, therefore there is a low serum calcium. Vitamin D also regulates **bone turnover**.

Secondary hyperparathyroidism occurs because the parathyroid glands react to the low serum calcium and high serum phosphate by excreting more parathyroid hormone. This leads to increased **osteoclast** activity. Osteoclast activity lead to the absorption of calcium from bone.

Osteomalacia occurs due to increased turnover of bones without adequate calcium supply.

Osteosclerosis occurs when the osteoblasts respond by increasing their activity to match the osteoclasts, creating new tissue in the bone. Due to the low calcium level this new tissue is not properly mineralised.

Osteoporosis can exist alongside the renal bone disease due to other risk factors such as age and use of steroids.

Management involves a combination of:
- Active forms of vitamin D (alfacalcidol and calcitriol)
- Low phosphate diet
- Bisphosphonates can be used to treat osteoporosis

Dialysis

Dialysis is a method for performing the filtration tasks of the kidneys artificially. It is used in patients with end stage renal failure or complications of renal failure. It involves removing excess fluid, solutes and waste products.

Indications for Acute Dialysis

The mnemonic **AEIOU** can be used to remember the indications for acute dialysis in patients with a severe AKI:
- **A** - **A**cidosis (severe and not responding to treatment)
- **E** - **E**lectrolyte abnormalities (severe and unresponsive hyperkalaemia)
- **I** - **I**ntoxication (overdose of certain medications)
- **O** - **O**edema (severe and unresponsive pulmonary oedema)
- **U** - **U**raemia symptoms such as seizures or reduced consciousness

Indications for Long Term Dialysis

- End stage renal failure (CKD stage 5)
- Any of the acute indications continuing long term

Options for Maintenance Dialysis

There are three main options for dialysis in patients requiring it long term:
- *Continuous ambulatory peritoneal dialysis*
- *Automated peritoneal dialysis*
- *Haemodialysis*

The decision about which form to use is based on:
- Patient preference
- Lifestyle factors
- Co-morbidities
- Individual differences regarding risks

Peritoneal Dialysis

Peritoneal dialysis uses the **peritoneal membrane** as a **filtration** membrane. A special **dialysis solution** containing dextrose is added to the **peritoneal cavity**. **Ultrafiltration** occurs from the blood, across the peritoneal membrane, into the dialysis solution. The dialysis solution is then replaced, taking away the waste products that have filtered out of the blood.

Peritoneal dialysis involves a **Tenckhoff catheter**. This is a plastic tube that is inserted into the peritoneal cavity with one end on the outside. It allows access to peritoneal cavity. This is used for inserting and removing the dialysis solution.

Continuous Ambulatory Peritoneal Dialysis
This is where the dialysis solution is in the peritoneum at all times. There are various regimes for changing the solution. One example is where 2 litres of fluid is inserted into the peritoneum and changed four times a day.

Automated Dialysis
This involves peritoneal dialysis occurring overnight. A machine continuously replaces the dialysis fluid in the abdomen overnight to optimise ultrafiltration. It takes 8-10 hours.

Complications of Peritoneal Dialysis

Bacterial peritonitis. Infusions of glucose solution make the peritoneum a great place for bacterial growth. Bacterial infection is a common and potentially serious complication of peritoneal dialysis.

Peritoneal sclerosis involves thickening and scarring of the peritoneal membrane.

Ultrafiltration failure can develop. This occurs when the patient starts to absorb the dextrose in the filtration solution. This reduces the filtration gradient making ultrafiltration less effective. This becomes more prominent over time.

Weight gain can occur as they absorb the carbohydrates in the dextrose solution.

Psychosocial effects. There are huge social and psychological effects of having to change dialysis solution and sleep with a machine every night.

Haemodialysis

With haemodialysis, patients have their blood filtered by a haemodialysis machine. Regimes can vary but a typical regime might be 4 hours a day for 3 days a week.

They need good access to an abundant blood supply. The options for this are:
- **Tunnelled cuffed catheter**
- **Arterio-venous fistula**

Tunnelled Cuffed Catheter

A tunnelled cuffed catheter is a tube inserted in to the **subclavian** or **jugular vein** with a tip that sits in the **superior vena cava** or **right atrium**. It has two lumens, one where blood exits the body (red) and one where blood enters the body (blue).

There is a ring called a "**Dacron cuff**" that surrounds of the catheter. It promotes healing and adhesion of tissue to the cuff, making the catheter more permanent and providing a barrier to bacterial infection. These can stay in long term and used for regular haemodialysis.

The main complications are **infection** and **blood clots** within the catheter.

Arteriovenous (AV) Fistula

An A-V fistula is an artificial connection between an artery and a vein. It bypasses the capillary system and allows blood to flow under high pressure from the artery directly into the vein. This provides a permanent, large, easy access blood vessel with high pressure arterial blood flow. Creating an A-V fistula requires a surgical operation and a 4 week to 4 month maturation period without use.

They are typically formed between an artery and vein in the patient's forearm:
- Radio-cephalic
- Brachio-cephalic
- Brachio-basilic (less common and more complex operation)

Examining an A-V fistula is a common exam question. Look for:
- Skin integrity
- Aneurysms
- Palpable thrill (a fine vibration felt over the anastomosis)
- Stereotypical "**machinery murmur**" on auscultation

A-V Fistula Complications

- Aneurysm
- Infection
- Thrombosis
- Stenosis
- STEAL syndrome
- High output heart failure

STEAL Syndrome
STEAL syndrome is where there is inadequate blood flow to the limb distal to the AV fistula. The AV fistula "steals" blood from the distal limb. The blood is diverted away from where it was supposed to supply and flows straight into the venous system. This causes distal ischaemia.

High Output Heart Failure
Blood is flowing very quickly from the arterial to the venous system through an A-V fistula. This means there is rapid return of blood to the heart. This increases the pre-load in the heart (how full the heart is before it pumps). This leads to hypertrophy of the heart muscle and heart failure.

TOM TIP: NEVER take blood from a fistula! This is a lifeline for the patient, providing access to dialysis. If it gets damaged it will set them back and you will be in big trouble.

Renal Transplant

Renal transplant is where a kidney is transplanted in to a patient with end stage renal failure. It typically adds 10 years to life compared with just using dialysis.

Donor Matching

Patients and donor kidneys are matched based on the **human leukocyte antigen** (HLA) type A, B and C on chromosome 6. They don't have to fully match. Recipients can receive treatment to desensitise them to the donor HLA when there is a living donor. The less they match, the more likely the transplant is to fail.

Procedure

The patient's own kidneys are left in place. The donor kidney's blood vessels are connected (**anastomosed**) with the patient's pelvic vessels, usually the external iliac vessels. The ureter of the donor kidney is anastomosed directly with the patient's bladder. The donor kidney is placed anteriorly in the abdomen and can usually be palpated in the iliac fossa area. They typically use a "**hockey stick incision**" and there will be a "**hockey stick scar**".

Post Renal Transplant

The new kidney will start functioning immediately.

Patients will require life long immunosuppression to reduce the risk of transplant rejection. The usual immunosuppressant regime is:
- Tacrolimus
- Mycophenolate
- Prednisolone

Other possible immunosuppressants:
- Cyclosporine
- Sirolimus
- Azathioprine

Complications

Complications relating to the transplant:
- Transplant rejection (hyperacute, acute and chronic)
- Transplant failure
- Electrolyte imbalances

Complications related to immunosuppressants:
- Ischaemic heart disease
- Type 2 diabetes (steroids)
- Infections are more likely and more severe
- Unusual infections can occur (PCP, CMV, PJP and TB)
- Non-Hodgkin lymphoma
- Skin cancer (particularly squamous cell carcinoma)

Glomerulonephritis

Important Definitions

The terminology around **intrinsic kidney disease** gets very confusing. It is really important to thoroughly understand the fundamentals or you risk getting very confused later.

Nephritis is a very generic term that means **inflammation** of the **kidneys**. It is a very non-specific descriptive term and is not a diagnosis or syndrome that has any criteria. It is easy to get confused and think that when a patient is described as having "**nephritis**" this is a diagnosis. It is not, they are simply saying that the patient has inflammation of the kidney.

Nephritic syndrome or **acute nephritic syndrome** refers to a group of symptoms, not a diagnosis. When we say a patient has "**nephritic syndrome**" it simply means they fit a clinical picture of having inflammation of their kidney and it does not represent a specific diagnosis or give the underlying cause. Unlike **nephrotic syndrome**, there are no set criteria, however there are the following features of **nephritic syndrome**:
- **Haematuria** means blood in the urine. This can be **microscopic** (not visible) or **macroscopic** (visible).
- **Oliguria** means there is a significantly reduced urine output.
- **Proteinuria** is protein in the urine. In nephritic syndrome there is less than 3g per 24 hours of urine. Any more and it starts being classified as nephrotic syndrome.
- **Fluid retention**

Nephrotic syndrome refers to a group of symptoms without specifying the underlying cause. Therefore **nephrotic syndrome** is not a disease, but is a way of saying "the patient has these symptoms". To have **nephrotic syndrome** a patient must fulfil the following criteria:
- **Peripheral oedema**
- **Proteinuria** (more than 3g per 24 hours)
- **Serum albumin** (less than 25g per litre)
- **Hypercholesterolaemia**

Glomerulonephritis is an umbrella term applied to conditions that cause inflammation of or around the **glomerulus**. Therefore, there are many conditions that can be described as a glomerulonephritis. Below there is a list of the types of glomerulonephritis. These are specific diseases and diagnoses that have their own pathophysiology.

Interstitial nephritis is term to describe a situation where there is inflammation of the space between cells and tubules (the **interstitium**) within the kidney. It is important not to confuse this with glomerulonephritis. Under the umbrella term of interstitial nephritis there are two key specific diagnoses: **acute interstitial nephritis** and **chronic tubulointerstitial nephritis**. These are discussed in a later section.

Glomerulosclerosis is a term to describe the pathological process of scarring of the tissue in the glomerulus. It is not a diagnosis in itself and is more a term used to describe the damage and scarring done by other diagnoses. ***Glomerulosclerosis*** can be caused by any type of **glomerulonephritis** or **obstructive uropathy** (blockage of urine outflow), and by a disease called *focal segmental glomerulosclerosis*.

Specific Types of Glomerulonephritis

Each disease listed has its own epidemiology, causes and treatments. It is easy to get overwhelmed and confused, since they are very similar names. I would suggest not trying to learn every detail until you really understand the basics. If you understand the basics you will be ahead of most of your colleagues. The types of glomerulonephritis are:
- Minimal change disease
- Focal segmental glomerulosclerosis
- Membranous glomerulonephritis
- IgA nephropathy (AKA mesangioproliferative glomerulonephritis or Berger's disease)
- Post streptococcal glomerulonephritis (AKA diffuse proliferative glomerulonephritis)
- Mesangiocapillary glomerulonephritis
- Rapidly progressive glomerulonephritis
- Goodpasture Syndrome

Key Facts

Here are some key facts that will allow you to answer almost all exam questions on glomerulonephritis without getting overwhelmed and confused trying to learn everything about kidneys.

Most types of glomerulonephritis are treated with:
- Immunosuppression (e.g. steroids)
- Blood pressure control by blocking the renin-angiotensin system (i.e. ACE inhibitors or angiotensin receptor blockers)

Nephrotic Syndrome
Nephrotic syndrome usually presents with oedema. Patients might notice frothy urine (proteinuria). Nephrotic syndrome predisposes patients to thrombosis, hypertension and high cholesterol.

The most common cause of nephrotic syndrome in children is **minimal change disease**. This is usually:
- Idiopathic (no identified cause)
- Treated successfully with steroids

The most common cause of nephrotic syndrome in adults is **focal segmental glomerulosclerosis**.

IgA nephropathy (AKA Berger's disease)
- The most common cause of **primary** glomerulonephritis
- Peak age at presentation is in the 20s
- Histology shows "IgA deposits and glomerular mesangial proliferation"

Membranous glomerulonephritis
- The most common type of glomerulonephritis overall
- There is a bimodal peak in age in the 20s and 60s.
- Histology shows "IgG and complement deposits on the basement membrane"
- The majority (~70%) are idiopathic
- Can be secondary to malignancy, rheumatoid disorders and drugs (e.g. NSAIDS)

Post streptococcal glomerulonephritis (AKA diffuse proliferative glomerulonephritis)
Patients are typically under 30 years old. It presents as:
- 1 to 3 weeks after a streptococcal infection (e.g. tonsillitis or impetigo)
- They develop a nephritic syndrome
- There is usually a full recovery

Goodpasture Syndrome
Anti-GBM (*glomerular basement membrane*) *antibodies* attack the glomerulus and pulmonary basement membranes. This causes *glomerulonephritis* and *pulmonary haemorrhage*. In your exam there may be a patient that presents with *acute kidney failure* and *haemoptysis* (coughing up blood).

Rapidly Progressive Glomerulonephritis
- Histology shows "crescentic glomerulonephritis"
- It presents with a very acute illness with sick patients but it responds well to treatment
- Often secondary to Goodpasture syndrome

Diabetic Nephropathy

Diabetic nephropathy is the most common cause of **glomerular pathology** and **chronic kidney disease** in the UK. The chronic high level of glucose passing through the glomerulus causes scarring. This is called **glomerulosclerosis.**

Proteinuria is a key feature of diabetic nephropathy. This is due to damage to the glomerulus allowing protein to be filtered from the blood to the urine.

Patients with diabetes should have regular screening for diabetic nephropathy by testing the **albumin:creatinine ratio** and **U&Es**.

Management

Treatment is through optimising blood sugar levels and blood pressure. **ACE inhibitors** are the treatment of choice in diabetics for blood pressure control. They should be started in patients with diabetic nephropathy even if they have a normal blood pressure.

Interstitial Kidney Disease

Interstitial nephritis is term to describe a situation where there is inflammation of the space between cells and tubules (the *interstitium*) within the kidney. This is different to glomerulonephritis, where there is inflammation around the glomerulus. There are two types of interstitial nephritis: *acute interstitial nephritis* and *chronic tubulointerstitial nephritis*.

Acute Interstitial Nephritis

Acute interstitial nephritis presents with *acute kidney injury* and *hypertension*. There is acute *inflammation* of the *tubules* and *interstitium*. This is usually caused by a *hypersensitivity reaction* to:

- Drugs (e.g. NSAIDS or antibiotics)
- Infection

Other features of a generalised hypersensitivity reaction can accompany the acute kidney injury:
- Rash
- Fever
- Eosinophilia

Management involves treating the underlying cause. Steroids have a role in reducing inflammation and improving recovery.

Chronic Tubulointerstitial Nephritis

Chronic tubulointerstitial nephritis involves **chronic inflammation** of the **tubules** and **interstitium**. It presents with **chronic kidney disease**.

It has a large number of underlying autoimmune, infectious, iatrogenic and granulomatous disease causes.

Management involves treating the underlying cause. Steroids have a role when guided by a specialist.

Acute Tubular Necrosis

Acute tubular necrosis is damage and death (**necrosis**) of the **epithelial cells** of the renal **tubules**. It is the most common cause of **acute kidney injury**. Damage to the kidney cells occurs due to **ischaemia** or **toxins**. The epithelial cells have the ability to regenerate making acute tubular necrosis reversible. It usually takes 7 to 21 days to recover.

Causes

Ischaemia can occur secondary to hypoperfusion in:
- Shock
- Sepsis
- Dehydration

Direct damage from toxins can occur due to:
- Radiology contrast dye
- Gentamicin
- NSAIDs
- Lithium
- Heroin

Urinalysis

"**Muddy brown casts**" found on urinalysis is a **pathognomonic** finding specific to acute tubular necrosis. There can also be renal tubular epithelial cells in the urine.

Management

Treatment is the same as other causes of acute kidney injury:
- Supportive management
- IV fluids
- Stop nephrotoxic medications
- Treat complications

Renal Tubular Acidosis

Renal tubular acidosis is where there is a *metabolic acidosis* due to pathology in the *tubules* of the *kidney*. The tubules are responsible for balancing the *hydrogen* and *bicarbonate ions* between the blood and urine and maintaining a normal *pH*. There are four types, each with different pathophysiology.

Type 1 and type 4 are the two that may come up in your exams and are most relevant to clinical practice.

Type 1 Renal Tubular Acidosis

Type 1 renal tubular acidosis is due to pathology in the *distal tubule*. The distal tubule is **unable to excrete hydrogen ions**.

There are many causes:
- Genetic. There are both autosomal dominant and recessive forms.
- Systemic lupus erythematosus
- Sjogrens syndrome
- Primary biliary cirrhosis
- Hyperthyroidism
- Sickle cell anaemia
- Marfan's syndrome

Presentation:
- Failure to thrive in children
- Hyperventilation to compensate for the metabolic acidosis
- Chronic kidney disease
- Bone disease (osteomalacia)

Results:
- Hypokalaemia
- Metabolic acidosis
- High urinary pH (above 6)

Treatment is with oral *bicarbonate*. This corrects the other electrolyte imbalances as well as the acidosis.

Type 2 Renal Tubular Acidosis

Type 2 renal tubular acidosis is due to pathology in the *proximal tubule*. The proximal tubule is **unable to reabsorb bicarbonate** from the urine to the blood. Excessive bicarbonate is excreted in the urine.

Fanconi's syndrome is the main cause. This is a genetic condition commonly associated with **Ashkenazi Jews**, that causes **bone marrow failure**, **acute myeloid leukaemia** and other cancers. There are certain features on examination such as **cafe au lait spots**, certain **facial features** and an **absence of the radius** bone bilaterally.

Results:
- Hypokalaemia
- Metabolic acidosis
- High urinary pH (above 6)

Treatment is with oral **bicarbonate**.

Type 3 Renal Tubular Acidosis

Type 3 renal tubular acidosis is a combination of type 1 and type 2 with pathology in the proximal and distal tubule. This is rare and unlikely to appear in your exams or clinical practice.

Type 4 Renal Tubular Acidosis

Type 4 renal tubular acidosis is caused by **reduced aldosterone**. Aldosterone is responsible for stimulating sodium reabsorption and potassium and hydrogen ion excretion in the distal tubules. Therefore, low aldosterone or low aldosterone function leads to insufficient potassium and hydrogen ion excretion, causing a **hyperkalaemic renal tubular acidosis**. Normally ammonia is produced in the distal tubules to balance the excretion of hydrogen ions and prevent the urine from become too acidotic (ammonia is a base). Hyperkalaemia suppresses the production of ammonia, so the urine is acidotic in type 4 RTA. This is the most common type of renal tubular acidosis and the most likely to turn up in your exams and clinical practice.

Low aldosterone or low aldosterone activity can be due to **adrenal insufficiency**, medications such as **ACE inhibitors** and **spironolactone** or systemic conditions that affect the kidneys such as **systemic lupus erythematosus**, **diabetes** or **HIV**.

Results:
- Hyperkalaemia
- High chloride
- Metabolic acidosis
- Low urinary pH (due to reduced ammonia production)

Management is with **fludrocortisone** (a **mineralocorticoid** steroid medication). **Sodium bicarbonate** and treatment of the **hyperkalaemia** may also be required.

Haemolytic Uraemic Syndrome

Haemolytic uraemic syndrome (HUS) occurs when there is **thrombosis** in **small blood vessels** throughout the body. This is usually triggered by a bacterial toxin called the **shiga toxin**. It leads to the classic triad of:
- Haemolytic anaemia
- Acute kidney injury
- Low platelet count (thrombocytopenia)

The most common cause is a toxin produced by the bacteria **e. coli 0157** called the **shiga toxin**. **Shigella** also produces this toxin. The use of antibiotics and anti-motility medications such as loperamide to treat gastroenteritis caused by these pathogens increases the risk of developing HUS.

Presentation

E. coli 0157 causes a brief **gastroenteritis**, often with bloody diarrhoea.

Around 5 days after the diarrhoea the person will start displaying symptoms of HUS:
- Reduced urine output
- Haematuria or dark brown urine
- Abdominal pain
- Lethargy and irritability
- Confusion
- Hypertension
- Bruising

Management

HUS is a **medical emergency** and has a 10% mortality. The condition is self limiting and **supportive management** is the mainstay of treatment:
- Antihypertensives
- Blood transfusions
- Dialysis

70 to 80% of patients make a full recovery.

Rhabdomyolysis

Rhabdomyolysis is a condition where skeletal muscle tissue breaks down and releases breakdown products into the blood. This is usually triggered by an event that causes the muscle to break down, such as extreme underuse or overuse or a traumatic injury.

The muscle cells (**myocytes**) undergo cell death (**apoptosis**). The cell death results in muscle cells releasing:
- **Myoglobin** (causing **myoglobinurea**)
- **Potassium**
- **Phosphate**
- **Creatine Kinase**

Potassium is the most immediately dangerous breakdown product, as **hyperkalaemia** can cause **cardiac arrhythmias** that can potentially result in a **cardiac arrest**.

These breakdown products are filtered by the kidney and cause injury to the kidney. **Myoglobin** in particular is toxic to the kidney in high concentrations. This results in **acute kidney injury**. The acute kidney injury results in the breakdown products accumulating further in the blood.

Causes

Anything that causes significant damage to muscle cells can cause rhabdomyolysis:
- **Prolonged immobility**, particularly frail patients that fall and spend time on the floor before being found.
- **Extremely rigorous exercise** beyond the person's fitness level (e.g. ultramaraton, triathalon or crossfit competition)
- **Crush injuries**
- **Seizures**

Signs and Symptoms

- Muscle aches and pain
- Oedema
- Fatigue
- Confusion (particularly in elderly frail patients)
- Red-brown urine

Investigations

Creatine Kinase (**CK**) blood test is a key investigation in establishing the diagnosis. It will be in the thousands to hundreds of thousands of Units/L. CK typically rises in the first 12 hours, then remains elevated for 1 to 3 days, then falls gradually. A higher CK increases the risk of kidney injury.

Myoglobinurea is **myoglobin** in the urine. It gives urine a **red-brown colour**. This will cause a **urine dipstick** to be positive for blood.

Urea and electrolytes (**U&E**) blood tests for **acute kidney injury** and **hyperkalaemia**.

ECG is important in assessing the heart's response to **hyperkalaemia**.

Management

Suspect rhabdomyolysis in patients with trauma, crush injury, prolonged immobilisation or excessive exercise.

IV fluids are the mainstay of treatment. The aim is to rehydrate the patient and encourage filtration of the breakdown products.

Consider IV **sodium bicarbonate**. This aims to make the urine more alkaline (pH ≥ 6.5), reducing the toxicity of the myoglobin on the kidneys. The evidence on this is not clear and there is some debate about whether to use it.

Consider IV **mannitol**. This aims to increase the **glomerular filtration rate** to help flush the breakdown products and to reduce **oedema** surrounding muscles and nerves. Hypovolaemia should be corrected before giving mannitol. The evidence on this is not clear and there is some debate about whether to use it.

Treat **complications**, particularly **hyperkalaemia**. **Hyperkalaemia** can be immediately life threatening as it can cause arrhythmias (particularly **ventricular fibrillation**).

Hyperkalaemia

Hyperkalaemia is a high **serum potassium**. It is important to remember the investigations and management of hyperkalaemia as it is a common exam and real life scenario. The main complication is **cardiac arrhythmias** such as **ventricular fibrillation**. These can be fatal.

Causes

Conditions
- Acute kidney injury
- Chronic kidney disease
- Rhabdomyolysis
- Adrenal insufficiency
- Tumour lysis syndrome

Medications
- Aldosterone antagonists (spironolactone and eplerenone)
- ACE inhibitors
- Angiotensin II receptor blockers
- NSAIDS
- Potassium supplements

Urea and Electrolytes

Hyperkalaemia is diagnosed on a formal **urea and electrolytes** (**U&E**) blood test. Pay attention to **creatinine**, **urea** and **eGFR**. Acute or chronic renal failure is important as they will need discussion with the renal team and consideration of **haemodialysis**.

Haemolysis (breakdown of red blood cells) during sampling can result in a falsely elevated potassium. The lab might indicate that they have noticed some haemolysis and require a repeat sample to confirm the correct potassium result.

ECG Signs

An ECG is required in all patients with a potassium above 6 mmol/L. It is worth memorising the ECG changes in hyperkalaemia:
- Tall peaked T waves
- Flattening or absence of P waves
- Broad QRS complexes

Management

Follow the local policy and protocol for treating hyperkalaemia. Get help from an experienced doctor. Patients with significant hyperkalaemia will need close ECG monitoring to detect changes and arrhythmias. Patients with significant renal impairment should be discussed with the renal physicians.

Patients with a **potassium ≤ 6 mmol/L** with otherwise stable renal function don't need urgent treatment and may just require a change in diet and medications (i.e. stopping their spironolactone or ACE inhibitor).

Patients with a **potassium ≥ 6 mmol/L and ECG changes** need urgent treatment.

Patients with a **potassium ≥ 6.5 mmol/L** need urgent treatment regardless of the ECG.

The mainstay of treatment is with an *insulin and dextrose infusion* and IV *calcium gluconate*:
- *Insulin* and *dextrose* drive carbohydrate into cells and take potassium with it, reducing the blood potassium.
- *Calcium gluconate* stabilises the cardiac muscle cells and reduces the risk of arrhythmias.

Other options for lowering the serum potassium:
- *Nebulised salbutamol* temporarily drives potassium into cells.
- *IV fluids* can be used to increase urine output, which encourages potassium loss from the kidneys (but don't fluid overload patients with renal failure).
- *Oral calcium resonium* draws potassium out of the gut and into stools. It works slowly and is suitable for milder cases of hyperkalaemia.
- *Sodium bicarbonate* (IV or oral) may be considered on the advice of a renal specialist in acidotic patients with renal failure. It drives potassium into cells as the acidosis is corrected.
- *Dialysis* may be required in severe or persistent cases associated with renal failure.

Polycystic Kidney Disease

Polycystic kidney disease is a *genetic condition* where the kidneys develop multiple fluid filled *cysts*. Kidney function is also significantly impaired. There are a number of associated findings outside the kidneys, such as *hepatic cysts* and *cerebral aneurysms*. Palpable, enlarged kidneys may be felt on examination.

There is an *autosomal dominant* and an *autosomal recessive* type. The autosomal dominant type of PKD is more common than the autosomal recessive type.

Diagnosis is by kidney *ultrasound scan* and *genetic testing*.

Autosomal Dominant Type

Autosomal Dominant Genes
- PKD-1: chromosome 16 (85% of cases)
- PKD-2: chromosome 4 (15% of cases)

Extra-Renal Manifestations
- Cerebral aneurysms
- Hepatic, splenic, pancreatic, ovarian and prostatic cysts
- Cardiac valve disease (mitral regurgitation)
- Colonic diverticula
- Aortic root dilatation

Complications
- *Chronic loin pain*
- *Hypertension*
- *Cardiovascular disease*
- *Gross haematuria* can occur with cyst rupture. This usually resolves within a few days.
- *Renal stones* are more common in patients with PKD
- *End stage renal failure* occurs at a mean age of 50 years

Autosomal Recessive Type

Autosomal recessive polycystic kidney disease (ARPKD) is caused by a gene on **chromosome 6**. It is more rare and more severe. It often presents in pregnancy with **oligohydramnios** as the fetus does not produce enough urine.

Features
The oligohydramnios leads to underdevelopment of the lungs, resulting in respiratory failure shortly after birth. Patients may require dialysis within the first few days of life. They can have dysmorphic features such as underdeveloped ear cartilage, low set ears and a flat nasal bridge. They usually have **end stage renal failure** before reaching adulthood.

Management

Tolvaptan (a vasopressin receptor antagonist) can slow the development of cysts and the progression of renal failure in autosomal dominant polycystic kidney disease. It is recommended by NICE in certain situations although it should be initiated and monitored by a specialist.

Management of polycystic kidney disease is mainly supportive of the complications:
- Antihypertensives for hypertension
- Analgesia for renal colic related to stones or cysts
- Antibiotics for infection. Drainage of infected cysts may be required.
- Dialysis for end stage renal failure
- Renal transplant for end stage renal failure

Other management steps:
- Genetic counselling
- Avoid contact sports due to the risk of cyst rupture
- Avoid anti-inflammatory medications and anticoagulants
- Regular ultrasound to monitor the cysts
- Regular bloods to monitor renal function
- Regular blood pressure to monitor for hypertension
- MR angiogram can be used to diagnose intracranial aneurysms in symptomatic patients or those with a family history

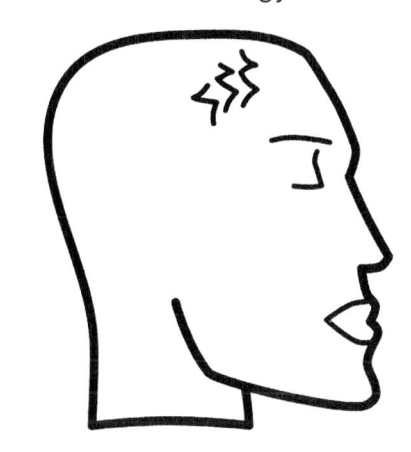

NEUROLOGY

9.1	Stroke	268
9.2	Intracranial Bleeds	270
9.3	Subarachnoid Haemorrhage	273
9.4	Multiple Sclerosis	274
9.5	Motor Neurone Disease	278
9.6	Parkinson's Disease	279
9.7	Benign Essential Tremor	282
9.8	Epilepsy	283
9.9	Neuropathic Pain	286
9.10	Facial Nerve Palsy	287
9.11	Brain Tumours	289
9.12	Huntington's Chorea	292
9.13	Myasthenia Gravis	293
9.14	Lambert-Eaton Myasthenic Syndrome	296
9.15	Charcot-Marie-Tooth Disease	296
9.16	Guillain-Barré Syndrome	297
9.17	Neurofibromatosis	298
9.18	Tuberous Sclerosis	300
9.19	Headaches	301
9.20	Migraines	304
9.21	Cluster Headaches	306

Stroke

Stroke is also referred to as *cerebrovascular accident* (*CVA*).

Cerebrovascular accidents are either:
- *Ischaemia* or *infarction* of brain tissue secondary to inadequate blood supply
- *Intracranial haemorrhage*

Disruption of blood supply can be caused by:
- Thrombus formation or embolus, for example in patients with atrial fibrillation
- Atherosclerosis
- Shock
- Vasculitis

Transient ischaemic attack (*TIA*) was originally defined as symptoms of a stroke that resolve within 24 hours. It has been updated based on advanced imaging to now be defined as transient neurological dysfunction secondary to *ischaemia* without *infarction*.

Transient ischaemic attacks often precede a full stroke. A *crescendo TIA* is where there are two or more TIAs within a week. This carries a high risk of progressing to a stroke.

Presentation

In neurology, suspect a vascular cause where there is a **sudden onset** of neurological symptoms.

Stoke symptoms are typically asymmetrical:
- Sudden weakness of limbs
- Sudden facial weakness
- Sudden onset dysphasia (speech disturbance)
- Sudden onset visual or sensory loss

Risk Factors

- Cardiovascular disease such as angina, myocardial infarction and peripheral vascular disease
- Previous stroke or TIA
- Atrial fibrillation
- Carotid artery disease
- Hypertension
- Diabetes
- Smoking
- Vasculitis
- Thrombophilia
- Combined contraceptive pill

FAST Tool for Identifying a Stroke in the Community

- **F** - **F**ace
- **A** - **A**rm
- **S** - **S**peech
- **T** - **T**ime (act fast and call 999)

ROSIER Tool for Recognition Of Stroke In Emergency Room

ROSIER is a scoring tool based on clinical features and duration. Stroke is likely if the patient scores anything above 0.

ABCD2 Score for Patients with a TIA

The ABCD2 score is used for assessing patients with a suspected TIA to estimate their risk of subsequently having a stoke. A higher score suggests a higher risk of stroke within the following 48 hours.

The ABCD2 score is based on:
- **A** - **A**ge (> 60 = 1)
- **B** - **B**lood pressure (> 140/90 = 1)
- **C** - **C**linical features (unilateral weakness = 2, dysphasia without weakness = 1)
- **D** - **D**uration (more than 60 minutes = 2, 10 to 60 minutes = 1, less than 10 minutes = 0)
- **D** - **D**iabetes = 1

Management of Stroke

This is adapted from the NICE guidelines updated in 2017 to help your learning. See the full guidelines before treating patients.
- Admit patients to a specialist stroke centre
- Exclude hypoglycaemia
- Immediate CT brain to exclude primary intracerebral haemorrhage
- Aspirin 300mg stat (after the CT) and continued for 2 weeks

Thrombolysis with alteplase can be used after the CT brain scan has excluded an intracranial haemorrhage. **Alteplase** is a **tissue plasminogen activator** that rapidly breaks down clots and can reverse the effects of a stroke if given in time. It is given based on local protocols by an experienced physician. It needs to be given within a defined window of opportunity, for example 4.5 hours. Patients need monitoring for post thrombolysis complications such as intracranial or systemic haemorrhage. This includes using repeated CT scans of the brain.

Generally blood pressure should not be lowered during a stroke because this risks reducing the perfusion to the brain.

Management of TIA

Start **aspirin 300mg daily**. Start **secondary prevention** measures for cardiovascular disease. If they have crescendo TIAs they should be seen within 24 hours by a specialist.

Perform an ABCD2 Score
- Score 3 or less: specialist assessment within 1 week
- Score more than 3: specialist assessment within 24 hours

Specialist Imaging

The aim of imaging is to establish the vascular territory that is affected. It is guided by specialist assessment.

Diffusion-weighted MRI is the gold standard imaging technique. CT is an alternative.

Carotid ultrasound can be used to assess for **carotid stenosis**. **Endarterectomy** to remove plaques or **carotid stenting** to widen the lumen should be considered if there is carotid stenosis.

Secondary Prevention of Stroke

- Clopidogrel 75mg once daily (alternatively dipyridamole 200mg twice daily)
- Atorvastatin 80mg should be started but not immediately
- Carotid endarterectomy or stenting in patients with carotid artery disease
- Treat modifiable risk factors such as hypertension and diabetes

Stroke Rehabilitation

Once patients have had a stroke they require a period of adjustment and rehabilitation. This is essential and central to stroke care. It involves a **multi disciplinary team** including:
- Nurses
- Speech and language (SALT)
- Nutrition and dietetics
- Physiotherapy
- Occupational therapy
- Social services
- Optometry and ophthalmology
- Psychology
- Orthotics

Intracranial Bleeds

Round 10 to 20% of strokes are caused by intracranial bleeds.

Risk Factors

- Head injury
- Hypertension
- Aneurysms
- Ischaemic stroke can progress to haemorrhage
- Brain tumours
- Anticoagulants such as warfarin

Presentation

Sudden onset headache is a key feature. They can also present with:

- Seizures
- Weakness
- Vomiting
- Reduced consciousness
- Other sudden onset neurological symptoms

Glasgow Coma Scale

The **Glasgow coma scale** (**GCS**) is a universal assessment tool for the level of consciousness. It is worth learning for your exams and every day practice as it frequently appears.

It is scored based on *eyes*, *verbal* response and *motor* response. The maximum score is 15/15, minimum is 3/15. When someone has a score of 8/15 or below then you need to consider securing their airway, as there is a risk they are not able to maintain it on their own.

Eyes
- Spontaneous = 4
- Speech = 3
- Pain – 2
- None = 1

Verbal response
- Orientated = 5
- Confused conversation = 4
- Inappropriate words = 3
- Incomprehensible sounds = 2
- None = 1

Motor response
- Obeys commands = 6
- Localises pain = 5
- Normal flexion = 4
- Abnormal flexion = 3
- Extends = 2
- None = 1

Subdural Haemorrhage

Subdural haemorrhage is caused by rupture of the **bridging veins** in the outermost meningeal layer. It occurs between the **dura mater** and **arachnoid mater**. On a CT scan they have a **crescent shape** and are not limited by the **cranial sutures** (they can cross over the sutures).

Subdural haemorrhages occur more frequently in elderly and alcoholic patients. These patients have more **atrophy** in their brains making vessels more likely to rupture.

Extradural Haemorrhage

Extradural haemorrhage is usually caused by rupture of the **middle meningeal artery** in the **temporo-parietal region**. It can be associated with a fracture of the **temporal bone**. It occurs between the **skull** and **dura mater**. On a CT scan they have a **bi-convex shape** and are limited by the **cranial sutures** (they can't cross over the sutures).

The typical history is a young patient with a traumatic head injury that has an ongoing headache. They have a period of improved neurological symptoms and consciousness followed by a rapid decline over hours as the haematoma gets large enough to compress the intracranial contents.

Intracerebral Haemorrhage

Intracerebral haemorrhage involves bleeding in the brain tissue. It presents similarly to an ischaemic stroke.

These can be anywhere in the brain tissue:
- Lobar intracerebral haemorrhage
- Deep intracerebral haemorrhage
- Intraventricular haemorrhage
- Basal ganglia haemorrhage
- Cerebellar haemorrhage

They can occur spontaneously or as the result of bleeding into an ischaemic infarct or tumour or rupture of an aneurysm.

Subarachnoid Haemorrhage

Subarachnoid haemorrhage involves bleeding in the **subarachnoid space**, where the **cerebrospinal fluid** is located, between the **pia mater** and the **arachnoid membrane**. This is usually the result of a ruptured **cerebral aneurysm**.

The typical history is a sudden onset **occipital headache** that occurs during strenuous activity such as weight lifting or sex. This occurs so suddenly and severely that it is known as a "**thunderclap headache**".

They are particularly associated with **cocaine** and **sickle cell anaemia**.

Principles of Management

- Immediate CT head to establish the diagnosis
- Check FBC and clotting
- Admit to a specialist stroke unit
- Discuss with a specialist neurosurgical centre to consider surgical treatment
- Consider intubation, ventilation and ICU care if they have reduced consciousness
- Correct any clotting abnormality
- Correct severe hypertension but avoid hypotension

Subarachnoid Haemorrhage

Subarachnoid haemorrhage involves bleeding in the **subarachnoid space**, where the **cerebrospinal fluid** is located, between the **pia mater** and the **arachnoid membrane**. This is usually the result of a ruptured **cerebral aneurysm**.

Subarachnoid haemorrhage has a very high **mortality** and **morbidity**. It is very important not to miss the diagnosis and you need to have a low suspicion to trigger full investigations. It needs to be discussed with the **neurosurgical unit** with a view to surgical intervention.

Thunderclap Headache

The typical history is a **sudden onset occipital headache** that occurs during strenuous activity such as weight lifting or sex. This occurs so suddenly and severely that it is known as a "**thunderclap headache**". It is described like being hit really hard on the back of the head. Other features are:
- Neck stiffness
- Photophobia
- Neurological symptoms such as visual changes, speech changes, weakness, seizures and loss of consciousness

Risk Factors

- Hypertension
- Smoking
- Excessive alcohol consumption
- Cocaine use
- Family history

Subarachnoid haemorrhage is more common in:
- Black patients
- Female patients
- Age 45 to 70

It is particularly associated with:
- Cocaine use
- Sickle cell anaemia
- Connective tissue disorders (such as Marfan syndrome or Ehlers-Danlos)
- Neurofibromatosis

Investigations

CT head is the first line investigation. Immediate CT head is required. Blood will cause **hyperattenuation** in the **subarachnoid space**. CT head may be normal and does not always exclude a subarachnoid haemorrhage.

Lumbar puncture is used to collect a sample of the **cerebrospinal fluid** if the CT head is negative. CSF can be tested for signs of subarachnoid haemorrhage:
- **Red cell count** will be raised. If the cell count is decreasing in number over the samples, this could be due to a traumatic lumbar puncture.
- **Xanthochromia** is a yellow colour to the CSF caused by bilirubin

Angiography (CT or MRI) can be used once a subarachnoid haemorrhage is confirmed to locate the source of the bleeding.

Management

Patients should be managed by a **specialist neurosurgical unit**. Patients with reduced consciousness may require intubation and ventilation. Supportive care as part of a multi-disciplinary team is important with good nursing, nutrition, physiotherapy and occupational therapy involved during the initial stages and recovery.

Surgical intervention may be used to treat aneurysms. The aim is to repair the vessel and prevent re-bleeding. This can be done by **coiling**, which involves inserting a catheter into the arterial system (taking an "***endovascular approach***"), placing platinum coils in the aneurysm and sealing it off from the artery. An alternative is ***clipping***, which involves cranial surgery and putting a clip on the aneurysm to seal it.

Nimodipine is a calcium channel blocker that is used to prevent ***vasospasm***. ***Vasospasm*** is a common complication that can result in brain ischaemia following a subarachnoid haemorrhage.

Lumbar puncture or insertion of a ***shunt*** may be required to treat ***hydrocephalus***.

Anti-epileptic medications can be used to treat ***seizures***.

Multiple Sclerosis

Multiple sclerosis (MS) is a chronic and progressive condition that involves **demyelination** of the **myelinated neurones** in the **central nervous system**. This is caused by an **inflammatory process** involving activation of **immune cells** against the **myelin**.

MS typically presents in young adults (under 50 years) and is more common in women. Symptoms tend to improving in pregnancy and the postpartum period.

Pathophysiology

Myelin covers the **axons** of **neurones** in the **central nervous system**. This myelin helps the electrical impulses move faster along the **axon**. Myelin is provided by cells that wrap themselves around the axons. These are **Schwann cells** in the **peripheral nervous system** and **oligodendrocytes** in the **central nervous system**.

Multiple sclerosis typically only affects the **central nervous system** (the **oligodendrocytes**). There is **inflammation** around myelin and infiltration of **immune cells** that cause damage to the myelin. This affects the way electrical signals travel along the nerve leading to the symptoms of multiple sclerosis.

When a patient presents with symptoms of a clinical "***attack***" of MS, for example an episode of ***optic neuritis***, there are usually other lesions of demyelination throughout the central nervous system, most of which are not causing symptoms.

In early disease, ***re-myelination*** can occur and symptoms resolve. In the later stages of the disease, re-myelination is incomplete and symptoms gradually become more permanent.

A characteristic features of MS is that lesions vary in their location over time, meaning that different nerves are affected and symptoms change over time. The key expression to remember to describe the way MS lesions change location over time is that they are "*disseminated in time and space*".

Causes

The cause of the demyelination is unclear, but there is growing evidence that it is influenced by a combination of:
- Multiple genes
- Epstein–Barr virus (EBV)
- Low vitamin D
- Smoking
- Obesity

Signs and Symptoms

Symptoms usually progress over more than 24 hours. At the first presentation symptoms tend to last days to weeks and then improve. There are a number of ways MS can present. These are described below.

Optic Neuritis
Optic neuritis is the most common presentation of multiple sclerosis. It involves demyelination of the optic nerve and loss of vision in one eye. This is discussed in more detail below.

Eye Movement Abnormalities
Patients may present with double vision due to lesions affecting the **sixth cranial nerve** (**abducens nerve**). There are two key phrases to remember to describe a sixth cranial nerve palsy: *internuclear ophthalmoplegia* and *conjugate lateral gaze disorder*.

Unilateral lesions in the sixth nerve causes a condition called *internuclear ophthalmoplegia*. *Internuclear* refers to the nerve fibres that connect between the *cranial nerve nuclei* that control eye movements (3rd, 4th and 6th cranial nerve nuclei). The internuclear nerve fibres are responsible for coordinating the eye movements to ensure the eyes move together. *Ophthalmoplegia* means a problem with the muscles around the eye.

Lesions in the sixth cranial nerve cause a *conjugate lateral gaze disorder*. *Conjugate* means connected. *Lateral gaze* is where both eyes move together to look laterally to the left or right. It is *disordered* in a sixth cranial nerve palsy. When looking laterally in the direction of the affected eye, the affected eye will not be able to abduct. For example, in a lesion affecting the left eye, when looking to the left, the right eye will *adduct* (move towards the nose) and the left eye will remain in the middle as the muscle responsible for making it move laterally is not functioning.

Focal Weakness
- Bells palsy
- Horners syndrome
- Limb paralysis
- Incontinence

Focal sensory symptoms
- Trigeminal neuralgia
- Numbness
- Paraesthesia (pins and needles)
- **Lhermitte's sign**

Lhermitte's sign is an electric shock sensation travels down the spine and into the limbs when flexing the neck. It indicates disease in the cervical spinal cord in the dorsal column. It is caused by stretching the demyelinated dorsal column.

Ataxia

Ataxia is a problem with coordinated movement. It can be **sensory** or **cerebellar**:
- **Sensory ataxia** is due to loss of the **proprioceptive sense**, which is the ability to sense the position of the joint (e.g. is the joint flexed or extended). This results in a positive **Romberg's test** and can cause **pseudoathetosis**.
- **Cerebellar ataxia** is the result of problems with the **cerebellum** coordinating movement. This suggests a cerebellar lesion.

Disease Patterns

The disease course is highly variable between individuals. Some patients have mild relapsing-remitting episodes for life whereas others have primary progressive MS that progresses without any improvement in symptoms. There are certain classifications used to describe the pattern of MS in an individual. These patterns are not separate conditions but part of a spectrum of disease activity.

Clinically Isolated Syndrome
This describes the first episode of demyelination and neurological signs and symptoms. MS cannot be diagnosed on one episode as the lesions have not been "***disseminated in time and space***". Patients with **clinically isolated syndrome** may never have another episode or may develop MS. If lesions are seen on MRI then they are more likely to progress to MS.

Relapsing-Remitting
Relapsing-remitting MS is the most common pattern at initial diagnosis. It is characterised by episodes of disease and neurological symptoms followed by recovery. In MS the symptoms occur in different areas with different episodes. This can be further classified based on whether the disease is **active** and/or **worsening**:
- **Active**: new symptoms are developing or new lesions are appearing on MRI
- **Not active**: no new symptoms or MRI lesions are developing
- **Worsening**: there is an overall worsening of disability over time
- **Not worsening**: there is no worsening of disability over time

Secondary Progressive
Secondary progressive MS is where there was relapsing-remitting disease at first, but now there is a progressive worsening of symptoms with incomplete remissions. Symptoms become more and more permanent. Secondary progressive MS can be further classified based on whether the disease is **active** and/or **progressing**.
- **Active**: new symptoms are developing or new lesions are appearing on MRI
- **Not active**: no new symptoms or MRI lesions are developing
- **Progressing**: there is an overall worsening of disease over time (regardless of relapses)
- **Not progressing**: there is no worsening of disease over time

Primary Progressive
Primary progressive MS is where there is a worsening of disease and neurological symptoms from the point of diagnosis without initial relapses and remissions. This can be further classified in a similar way to secondary progressive based on whether it is **active** and/or **progressing**.

Diagnosis

Diagnosis is made by a neurologist based on the clinical picture and symptoms suggesting lesions that change location over time. Symptoms have to be progressive over a period of 1 year to diagnose primary progressive MS. Other causes for the symptoms need to be excluded.

Investigations can support the diagnosis:
- **MRI scans** can demonstrate typical lesions
- **Lumbar puncture** can detect "**oligoclonal bands**" in the cerebrospinal fluid (CSF)

Optic Neuritis

Optic neuritis presents with unilateral reduced vision developing over hours to days. Key features are:
- **Central scotoma**. This is an **enlarged blind spot**.
- **Pain** on eye movement
- Impaired **colour vision**
- Relative afferent pupillary defect

Multiple sclerosis is the main cause of optic neuritis, however it can also be caused by:
- Sarcoidosis
- Systemic lupus erythematosus
- Diabetes
- Syphilis
- Measles
- Mumps
- Lyme disease

Patients presenting with acute loss of vision should be seen urgently by an **ophthalmologist** for assessment. It is treated with steroids and recovery takes 2-6 weeks. Around 50% of patients with a single episode of optic neuritis will go on to develop MS over the next 15 years. Changes on an MRI scan help to predict which patients will go on to develop MS.

Management

Multiple sclerosis is managed by a specialist **multidisciplinary team** (**MDT**) including neurologists, specialist nurses, physiotherapy, occupational therapy and others. Patient should be fully educated about their condition and treatment.

Disease Modification
Treatment with **disease modifying drugs** and **biologic therapy** has changed the management of multiple sclerosis so that the aim of treatment is now to induce long term remission with no evidence of disease activity. There are many options that target various mechanisms such as **interleukins**, inflammatory **cytokines** and various **immune cells**. Going in to detail about these drugs is beyond what would be expected in your exams. Disease modifying drug treatment will be coordinated by specialists in multiple sclerosis.

Treating Relapses
Relapses can be treated with steroids. NICE recommend **methylprednisolone**:
- 500mg orally daily for 5 days
- 1g intravenously daily for 3–5 days where oral treatment has failed previously or where relapses are severe

Symptomatic Treatments

It is important to treat the symptom that result from the disease process along with treating the disease process itself:
- **Exercise** to maintain activity and strength
- **Neuropathic pain** can be managed with medication such as amitriptyline and gabapentin
- **Depression** can be managed with antidepressants such as SSRIs
- **Urge incontinence** can be managed with anticholinergic medications such as tolterodine or oxybutynin (although be aware these can cause or worsen cognitive impairment)
- **Spasticity** can be managed with baclofen, gabapentin and physiotherapy

Motor Neurone Disease

Motor neurone disease is an umbrella term that encompasses a variety of specific diagnoses. Motor neurone disease is a progressive, ultimately fatal condition where the motor neurones stop functioning. There is no effect on the sensory neurones and patients should not experience any sensory symptoms.

Amylotropic lateral sclerosis (**AML**) is the most common and well known specific type of **motor neurone disease**. Stephen Hawking had amylotropic lateral sclerosis.

Progressive bulbar palsy is the second most common form of **motor neurone disease**. It affects primarily the muscles of talking and swallowing.

Other types of motor neurone disease to be aware of are **progressive muscular atrophy** and **primary lateral sclerosis**.

Pathophysiology

There is progressive degeneration of both **upper** and **lower motor neurones**. The **sensory neurones** are spared.

The exact cause is unclear although several mechanisms have been considered. There is a **genetic** component and many genes have been linked with an increased risk of developing the condition. Taking a good **family history** is important as around 5-10% of cases are inherited. There also seems to be an increased risk with **smoking**, exposure to **heavy metals** and certain **pesticides**.

Presentation

The typical patient is a late middle aged (e.g. 60) man, possibly with an affected relative. There is an insidious, progressive weakness of the muscles throughout the body affecting the limbs, trunk, face and speech. The weakness is often first noticed in the upper limbs. There may be increased fatigue when exercising. They may complain of clumsiness, dropping things more often or tripping over. They can develop slurred speech (**dysphasia**).

Signs of **lower motor neurone disease**:
- Muscle wasting
- Reduced tone
- Fasciculations (twitches in the muscles)
- Reduced reflexes

Signs of *upper motor neurone disease*:
- Increased tone or spasticity
- Brisk reflexes
- Upgoing plantar reflex

Diagnosis

The diagnosis of motor neurone disease needs to be made very carefully. It is based on the clinical presentation and excluding other conditions that can cause motor neurone symptoms. It should only be made by a specialist when there is certainty. Unfortunately the diagnosis is often delayed, which causes considerable anxiety and stress.

Management

Unfortunately there are no effective treatments for halting or reversing the progression of the disease

Riluzole can slow the progression of the disease and extend survival by a few months in AML. It is licensed in the UK and should be initiated by a specialist.

Edaravone is currently used in the United States but not the UK. Recent studies suggest it may have the potential to slow the progression of the disease and it may come in to use in the future.

Non-invasive ventilation (*NIV*) used at home to support breathing at night improves survival and quality of life.

The key to management of the condition is supporting the person and their family.
- Effectively **breaking bad news**
- Involving the **multidisciplinary team** (**MDT**) in supporting and maintaining their quality of life
- **Advanced directives** to document the patients wishes as the disease progresses
- **End of life care** planning
- Patients usually die of respiratory failure or pneumonia

Parkinson's Disease

Parkinson's disease is a condition where there is a progressive reduction of *dopamine* in the *basal ganglia* of the brain, leading to disorders of movement. The symptoms are characteristically asymmetrical, with one side affected more than the other.

There is a *classic triad* of features in Parkinson's disease:
- *Resting tremor*
- *Rigidity*
- *Bradykinesia*

Pathophysiology

The *basal ganglia* are a group of structures situated in the middle of the brain. They are responsible for coordinating habitual movements such as walking or looking around, controlling voluntary movements and learning specific movement patterns. Part of the *basal ganglia* called the *substantia nigra* produces a *neurotransmitter* called *dopamine*. Dopamine is essential for the correct functioning of the basal ganglia. In Parkinson's disease, there is a gradual but progressive fall in the production of dopamine.

Presentation

The typical patient is an older aged man around the age of 70.

Unilateral Tremor
The tremor in Parkinsons has a frequency of 4-6 Hz, meaning it occurs 4 to 6 times a second. This is described as a "*pill rolling tremor*" because it looks like they are rolling a pill between their fingertips and thumb. It is more pronounced when resting and improves on voluntary movement. The tremor is worsened if the patient is distracted. Asking them to do a task with the other hand, such as miming the motion of painting a fence, can exaggerate the tremor.

"Cogwheel" Rigidity
Rigidity is a resistance to passive movement of a joint. If you take their hand and passively flex and extend their arm at the elbow, you will feel a tension in their arm that gives way to movement in small increments (like little jerks). This is what leads to the *cogwheel* description.

Bradykinesia
Bradykinesia describes how their movements get slower and smaller. This presents in a number of ways:
- Their handwriting gets smaller and smaller (this is a classic presenting complaint in exams)
- They can only take small steps when walking ("*shuffling gait*")
- They have difficulty initiating movement (e.g. from standing still to walking)
- They have difficulty in turning around when standing, having to take lots of little steps
- They have reduced facial movements and facial expressions (*hypomimia*)

Other Features
There are a number of other features that often affect patients with Parkinson's disease:
- Depression
- Sleep disturbance and insomnia
- Loss of the sense of smell (*anosmia*)
- Postural instability
- Cognitive impairment and memory problems

TOM TIP: A common exam task challenges you to distinguish between the tremor of Parkinson's disease and benign essential tremor. The table below gives some tips on this:

Parkinson's Tremor	Benign Essential Tremor
Asymmetrical	Symmetrical
4-6 hertz	5-8 hertz
Worse at rest	Improves at rest
Improves with intentional movement	Worse with intentional movement
Other Parkinson's features	No other Parkinson's features
No change with alcohol	Improves with alcohol

Parkinson's-plus Syndromes

Multiple System Atrophy
This is a rare condition where the neurones of multiple systems in the brain degenerate. It affects the basal ganglia as well as multiple other areas. The degeneration of the basal ganglia lead to a Parkinson's presentation. The degeneration in other areas lead to **autonomic dysfunction** (causing postural hypotension, constipation, abnormal sweating and sexual dysfunction) and **cerebellar dysfunction** (causing ataxia).

Dementia with Lewy Bodies
This is a type of dementia associated with features of Parkinsonism. It causes a progressive cognitive decline. There are associated symptoms of visual hallucinations, delusions, disorders of REM sleep and fluctuating consciousness.

Others
Two other Parkinson's-plus syndromes exist that involves a number of complex progressive neurological features:
- **Progressive Supranuclear Palsy**
- **Corticobasal Degeneration**

Diagnosis

Parkinson's disease is diagnosed clinically based on symptoms and examination. The diagnosis should be made by a specialist with experience in diagnosing Parkinson's. NICE recommend using the **UK Parkinson's Disease Society brain bank clinical diagnostic criteria**.

Management

Treatment is initiated and guided by a specialist, and is tailored to each individual patient and their response to different medications. There is no cure, so treatment is focused on controlling symptoms and minimising side effects.

Patients describe themselves as "**on**" when the medications are acting and they are moving freely, and "**off**" when the medications wear out, they have significant symptoms and their next dose is due.

Levodopa
This is **synthetic dopamine** given orally to boost dopamine levels. It is usually combined with a drug that stops levodopa being broken down in the body before it gets the chance to enter the brain. These are **peripheral decarboxylase inhibitors**. Examples are **carbidopa** and **benserazide**.

Combination drugs are:
- Co-benyldopa (**levodopa** and **benserazide**)
- Co-careldopa (**levodopa** and **carbidopa**)

Levodopa is the most effective treatment for symptoms but becomes less effective over time. It is often reserved for when other treatments are not managing to control symptoms.

The main side effect of dopamine is when the dose is too high patients develop **dyskinesias**. Theses are abnormal movements associated with **excessive motor activity**. Examples are:
- **Dystonia**: This is where excessive muscle contraction leads to abnormal postures or exaggerated movements.
- **Chorea**: These are abnormal involuntary movements that can be jerking and random.
- **Athetosis**: These are involuntary twisting or writhing movements usually in the fingers, hands or feet.

COMT Inhibitors

The main example of this is **entacapone**. These are inhibitors of **catechol-o-methyltransferase** (**COMT**). The **COMT enzyme** metabolises levodopa in both the body and brain. Entacapone is taken with levodopa (and a decarboxylase inhibitor) to slow breakdown of the levodopa in the brain. It extends the effective duration of the levodopa.

Dopamine Agonists

These mimic dopamine in the basal ganglia and stimulate the **dopamine receptors**. They are less effective than levodopa in reducing symptoms. They are usually used to delay the use of levodopa and are then used in combination with levodopa to reduce the dose of levodopa that is required to control symptoms. One notable side effect with prolonged use is **pulmonary fibrosis**. Examples are:
- Bromocryptine
- Pergolide
- Carbergoline

Monoamine Oxidase-B Inhibitors

Monoamine oxidase **enzymes** break down **neurotransmitters** such as **dopamine**, **serotonin** and **adrenaline**. The **monoamine oxidase-B** enzyme is more specific to dopamine and does not act on serotonin or adrenalin. These medications block this enzyme and therefore help increase the circulating dopamine. Similarly to dopamine agonists, they are usually used to delay the use of levodopa and then in combination with levodopa to reduce the required dose. Examples are:
- Selegiline
- Rasagiline

Benign Essential Tremor

Benign essential tremor is a relatively common condition associated with older age. It is characterised by a **fine tremor** affecting all the **voluntary** muscles. It is most notable in the hands but affects many other areas, for example causing a head tremor, jaw tremor and vocal tremor.

Features

- Fine tremor
- Symmetrical
- More prominent on voluntary movement
- Worse when tired, stressed or after caffeine
- Improved by alcohol
- Absent during sleep

Differential Diagnosis of Tremor

Benign essential tremor is diagnosed clinically based on the presenting features. It is important to look for features to exclude other causes of a tremor.

The key differential diagnoses of a tremor are:
- Parkinson's disease
- Multiple sclerosis
- Huntington's chorea
- Hyperthyroidism
- Fever
- Medications (e.g. antipsychotics)

Management

There is no definitive treatment for benign essential tremor. The tremor is not harmful and does not require treatment if not causing functional or psychological problems.

Medications that can be tried to improve symptoms are:
- **Propranolol** (a non-selective beta blocker)
- **Primidone** (a barbiturate anti-epileptic medication)

Epilepsy

Epilepsy is an umbrella term for a condition where there is a tendency to have seizures. Seizures are transient episodes of **abnormal electrical activity** in the brain. There are many different types of seizure.

A diagnosis of epilepsy is made by a specialist based on the characteristics of the seizure episodes.

Investigations

An **electroencephalogram** (**EEG**) can show typical patterns in different forms of epilepsy and support the diagnosis.

An **MRI brain** can be used to visualise the structure of the brain. It is used to diagnose structural problems that may be associated with seizures and other pathology such as tumours.

Other investigations can be used to exclude other pathology, particularly an **ECG** to exclude problems in the heart.

Types of Seizures

There are many types of seizures. There are different treatments for epilepsy based on the type of seizures. The aim of treatment is to be seizure free on the minimum anti-epileptic medications. Ideally they should be on monotherapy with a single anti-epileptic drug. Treatment is initiated and guided by a specialist.

Generalised Tonic-Clonic Seizures
These are what most people think of with an epileptic seizure. There is loss of consciousness and **tonic** (muscle tensing) and **clonic** (muscle jerking) episodes. Typically the tonic phase comes before the clonic phase. There may be associated tongue biting, incontinence, groaning and irregular breathing.

After the seizure there is a prolonged **post-ictal period** where the person is confused, drowsy and feels irritable or depressed.

Management of tonic-clonic seizures is with:
- First line: **sodium valproate**
- Second line: **lamotrigine** or **carbamazepine**

Focal Seizures
Focal seizures start in the **temporal lobes**. They affect hearing, speech, memory and emotions. There are various ways that focal seizures can present:
- Hallucinations
- Memory flashbacks
- Déjà vu
- Doing strange things on autopilot

One way to remember the treatment is that they are the reverse of tonic-clonic seizures:
- First line: **carbamazepine** or **lamotrigine**
- Second line: **sodium valproate** or **levetiracetam**

Absence Seizures
Absence seizures typically happen in children. The patient becomes blank, stares into space and then abruptly returns to normal. During the episode they are unaware of their surroundings and won't respond. These typically only lasts 10 to 20 seconds. Most patients (> 90%) stop having absence seizures as they get older. Management is:
- First line: **sodium valproate** or **ethosuximide**

Atonic Seizures
Atonic seizures are also known as "**drop attacks**". They are characterised by brief lapses in muscle tone. These don't usually last more than 3 minutes. They typically begin in childhood. They may be indicative of **Lennox-Gastaut syndrome**. Management is:
- First line: **sodium valproate**
- Second line: **lamotrigine**

Myoclonic Seizures
Myoclonic seizures present as sudden brief muscle contractions, like a sudden "jump". The patient usually remains awake during the episode. They occur in various forms of epilepsy but typically happen in children as part of **juvenile myoclonic epilepsy**. Management is:
- First line: **sodium valproate**
- Other options: **lamotrigine**, **levetiracetam** or **topiramate**

Infantile Spasms
This is also known as **West syndrome**. It is a rare (1 in 4000) disorder starting in infancy at around 6 months of age. It is characterised by clusters of full body spasms. There is a poor prognosis: 1/3 die by age 25, however 1/3 are seizure free. It can be difficult to treat but first line treatments are:
- *Prednisolone*
- *Vigabatrin*

Epilepsy Maintenance Medication

Sodium Valproate
This is a first line option for most forms of epilepsy (except focal seizures). It works by increasing the activity of GABA, which has a relaxing effect on the brain.

Notable side effects:
- **Teratogenic** so patients need careful advice about contraception
- Liver damage and hepatitis
- Hair loss
- Tremor

There are a lot of warning about the **teratogenic** effects of **sodium valproate** and NICE updated their guidelines in 2018 to reflect this. It must be avoided in girls or women unless there are no suitable alternatives and strict criteria are met to ensure they do not get pregnant.

Carbamazepine
This is first line for focal seizures. Notable side effects are:
- Agranulocytosis
- Aplastic anaemia
- Induces the P450 system so there are many drug interactions

Phenytoin
Notable side effects:
- Folate and vitamin D deficiency
- Megaloblastic anaemia (folate deficiency)
- Osteomalacia (vitamin D deficiency)

Ethosuximide
Notable side effects:
- Night terrors
- Rashes

Lamotrigine
Notable side effects:
- Stevens-Johnson syndrome or DRESS syndrome. These are life threatening skin rashes.
- Leukopenia

Status Epilepticus

Status epilepticus is an important condition you need to be aware of and how to treat. It is a medical emergency. It is defined as seizures lasting **more than 5 minutes** or **more than 3 seizures in one hour**.

Management of status epileptics in the hospital (take an ABCDE approach):
- Secure the airway
- Give high-concentration oxygen
- Assess cardiac and respiratory function
- Check blood glucose levels
- Gain intravenous access (insert a cannula)
- IV **lorazepam** 4mg, repeated after 10 minutes if the seizure continues
- If seizures persist: IV **phenobarbital** or **phenytoin**

Medical options in the community:
- Buccal midazolam
- Rectal diazepam

Neuropathic Pain

Neuropathic pain is caused by abnormal functioning of the sensory nerves, delivering abnormal and painful signals to the brain. Abnormal sensations from the skin, such as burning, tingling, pins and needles and numbness, is called **paresthesia**.

Presentation

Neuropathic pain can affect a wide variety of areas with number of different causes:
- **Post-herpetic neuralgia** from **shingles** is in the distribution of a **dermatome** and usually on the trunk
- Nerve damage from surgery
- Multiple sclerosis
- Diabetic neuralgia typically affects the feet
- Trigeminal neuralgia
- **Complex regional pain syndrome** (**CRPS**)

Typical Features

- Burning
- Tingling
- Pins and needles
- Electric shocks
- Loss of sensation to touch of the affected area

DN4 Questionnaire

This is used to assess the characteristics of the pain to determine whether it is likely to be neuropathic. It involves a combination of symptoms and examination. They are scored out of 10. A score of 4 or more indicates neuropathic pain.

Management

There are four first line treatments for neuropathic pain:
- **Amitriptyline** is a tricyclic antidepressant
- **Duloxetine** is an SNRI antidepressant
- **Gabapentin** is an anticonvulsant
- **Pregabalin** is an anticonvulsant

NICE recommend using one of these four medications to control neuropathic pain. If that does not work then stop it and start an alternative. Repeat this until all four have been tried.

Other options
- Tramadol ONLY as a rescue for short term control of flares
- Capsaicin cream (chilli pepper cream) for localised areas of pain
- Physiotherapy to maintain strength
- Psychological input to help with understanding and coping

Trigeminal neuralgia is a type of neuropathic pain however NICE recommend *carbamazepine* as first line for trigeminal neuralgia and if that does not work to refer to a specialist.

Complex Regional Pain Syndrome

This is a condition where areas are affected by abnormal nerve functioning, causing neuropathic pain and abnormal sensations. It is usually isolated to one limb. Often it is triggered by an injury to the area.

The area can become very painful and hypersensitive even to simple inputs such as wearing clothing. It can also intermittently swell, change colour, change temperature, flush with blood and have abnormal sweating.

Treatment is often guided by a pain specialist and is similar to other neuropathic pain.

Facial Nerve Palsy

Facial nerve palsy refers to isolated dysfunction of the *facial nerve*. This typically presents with a *unilateral facial weakness*. It is important to understand some basics about the pathway of the facial nerve and the function of the facial nerve to consider the causes and management.

Facial Nerve Pathway

The facial nerve exits the *brainstem* at the *cerebellopontine angle*. On its journey to the face it passes through the *temporal bone* and *parotid gland*.

It then divides in to five branches that supply different areas of the face:
- *Temporal*
- *Zygomatic*
- *Buccal*
- *Marginal mandibular*
- *Cervical*

Facial Nerve Function

There are three functions of the facial nerve: *motor*, *sensory* and *parasympathetic*.

Motor: It supplies the muscles of *facial expression*, the *stapedius* in the inner ear and the *posterior digastric*, *stylohyoid* and *platysma* muscles in the neck.

Sensory: It carries *taste* from the *anterior 2/3* of the tongue.

Parasympathetic: It provides the parasympathetic supply to the *submandibular* and *sublingual salivary glands* and the *lacrimal gland* (stimulating tear production).

Upper vs Lower Motor Neurone Lesion

A very common exam task is to distinguish between an **upper motor neurone** and **lower motor neurone** facial nerve palsy. It is essential to be able to make this distinction, because in a patient with a new onset **upper motor neurone facial nerve palsy** you should be referring urgently with a suspected **stroke**, whereas patients with lower motor neurone facial nerve palsy can be reassured and managed in the community.

Each side of the forehead has **upper motor neurone innervation** by **both sides** of the brain. Each side of the forehead only has **lower motor neurone innervation** from **one side** of the brain.

In an **upper motor neurone lesion**, the **forehead will be spared** and the patient can move their forehead on the affected side.

In a **lower motor neurone lesion**, the **forehead will NOT be spared** and the patient cannot move their forehead on the affected side.

Upper Motor Neurone Lesions

Unilateral upper motor neurone lesions occur in:
- **Cerebrovascular accidents** (strokes)
- **Tumours**

Bilateral upper motor neurone lesions are rare. They may occur in:
- **Pseudobulbar palsies**
- **Motor neurone disease**

Bell's Palsy

Bell's palsy is a relatively common condition. It is **idiopathic**, meaning there is no clear cause. It presents as a unilateral lower motor neurone facial nerve palsy. The majority of patients fully recover over several weeks, but recovery may take up to 12 months. A third are left with some residual weakness.

If patients present within 72 hours of developing symptoms, NICE guidelines recommend considering **prednisolone** as treatment, either:
- 50mg for 10 days
- 60mg for 5 days followed by a 5 day reducing regime of 10mg a day

Patients also require **lubricating eye drops** to prevent the eye on the affected drying out and being damaged. If they develop pain in the eye they need ophthalmology review for **exposure keratopathy**. Tape can be used to keep the eye closed at night.

Ramsay-Hunt Syndrome

Ramsay-Hunt syndrome is caused by the **herpes zoster virus**. It presents as a unilateral lower motor neurone facial nerve palsy. Patients stereotypically have a painful and tender **vesicular rash** in the ear canal, pinna and around the ear on the affected side. This rash can extend to the anterior two thirds of the tongue and hard palate.

Treatment should ideally be initiated within 72 hours. Treatment is with:
- **Prednisolone**
- **Aciclovir**

Patients also require **lubricating eye drops**.

TOM TIP: Ramsay-Hunt syndrome is a very popular presentation in your MCQ exams. Look out for that patient with a vesicular rash around their ear and a facial nerve palsy.

Other Causes of Lower Motor Neurone Facial Nerve Palsy

Infection:
- Otitis media
- Malignant otitis externa
- HIV
- Lyme's disease

Systemic disease:
- Diabetes
- Sarcoidosis
- Leukaemia
- Multiple sclerosis
- Guillain–Barré syndrome

Tumours:
- Acoustic neuroma
- Parotid tumours
- Cholesteatomas

Trauma:
- Direct nerve trauma
- Damage during surgery
- Base of skull fractures

Brain Tumours

Brain tumours are abnormal growths in the brain. There are many different types of brain tumour. They vary from benign tumours (e.g. *meningiomas*) to highly malignant (e.g. *glioblastomas*).

Presentation

Often brain tumours do not have any symptoms, particularly when they are small. As they develop they present with *focal neurological symptoms* depending on the location of the lesion.

Brain tumours often present with symptoms and signs of *raised intracranial pressure*. As a tumour grows within the skull it takes up space. This leaves less space for the other contents of the skull (such as the cerebrospinal fluid) and leads to a rise in the pressure within the intracranial space.

TOM TIP: A common exam question asks the location of the lesion based on the neurology. They often describe a patient that has had an unusual change in personality and behaviour. This indicates a tumour in the frontal lobe. Remember that the frontal lobe is responsible for personality and higher level decision making.

Raised Intracranial Pressure

Anything that takes up additional space within the skull will increase the pressure in the intracranial space. Raised intracranial pressure causes symptoms that can lead to a diagnosis of a brain tumour. **Papilloedema** is a key finding on *fundoscopy* in patients with raised intracranial pressure.

Causes
- Brain tumours
- Intracranial haemorrhage
- Idiopathic intracranial hypertension
- Abscesses or infection

Presentation
Concerning features of a headache that should prompt further examination and investigation include:
- Constant
- Nocturnal
- Worse on waking
- Worse on coughing, straining or bending forward
- Vomiting

Other presenting features of raised intracranial pressure may be:
- Altered mental state
- Visual field defects
- Seizures (particularly focal)
- Unilateral ptosis
- Third and sixth nerve palsies
- Papilloedema (on fundoscopy)

Papilloedema

Papilloedema is a swelling of the **optic disc** secondary to **raised intracranial pressure**. *Papill-* refers to a small rounded raised area (the optic disc) and *-oedema* refers to the swelling. The **sheath** around the **optic nerve** is connected with the **subarachnoid space**. Therefore it is possible for CSF under high pressure to flow in to the **optic nerve sheath**. This increases the pressure around the optic nerve where it connects with the back of the eye at the optic disc, causing optic disc swelling. This can be seen on *fundoscopy* examination as:
- Blurring of the optic disc margin
- Elevated optic disc (look for the way the retinal vessels flow across the disc to see the elevation)
- Loss of venous pulsation
- Engorged retinal veins
- Haemorrhages around optic disc
- **Paton's lines**, which are creases in the retina around the optic disc

TOM TIP: It can be tricky to learn to recognise papilloedema. When looking for elevation of the optic disc, look at the way the retinal vessels flow across the disc. Vessels are able to flow straight across a flat surface, whereas they will curve over a raised disc.

Types of Brain Tumour

Secondary Metastases
The common cancers that metastasise to the brain are:
- Lung
- Breast
- Colorectal
- Prostate

Gliomas
Gliomas are tumours of the **glial cells** in the brain or spinal cord. Gliomas are graded from 1 to 4. Grade 1 are the most benign (possibly curable with surgery). Grade 4 are the most malignant (glioblastomas). There are three types to remember (listed from most to least malignant):
- Astrocytoma (**glioblastoma multiforme** is the most common)
- Oligodendroglioma
- Ependymoma

Meningiomas
Meningiomas are tumours growing from the cells of the **meninges** in the brain and spinal cord. They are usually benign, however they take up space and this mass effect can lead to raised intracranial pressure and neurological symptoms.

Pituitary Tumours
Pituitary tumours tend to be benign. If they grow large enough they can press on the **optic chiasm** causing a specific visual field defect called a **bitemporal hemianopia**. This causes loss of the outer half of the visual fields in both eyes. They have the potential to cause **hormone deficiencies** (**hypopituitarism**) or to release **excessive hormones** leading to:
- Acromegaly (excessive growth hormone)
- Hyperprolactinaemia (excessive prolactin)
- Cushing's disease (excessive ACTH and cortisol)
- Thyrotoxicosis (excessive TSH and thyroid hormone)

Acoustic Neuroma (AKA Vestibular Schwannoma)
Acoustic neuromas are tumours of the **Schwann cells** surrounding the **auditory nerve** that innervates the inner ear. They occur around the "**cerebellopontine angle**" and are sometimes referred to as **cerebellopontine angle tumours**. They are slow growing but eventually grow large enough to produce symptoms and become dangerous.

Acoustic neuromas are usually unilateral. Bilateral acoustic neuromas are associated with **neurofibromatosis type 2**.

Classic symptoms of an **acoustic neuroma** are:
- Hearing loss
- Tinnitus
- Balance problems

They can also be associated with a facial nerve palsy.

Managing Brain Tumours

There is massive variation in brain tumours from completely benign to extremely malignant. Surgery is dependent on the grade and behaviour of the brain tumour.

Management options include:
- Palliative care
- Chemotherapy
- Radiotherapy
- Surgery

Treatment of Pituitary Tumours

- Trans-sphenoidal surgery
- Radiotherapy
- **Bromocriptine** to block **prolactin** secreting tumours
- Somatostatin analogues (e.g. **ocreotide**) to block **growth hormone** secreting tumours

Huntington's Chorea

Huntington's chorea is an **autosomal dominant** genetic condition that causes a progressive deterioration in the nervous system. Patients are usually asymptomatic until symptoms begin around aged 30 to 50.

Huntington's chorea is a "**trinucleotide repeat disorder**" that involves a genetic mutation in the **HTT gene** on **chromosome 4**.

Anticipation

Huntington's chorea displays something called genetic "**anticipation**". Anticipation is a feature of **trinucleotide repeat disorders**. This is where successive generations have more **repeats** in the gene, resulting in:
- Earlier age of onset
- Increased severity of disease

TOM TIP: Anticipation is a common topic of exam questions. It is worth remembering the features and connection with Huntington's for your exams.

Presentation

Huntington's chorea usually presents with an insidious, progressive worsening of symptoms. It typically begins with **cognitive**, **psychiatric** or **mood problems**. These are followed by the development of movement disorders.
- **Chorea** (involuntary, abnormal movements)
- **Eye movement disorders**
- Speech difficulties (**dysarthria**)
- Swallowing difficulties (**dysphagia**)

Diagnosis

Diagnosis is made in a specialist genetic centre using a genetic test for the faulty gene. It involves pre-test and post-test counselling regarding the implications of the results.

Management

There are currently no treatment options for slowing or stopping the progression of the disease.

The key to management of the condition is supporting the person and their family.
- Effectively **breaking bad news**
- Involvement of a **multidisciplinary team** in supporting and maintaining their quality of life (e.g. occupational therapy, physiotherapy and psychology)
- **Speech and language therapy** where there are speech and swallowing difficulties
- **Genetic counselling** regarding relatives, pregnancy and children
- **Advanced directives** to document the patients wishes as the disease progresses
- **End of life** care planning

Medical treatment is based on symptomatic relief. As the disease progresses medication requirements may change. It is important to discontinue unnecessary medication to minimise adverse effects.

Medications that can suppress the disordered movement:
- Antipsychotics (e.g. olanzapine)
- Benzodiazepines (e.g. diazepam)
- Dopamine-depleting agents (e.g. tetrabenazine)

Depression can be treated with antidepressants.

Prognosis

Huntington's chorea is a progressive condition. Life expectance is around 15-20 years after the onset of symptoms. As the disease progresses patients become more susceptible and less able to fight off illnesses. Death is often due to respiratory disease (e.g. pneumonia). **Suicide** is a more common cause of death than in the general population.

Myasthenia Gravis

Myasthenia gravis is an **autoimmune** condition that causes muscle weakness that gets progressively worse with activity and improves with rest.

Interestingly myasthenia gravis affects men and women at different ages. Typical patients are either a woman under the age of 40 or a man over the age of 60.

There is a strong link between **thymoma** (tumours of the **thymus gland**) and myasthenia gravis. 10 to 20% of patients with myasthenia gravis have a thymoma. 20 to 40% of patients with a thymoma develop myasthenia gravis.

Pathophysiology

Motor nerves communicate with **muscles** at **neuromuscular junctions**. At the neuromuscular junction, **axons** of motor nerves are situated across a **synapse** from the **post-synaptic membrane** on the **muscle cell**. The axons release a **neurotransmitter** from the **pre-synaptic membrane**. The neurotransmitter at these junctions is called **acetylcholine**. The acetylcholine travels across the synapse and attaches to **receptors** on the post-synaptic membrane. They stimulate the receptors, and this signal leads to **muscle contraction**.

In around 85% of patients with myasthenia gravis, **acetylcholine receptor antibodies** are produced by the immune system. These bind to the **postsynaptic** neuromuscular junction **receptors**. This blocks the receptor and prevents the acetylcholine from being able to stimulate the receptor and trigger muscle contraction. As the receptors are used more during muscle activity, more of them become blocked up. This leads to less effective stimulation of the muscle with increased activity. There is more muscle weakness the more the muscles are used. This improves with rest as more receptors are freed up for use again.

These antibodies also activate the **complement system** within the neuromuscular junction, leading to damage to cells at the **postsynaptic membrane**. This further worsens the symptoms.

There are two other antibodies that cause the other 15% of cases of myasthenia gravis. These are antibodies against **muscle-specific kinase** (**MuSK**) and antibodies against **low-density lipoprotein receptor-related protein 4** (**LRP4**). **MuSK** and **LRP4** are important proteins for the creation and organisation of the **acetylcholine receptor**. Destruction of these proteins by **autoantibodies** leads to inadequate **acetylcholine receptors**. This causes the symptoms of myasthenia gravis.

Presentation

The severity of symptoms can vary dramatically between patients. They can be mild and subtle or life threateningly severe. The characteristic feature is weakness that gets worse with muscle use and improves with rest. Symptoms are typically minimal in the morning and worst at the end of the day.

The symptoms most affect the **proximal muscles** and small muscles of the head and neck. It leads to:
- Extraocular muscle weakness causing double vision (**diplopia**)
- Eyelid weakness causing drooping of the eyelids (**ptosis**)
- Weakness in facial movements
- Difficulty with swallowing
- Fatigue in the jaw when chewing
- Slurred speech

Examination

There are a few ways to elicit fatiguability in the muscles:
- Repeated blinking will exacerbate ptosis
- Prolonged upward gazing will exacerbate diplopia on further eye movement testing
- Repeated abduction of one arm 20 times will result in unilateral weakness when comparing both sides

Check for a **thymectomy scar**.

Test the **forced vital capacity** (**FVC**).

Diagnosis

Diagnosis can be made by testing directly for the relevant antibodies:
- **Acetylcholine receptor (ACh-R) antibodies** (85% of patients)
- **Muscle-specific kinase (MuSK) antibodies** (10% of patients)
- **LRP4 (low-density lipoprotein receptor-related protein 4) antibodies** (less than 5%)

A **CT** or **MRI** of the **thymus** gland is used to look for a thymoma.

The **edrophonium test** can be helpful where there is doubt about the diagnosis.

Edrophonium Test

Patients are given an IV dose of **edrophonium chloride** (or **neostigmine**). There are **cholinesterase enzymes** in the **neuromuscular junction** that break down **acetylcholine**. Edrophonium block these enzymes and stop the breakdown of acetylcholine. As a result the level of acetylcholine at the neuromuscular junction increases. This briefly and temporarily relieves the weakness. This establishes a diagnosis of myasthenia gravis.

Treatment options

- **Reversible acetylcholinesterase inhibitors** (usually **pyridostigmine** or **neostigmine**) increases the amount of acetylcholine in the neuromuscular junction and improve symptoms
- **Immunosuppression** (e.g. prednisolone or azathioprine) suppresses the production of antibodies
- **Thymectomy** can improve symptoms even in patients without a thymoma

Monoclonal antibodies
- **Rituximab** is a monoclonal antibody that targets B cells and reduces the production of antibodies. It is available on the NHS if standard treatment is not effective and certain criteria are met.
- **Eculizumab** is a monoclonal antibody that targets **complement protein C5**. This could potentially prevent the complement activation and destruction of acetylcholine receptors. There is ongoing research and debate about whether the evidence is strong enough to offer it on the NHS. It is currently not recommended by NICE.

Myasthenic Crisis

Myasthenic crisis is a severe complication of myasthenia gravis. It can be life threatening. It causes an acute worsening of symptoms, often triggered by another illness such as a respiratory tract infection. This can lead to respiratory failure as a result of weakness in the muscles of respiration. Patients may require **non-invasive ventilation** with **BiPAP** or full **intubation and ventilation**.

Medical treatment of myasthenic crisis is with **immunomodulatory therapies** such as **IV immunoglobulins** and **plasma exchange**.

Lambert-Eaton Myasthenic Syndrome

Lambert-Eaton myasthenic syndrome has a similar set of features to **myasthenia gravis**. It causes progressive muscle weakness with increased use as a result of damage to the neuromuscular junction. The symptoms tend to be more insidious and less pronounced than in myasthenia gravis.

Lambert-Eaton syndrome typically occurs in patients with **small cell lung cancer**. It is a result of antibodies produced by the immune system against **voltage-gated calcium channels** in **small cell lung cancer** (**SCLC**) cells. These antibodies also target and damage **voltage-gated calcium channels** in the **presynaptic terminals** of the **neuromuscular junction** where **motor nerves** communicate with **muscle cells**.

These **voltage-gated calcium channels** are responsible for assisting in the release of **acetylcholine** into the **synapse** of the **neuromuscular junction**. This acetylcholine then binds to the **acetylcholine receptors** and stimulates a muscle contraction. When these channels are destroyed, less acetylcholine is release into the synapse.

Presentation

The symptoms of Lambert-Eaton syndrome tend to develop slowly. The **proximal muscles** are most notably affected, causing proximal muscle weakness. It can also affect the **intraocular muscles** causing double vision (**diplopia**), the **levator muscles** in the eyelid causing eyelid drooping (**ptosis**) and the **oropharyngeal muscles** causing slurred speech and swallowing problems (**dysphagia**). This weakness is worse with prolonged used of the muscles.

Treatment

It is important to diagnose and manage any underlying malignancy. In older smokers with symptoms of Lambert-Eaton syndrome consider investigating for **small cell lung cancer**.

Amifampridine is a medication that allows more acetylcholine to be released in the neuromuscular junction synapses. It works by blocking voltage-gated potassium channels in the presynaptic cells, which in turn prolongs the depolarisation of the cell membrane and assists calcium channels in carrying out their action. This improves symptoms in Lambert-Eaton syndrome.

Other options:
- Immunosuppressants (e.g. prednisolone or azathioprine)
- IV immunoglobulins
- Plasmapheresis

Charcot-Marie-Tooth Disease

Charcot-Marie-Tooth disease is an **inherited disease** that affects the peripheral **motor** and **sensory** nerves. There are various types of Charcot-Marie-Tooth, with different genetic mutations and different pathophysiology. They cause dysfunction in the **myelin** or the **axons**. The majority of mutations are inherited in an **autosomal dominant** pattern. Symptoms usually start to appear before the age of 10 years but the onset of symptoms can be delayed until 40 or later.

Classical Features

There are some classical features of Charcot-Marie-Tooth to look out for when examining patient. Not all of these features will apply to all patients with the condition but they are a helpful set of features to look out for, particularly in your OSCEs:
- High foot arches (*pes cavus*)
- Distal muscle wasting causing "*inverted champagne bottle legs*"
- Weakness in the lower legs, particularly loss of **ankle dorsiflexion**
- Weakness in the hands
- Reduced tendon reflexes
- Reduced muscle tone
- Peripheral sensory loss

Causes of Peripheral Neuropathy

- **A** - **A**lcohol
- **B** - **B**12 deficiency
- **C** - **C**ancer and **C**hronic Kidney Disease
- **D** - **D**iabetes and **D**rugs (e.g. *isoniazid*, *amiodarone* and *cisplatin*)
- **E** - **E**very vasculitis

TOM TIP: This is a common OSCE scenario. You will have to perform a neurological examination on a patient that has peripheral neuropathy. Charcot-Marie-Tooth is a relatively common (1 in 2,500 people) condition with good signs that has a high chance of appearing in your exams. Look for the other features, suggest the diagnosis, then run through the ABCDE mnemonic to suggest the possible other causes of a peripheral neuropathy.

Management

There is no treatment to alter the underlying disease or prevent it progressing. Management is purely supportive with input from various members of the multidisciplinary team:
- *Neurologists* and *geneticists* to make the diagnosis
- *Physiotherapists* to maintain muscle strength and joint range of motion
- *Occupational therapists* to assist with activities of living
- *Podiatrists* to help with foot symptoms and suggest insoles and other orthoses to improve symptoms
- *Orthopaedic surgeons* to correct disabling joint deformities

Guillain-Barré Syndrome

Guillain-Barré syndrome is an "*acute paralytic polyneuropathy*" that affects the peripheral nervous system. It causes acute, symmetrical, ascending weakness and can also cause sensory symptoms. It is usually triggered by an infection and is particularly associated with to *campylobacter jejuni*, *cytomegalovirus* and *Epstein-Barr virus*.

Pathophysiology

Guillain-Barré is thought to occur due to a process called *molecular mimicry*. The **B cells** of the immune system create **antibodies** against the **antigens** on the **pathogen** that causes the preceding infection. These antibodies also match proteins on the nerve cells. They may target proteins on the **myelin sheath** of the motor nerve cell or the **nerve axon** itself.

Presentation

- Symmetrical ascending weakness (starting at the feet and moving up body)
- Reduced reflexes
- There may be peripheral loss of sensation or neuropathic pain
- It may progress to the cranial nerves and cause facial nerve weakness

Clinical Course

Symptoms usually start within 4 weeks of the preceding infection. The symptoms typically start in the feet and progresses upward. Symptoms peak within 2 to 4 weeks, then there is a recovery period that can last months to years.

Diagnosis

A diagnosis of Guillain-Barré syndrome is made clinically. The **Brighton criteria** can be used for diagnosis. Diagnosis can be supported by investigations:

- **Nerve conduction studies** (reduced signal through the nerves)
- **Lumbar puncture** for **CSF** (**raised protein** with a normal cell count and glucose)

Management

- IV immunoglobulins
- Plasma exchange
- Supportive care
- VTE prophylaxis (**pulmonary embolism** is a leading cause of death)

In severe cases with **respiratory failure** patients may need intubation, ventilation and admission to the intensive care unit.

Prognosis

- 80% will fully recover
- 15% will be left with some neurological disability
- 5% will die

Neurofibromatosis

Neurofibromatosis is a genetic condition that causes nerve tumours (*neuromas*) to develop throughout the nervous system. These tumours are benign, however they do cause neurological and structural problems. There are two types of neurofibromatosis with different features. **Neurofibromatosis type 1** is more common than **type 2**. The majority of this section focuses on type 1.

NF1 Gene

The neurofibromatosis type 1 gene is found on **chromosome 17**. It codes for a protein called **neurofibromin**, which is a **tumour suppressor protein**. **Inheritance** of mutations in this gene is **autosomal dominant**.

Criteria

There are clear diagnostic criteria for NF1 based on the classical features of the condition. There must be **at least 2** of the 7 features to indicate a diagnosis. You can remember this with the mnemonic **CRABBING**.

- C - *Café-au-lait spots* (6 or more) measuring ≥ 5mm in children or ≥ 15mm in adults
- R - **R**elative with NF1
- A - **A**xillary or inguinal freckles
- BB - **B**ony dysplasia such as **B**owing of a long bone or sphenoid wing dysplasia
- I - *Iris hamartomas* (*Lisch nodules*) (2 or more) are yellow brown spots on the iris
- N - **N**eurofibromas (2 or more) **or** 1 plexiform neurofibroma
- G - **G**lioma of the optic nerve

Investigations

Diagnosis is based on clinical criteria and no investigations are required to make a definitive diagnosis.

Genetic testing can be used where there is doubt.

Xrays can be used to investigate bone pain and bone lesions.

Imaging with **CT** and **MRI** scans can be used to investigate lesions in the brain, spinal cord and elsewhere in the body.

Management

There is no treatment of the underlying disease process or ways to prevent the development of neurofibromas or complications. Management is to control symptoms, monitor the disease and treat complications.

Complications

- Migraines
- Epilepsy
- **Renal artery stenosis** causing **hypertension**
- Learning and behavioural problems (e.g. ADHD)
- Scoliosis of the spine
- Vision loss (secondary to optic nerve gliomas)
- **Malignant peripheral nerve sheath tumours**
- **Gastrointestinal stromal tumour** (a type of sarcoma)
- Brain tumours
- Spinal cord tumours with associated neurology (e.g. paraplegia)
- Increased risk of cancer (e.g. breast cancer)
- Leukaemia

Neurofibromatosis Type 2

The neurofibromatosis type 2 gene is found on **chromosome 22**. It codes for a protein called **merlin**, which is a **tumour suppressor protein** particularly important in **Schwann cells**. Mutations in this gene lead to the development of **schwannomas** (benign nerve sheath tumours of the Schwann cells). Inheritance is **autosomal dominant**.

Neurofibromatosis type 2 is most associated with **acoustic neuromas**. These are tumours of the **auditory nerve** innervating the inner ear. Symptoms of an **acoustic neuroma** are:
- Hearing loss
- Tinnitus
- Balance problems

Schwannomas can also develop in the brain and spinal cord with symptoms based on the location of the lesion.

Surgery can be used to resect tumours, although there is a risk of permanent nerve damage.

TOM TIP: Bilateral acoustic neuromas almost certainly indicate neurofibromatosis type 2. This is a popular association in exams so worth remembering.

Tuberous Sclerosis

Tuberous sclerosis is a **genetic condition** that causes features in multiple systems. The characteristic feature is the development of **hamartomas**. These are benign neoplastic growths of the tissue that they originate from. **Hamartomas** cause problems based on the location of the lesion. They commonly affect the:
- Skin
- Brain
- Lungs
- Heart
- Kidneys
- Eyes

Tuberous sclerosis is caused by mutations in one of two genes:
- **TSC1 gene** on **chromosome 9**, which codes for **hamartin**
- **TSC2 gene** on **chromosome 16**, which codes for **tuberin**

Hamartin and **tuberin** interact with each other to control the size and growth of cells. Abnormalities in one of these proteins leads to abnormal cell size and growth.

Skin Signs

- **Ash leaf spots** are depigmented areas of skin shaped like an ash leaf
- **Shagreen patches** are thickened, dimpled, pigmented patches of skin
- **Angiofibromas** are small skin coloured or pigmented papules that occur over the nose and cheeks
- **Subungual fibromata** are fibromas growing from the nail bed. They are usually circular painless lumps that grow slowly and displace the nail
- **Cafe-au-lait spots** are light brown "**coffee and milk**" coloured flat pigmented lesions on the skin
- **Poliosis** is an isolated patch of white hair on the head, eyebrows, eyelashes or beard

Neurological Features

- Epilepsy
- Learning disability and developmental delay

Other Features

- Rhabdomyomas in the heart
- Gliomas (tumours of the brain and spinal cord)
- Polycystic kidneys
- **Lymphangioleimyomatosis** are abnormal growth in smooth muscle cells, often affecting the lungs. These can cause cough, shortness of breath, chest pain, haemoptysis and pneumothorax.
- Retinal hamartomas

Presentation

The classical presentation is a child presenting with epilepsy found to have skin features of tuberous sclerosis. It can also present in adulthood.

Management

Management is supportive with monitoring and treating complications such as epilepsy. There is no treatment for the underlying gene defect.

Headaches

Headaches are a very common presentation with a large number of differential diagnoses.

Differential Diagnosis

- Tension headaches
- Migraines
- Cluster headaches
- Secondary headaches
- Sinusitis
- Giant cell arteritis
- Glaucoma
- Intracranial haemorrhage
- Subarachnoid haemorrhage
- Analgesic headache
- Hormonal headache
- Cervical spondylosis
- Carbon monoxide poisoning
- Trigeminal neuralgia
- Raised intracranial pressure
- Brain tumours
- Meningitis
- Encephalitis

Red Flags

It is important to consider **red flags** for serious conditions (such as **raised intracranial pressure** and **intracranial haemorrhage**) when taking a history and managing a patient with a headache. The **NICE Clinical Knowledge Summaries** on headache have a good summary of how to assess a headache. This is not an exhaustive list but includes key symptoms to look out for:

- Fever, photophobia or neck stiffness (meningitis or encephalitis)
- New neurological symptoms (haemorrhage, malignancy or stroke)
- Dizziness (stroke)
- Visual disturbance (giant cell arteritis or glaucoma)
- Sudden onset occipital headache (subarachnoid haemorrhage)
- Worse on coughing or straining (raised intracranial pressure)
- Postural, worse on standing, lying or bending over (raised intracranial pressure)
- Severe enough to wake the patient from sleep

- Vomiting (raised intracranial pressure or carbon monoxide poisoning)
- History of trauma (intracranial haemorrhage)
- Pregnancy (pre-eclampsia)

Fundoscopy examination to look for **papilloedema** is an important part of assessment of a headache. Papilloedema indicates raised intracranial pressure, which may be due to a **brain tumour**, **benign intracranial hypertension** or an **intracranial bleed**.

TOM TIP: Practice asking red flag questions so you can demonstrate in an exam that you are thinking about serious causes. This will score extra points in exams and help you document well when you start seeing patients.

Tension Headaches

Tension headaches are very common. Classically they produce a mild ache across the forehead and in a band-like pattern around the head. This may be due to muscle ache in the **frontalis**, **temporalis** and **occipitalis** muscles. Tension headaches comes on and resolve gradually and don't produce visual changes.

Associations
- Stress
- Depression
- Alcohol
- Skipping meals
- Dehydration

Treatment
- Reassurance
- Basic analgesia
- Relaxation techniques
- Hot towels to local area

Secondary Headaches

Secondary headaches give a similar presentation to a tension headache but with a clear cause. They produce a non-specific headache secondary to:
- Underlying medical conditions such as infection, obstructive sleep apnoea or pre-eclampsia
- Alcohol
- Head injury
- Carbon monoxide poisoning

Sinusitis

Sinusitis causes a headache associated with **inflammation** in the **ethmoidal**, **maxillary**, **frontal** or **sphenoidal** sinuses. This usually produces **facial pain** behind the nose, forehead and eyes. There is often tenderness over the effected sinus, which helps to establish the diagnosis.

Sinusitis usually resolves within 2-3 weeks. Most sinusitis is viral. Nasal irrigation with saline can be helpful. Prolonged symptoms can be treated with steroid nasal spray. Antibiotics are occasionally required.

Analgesic Headache

An analgesic headache is a headache caused by long term analgesia use. It gives similar non-specific features to a tension headache. They are secondary to continuous or excessive use of analgesia. Withdrawal of the analgesia is important in treating the headache, although this can be challenging in patients with long term pain and those that believe the analgesia is necessary to treat the headache.

Hormonal Headache

Hormonal headaches are related to **oestrogen**. The produce a generic, non-specific, tension-like headache. They tend to be related to **low oestrogen**:
- Two days before and the first three days of the menstrual period
- Around the menopause
- Pregnancy. It is worse in the first few weeks and improves in the last 6 months. Headaches in the second half of pregnancy should prompt investigations for pre-eclampsia.

The oral contraceptive pill can improve hormonal headaches.

Cervical Spondylosis

Cervical spondylosis is a common condition caused by degenerative changes in the cervical spine. It causes neck pain, usually made worse by movement. It often presents with headaches.

It is important to exclude other causes of neck pain such as inflammation, malignancy and infection. It is also important to exclude spinal cord or nerve root lesions.

Trigeminal Neuralgia

The trigeminal nerve is made up of three branches:
- Ophthalmic (V_1)
- Maxillary (V_2)
- Mandibular (V_3)

Trigeminal neuralgia can affect any combination of the branches. The cause is unclear but it is thought to be caused by compression of the nerve. 90% of cases are unilateral, 10% are bilateral. Around 5 to 10% of people with **multiple sclerosis** have trigeminal neuralgia.

It presents with intense **facial pain** that comes on spontaneously and last anywhere between a few seconds to hours. It is often described as an electricity-like shooting pain. Attacks often worsen in severity over time.

There are a number of possible triggers for the pain in patients with trigeminal neuralgia. These include things like cold weather, spicy food, caffeine and citrus fruits.

Treatment
NICE recommend **carbamazepine** as first line for trigeminal neuralgia. Surgery to decompress or intentionally damage the trigeminal nerve is an option.

Migraines

Migraines are a complex neurological condition that cause headache and other associated symptoms. They occur in "attacks" that often follow a typical pattern.

There are several types of migraine:
- **Migraine without aura**
- **Migraine with aura**
- **Silent migraine** (migraine with aura but without a headache)
- **Hemiplegic migraine**

The pathophysiology of migraine has been studied for decades. Various mechanisms and theories have developed. There is no simple explanation for why migraines occur and it may be a combination of structural, functional, chemical, vascular and inflammatory factors.

Typical Headache Symptoms

Headaches last between 4 and 72 hours. Typical features are:
- Moderate to severe intensity
- Pounding or throbbing in nature
- Usually unilateral but can be bilateral
- Discomfort with lights (**photophobia**)
- Discomfort with loud noises (**phonophobia**)
- With or without **aura**
- Nausea and vomiting

Aura

Aura is the term used to describe the **visual changes** associated with migraines. There can be multiple different types of aura:
- Sparks in vision
- Blurred vision
- Lines across vision
- Loss of different visual fields

Hemiplegic Migraine

Hemiplegic migraines can mimic **stroke**. It is essential to act fast and exclude a stroke in patients presenting with symptoms of hemiplegic migraine.

Symptoms of a hemiplegic migraine can vary significantly. They can include:
- Typical migraine symptoms
- Sudden or gradual onset
- **Hemiplegia** (unilateral weakness of the limbs)
- **Ataxia**
- Changes in consciousness

Triggers

Migraines can have specific triggers that are individual to the person. Often it is not possible to identify triggers. Potential triggers are:
- Stress
- Bright lights
- Strong smells
- Certain foods (e.g. chocolate, cheese and caffeine)
- Dehydration
- Menstruation
- Abnormal sleep patterns
- Trauma

Five stages

The course of a migraine can be described in 5 stages. These stages are not typical of everyone and will vary between patients. Some patients may only experience one or two of the stages. The prodromal stage can involve several days of subtle symptoms such as yawning, fatigue or mood change prior to the onset of the migraine.
- *Premonitory* or *prodromal* stage (can begin 3 days before the headache)
- *Aura* (lasting up to 60 minutes)
- *Headache* stage (lasts 4 to 72 hours)
- *Resolution* stage (the headache can fade away or be relieved completely by vomiting or sleeping)
- *Postdromal* or *recovery* phase

Acute Management

Patients can develop their own patterns for helping to relieve their symptoms. Often patients will go to a dark quiet room and sleep.

Options for medical management are:
- *Paracetamol*
- *Triptans* (e.g. sumatriptan 50mg as the migraine starts)
- *NSAIDs* (e.g ibuprofen or naproxen)
- *Antiemetics* if vomiting occurs (e.g. metoclopramide)

Triptans

Triptans are used to abort migraines when they start to develop. They are **5HT receptors agonists** (**serotonin receptor agonists**). They have various mechanisms of action and it is not clear which mechanisms are responsible for their effects on migraines. They act on:
- Smooth muscle in arteries to cause vasoconstriction
- Peripheral pain receptors to inhibit activation of pain receptors
- Reduce neuronal activity in the central nervous system

Migraine Prophylaxis

Keeping a headache diary can be helpful in identifying the triggers. Avoiding triggers can reduce the frequency of the migraine. A headache diary is also useful in demonstrating the response to treatment.

Certain medications can be used long term to reduce the frequency and severity of attacks:
- **Propranolol**
- **Topiramate** (this is teratogenic and can cause a cleft lip and palate, so patients should not get pregnant)
- **Amitriptyline**

Acupuncture is an option recommended by NICE recommend for the treatment of migraines. It is reported to be as effective as prophylactic medications.

Supplementation with vitamin B2 (*riboflavin*) may reduce frequency and severity.

In migraine specifically triggered around menstruation prophylaxis with **NSAIDS** (e.g. **mefanamic acid**) or **triptans** (*frovatriptan* or *zolmitriptan*) can be used around menstruation as a preventative measure.

Migraines tend to get better over time and people often go in to remission from their symptoms.

Cluster Headaches

Cluster headaches cause severe and unbearable *unilateral* headaches, usually around the eye. They are called cluster headaches as they come in clusters of attacks and then disappear for a while. For example, a patient may suffer 3 to 4 attacks a day for weeks or months followed by a pain free period lasting 1 to 2 years. Attacks last between 15 minutes and 3 hours. They can be triggered by things like alcohol, strong smells and exercise.

A typical patient with cluster headaches in your exams is a 30 to 50 year old male smoker.

Symptoms

Cluster headaches are often described as one of the most severe and intolerable pains in the world. They are sometimes referred to as "*suicide headaches*" due to the severity of the pain.

Symptoms are typically all unilateral:
- Red, swollen and watering eye
- Pupil constriction (*miosis*)
- Eyelid drooping (*ptosis*)
- Nasal discharge
- Facial sweating

Treatment options

Acute management:
- Triptans (e.g. sumatriptan 6mg injected subcutaneously)
- High flow 100% oxygen for 15 to 20 minutes (can be given at home)

Prophylaxis options:
- Verapamil
- Lithium
- Prednisolone (a short course for 2 to 3 weeks can be used to break the cycle during clusters)

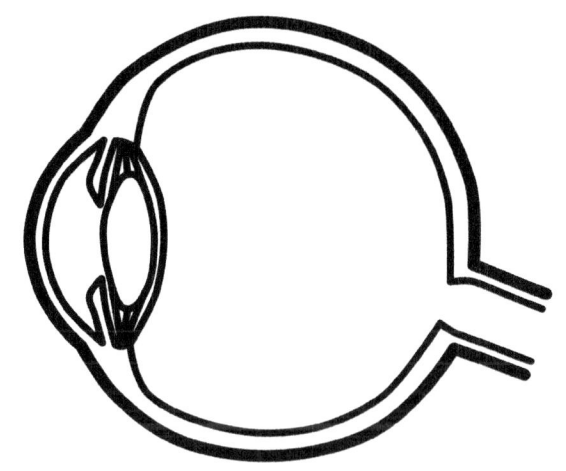

OPHTHALMOLOGY

10.1	Open Angle Glaucoma	308
10.2	Acute Angle Closure Glaucoma	310
10.3	Age Related Macular Degeneration	311
10.4	Diabetic Retinopathy	313
10.5	Hypertensive Retinopathy	314
10.6	Cataracts	315
10.7	Pupil Disorders	316
10.8	Eyelid Disorders	320
10.9	Conjunctivitis	322
10.10	Anterior Uveitis	323
10.11	Episcleritis	324
10.12	Scleritis	325
10.13	Corneal Abrasions	326
10.14	Herpes Keratitis	327
10.15	Subconjunctival Haemorrhage	328
10.16	Posterior Vitreous Detachment	329
10.17	Retinal Detachment	329
10.18	Retinal Vein Occlusion	330
10.19	Central Retinal Artery Occlusion	331
10.20	Retinitis Pigmentosa	332

Open Angle Glaucoma

Glaucoma refers to the **optic nerve** damage caused by a significant rise in **intraocular pressure.** Raised intraocular pressure is caused by a blockage in **aqueous humour** trying to escape the eye. There are two types of glaucoma: **open angle** and **closed angle**.

Basic Anatomy and Physiology

The **vitreous chamber** of the eye is filled with **vitreous humour**. The **anterior chamber** between the **cornea** and **iris** and the **posterior chamber** between the **lens** and **iris** are filled with **aqueous humour** that supplies nutrients to the cornea. The **aqueous humour** is produced by the **ciliary body**. This flows around the **iris** to the **anterior chamber** where it drains through the **trabecular meshwork** at the angle between the **cornea** and the **iris**.

The aqueous humour flows from the **ciliary body**, around the **lens** and under the **iris**, through the **anterior chamber**, through the **trabecular meshwork** and into the **canal of Schlemm**. From the **canal of Schlemm** it eventually enters the general circulation.

The normal **intraocular pressure** is 10 to 21 mmHg. This pressure is created by the **resistance** to flow through the **trabecular meshwork**.

Pathophysiology

In **open angle glaucoma** there is a gradual increase in **resistance** through the **trabecular meshwork**. This makes it more difficult for aqueous humour to flow through the meshwork and exit the eye. Therefore, the pressure slowly builds within the eye and this gives a slow and chronic onset of glaucoma.

In **acute angle closure glaucoma** the **iris** bulges forward and seals off the **trabecular meshwork** from the **anterior chamber** preventing aqueous humour being able to drain away. This leads to a continual build up of pressure. This is an **ophthalmology emergency**.

Increased pressure in the eye causes **cupping** of the **optic disc**. In the centre of a normal **optic disc** is the **optic cup**. This is a small indent in the optic disc. It is usually less than half the size of the optic disc. When there is raised intraocular pressure, this indent becomes larger as the pressure in the eye puts pressure on that indent, making it wider and deeper. This is called "**cupping**". An optic cup greater than 0.5 the size of the optic disc is abnormal.

Risk Factors

- Increasing age
- Family history
- Black ethnic origin
- Nearsightedness (**myopia**)

Presentation of Open Angle Glaucoma

Often the rise in intraocular pressure is asymptomatic for a long period of time. It is diagnosed by routine screening when attending optometry for an eye check.

Glaucoma affects the **peripheral vision** first. Gradually the peripheral vision closes in until they experience **tunnel vision**.

It can present with gradual onset of fluctuating pain, headaches, blurred vision and halos appearing around lights, particularly at night time.

Measuring Intraocular Pressure

Non-contact tonometry is the commonly used machine for estimating intraocular pressure by opticians. It involves shooting a "puff of air" at the cornea and measuring the corneal response to that air. It is less accurate but gives a helpful estimate for general screening purposes.

Goldmann applanation tonometry is the gold standard way to measure intraocular pressure. This involves a special device mounted on a slip lamp that makes contact with the cornea and applies different pressures to the front of the cornea to get an accurate measurement of the intraocular pressure.

Diagnosis

Goldmann applanation tonometry can be used to check the intraocular pressure.

Fundoscopy assessment to check for optic disc cupping and optic nerve health.

Visual field assessment to check for peripheral vision loss.

Management of Open Angle Glaucoma

Management of glaucoma aims to reduce the intraocular pressure. Treatment is usually started at an intraocular pressure of 24 mmHg or above. Patients are followed up closely to assess the response to treatment.

Prostaglandin analogue eyedrops (e.g. **latanoprost**) are first line. These increase **uveoscleral outflow**. Notable side effects are eyelash growth, eyelid pigmentation and iris pigmentation (browning).

Other options:
- **Beta blockers** (e.g. **timolol**) reduce the production of aqueous humour
- **Carbonic anhydrase inhibitors** (e.g. **dorzolamide**) reduce the production of aqueous humour
- **Sympathomimetics** (e.g. **brimonidine**) reduce the production of aqueous fluid and increase uveoscleral outflow

Trabeculectomy surgery may be required where eye drops are ineffective. This involves creating a new channel from the anterior chamber, through the **sclera** to a location under the **conjunctiva**. It causes a "**bleb**" under the conjunctiva where the aqueous humour drains. It is then reabsorbed from this bleb into the general circulation.

Acute Angle Closure Glaucoma

Glaucoma refers to the **optic nerve damage** caused by a significant rise in **intraocular pressure**. The raised intraocular pressure is caused by a blockage in aqueous humour trying to escape the eye.

Acute angle closure glaucoma occurs when the **iris** bulges forward and seals off the **trabecular meshwork** from the **anterior chamber**, preventing **aqueous humour** being able to **drain away**. This leads to a continual build up of pressure in the eye. The pressure builds up particularly in the **posterior chamber**, which causes pressure behind the **iris** and worsens the closure of the angle.

Acute angle closure glaucoma is an **ophthalmology emergency**. Emergency treatment is required to prevent permanent loss of vision.

Risk Factors

The risk factors are slightly different to open angle glaucoma:
- Increasing age
- Females are affected around 4 times more often than males
- Family history
- Chinese and East Asian ethnic origin. Unlike open angle glaucoma it is rare in people of black ethnic origin.
- Shallow anterior chamber

Certain medications can precipitate acute angle closure glaucoma:
- **Adrenergic medications** such as **noradrenalin**
- **Anticholinergic medications** such as **oxybutynin** and **solifenacin**
- **Tricyclic antidepressants** such as **amitriptyline**, which have anticholinergic effects

Presentation

The patient will generally appear unwell in themselves. They have a short history of:
- Severely painful red eye
- Blurred vision
- Halos around lights
- Associated headache, nausea and vomiting

Examination

- Red eye
- Teary
- Hazy cornea
- Decreased visual acuity
- Dilatation of the affected pupil
- Fixed pupil size
- Firm eyeball on palpation

Initial Management

NICE CKS (2019) say patients with potentially life threatening causes of red eye should be referred for same day assessment by an ophthalmologist. If there is a delay in admission, whilst waiting for an ambulance:
- Lie patient on their back without a pillow
- Give **pilocarpine eye drops** (2% for blue, 4% for brown eyes)
- Give **acetazolamide** 500 mg orally
- Given analgesia and an antiemetic if required

Pilocarpine acts on the **muscarinic receptors** in the sphincter muscles in the iris and causes constriction of the pupil. It is a **miotic agent**. It also causes **ciliary muscle** contraction. These two effects cause the pathway for the flow of aqueous humour from the ciliary body, around the iris and into the trabecular meshwork to open up.

Acetazolamide is a **carbonic anhydrase inhibitor**. This reduces the production of aqueous humour.

Secondary Care Management

Various medical options can be tried to reduce the pressure:
- **Pilocarpine**
- **Acetazolamide** (oral or IV)
- **Hyperosmotic agents** such as **glycerol** or **mannitol** increase the osmotic gradient between the blood and the fluid in the eye
- **Timolol** is a **beta blocker** that reduces the production of aqueous humour
- **Dorzolamide** is a **carbonic anhydrase inhibitor** that reduces the production of aqueous humour
- **Brimonidine** is a **sympathomimetics** that reduces the production of aqueous fluid and increase uveoscleral outflow

Laser iridotomy is usually required as a definitive treatment. This involves using a laser to make a hole in the iris to allow the aqueous humour to flow from the posterior chamber to the anterior chamber. This relieves the pressure that was pushing the iris against the cornea and allows the humour the drain.

Age Related Macular Degeneration

Age related macular degeneration is a condition where there is **degeneration** in the **macular** that cause a progressive deterioration in vision. In the UK it is the most common cause of blindness. A key finding associated with macular degeneration is **drusen** seen during **fundoscopy**.

There are two types, **wet** and **dry**. 90% of cases are dry and 10% are wet. **Wet age related macular degeneration** carries a worse prognosis.

The **macular** is made of four key layers. At the bottom there is the **choroid layer**, which contains blood vessels that provide the blood supply to the macula. Above that is **Bruch's membrane**. Above Bruch's membrane there is the **retinal pigment epithelium** and above that are the **photoreceptors**.

Drusen are yellow deposits of **proteins** and **lipids** that appear between the **retinal pigment epithelium** and **Bruch's membrane**. Some drusen can be normal. Normal drusen are small (less than 63 micrometres) and hard. Larger and greater numbers of drusen can be an early sign of **macular degeneration**. They are common to both wet and dry AMD.

Other features that are common to wet and dry AMD are:
- **Atrophy** of the **retinal pigment epithelium**
- **Degeneration** of the **photoreceptors**

In **wet AMD** there is development of **new vessels** growing from the **choroid layer** in to the **retina**. These vessels can leak fluid or blood and cause **oedema** and more rapid loss of vision. A key chemical that stimulates the development of new vessels is **vascular endothelial growth factor** (**VEGF**). This is the target of medications to treat **wet AMD**.

Risk factors

- Age
- Smoking
- White or Chinese ethnic origin
- Family history
- Cardiovascular disease

Presentation

There are some key visual changes to remember for spotting AMD in your exams:
- Gradual worsening **central visual field loss**
- Reduced **visual acuity**
- **Crooked or wavy appearance to straight lines**

Wet age related macular degeneration presents more acutely. It can present with a loss of vision over days and progress to full loss of vision over 2 to 3 years. It often progresses to bilateral disease.

Examination

- Reduced acuity using a **Snellen chart**
- **Scotoma** (a central patch of vision loss)
- **Amsler grid test** can be used to assess distortion of straight lines
- **Fundoscopy**. Drusen are the key finding.

Slit-lamp biomicroscopic fundus examination by a specialist can be used to diagnose AMD.

Optical coherence tomography is a technique used to gain a cross sectional view of the layers of the retina. It can be used to diagnose wet AMD.

Fluorescein angiography involves giving a fluorescein contrast and photographing the retina to look in detail at the blood supply to the retina. It is useful in revealing **oedema** and **neovascularisation**. It is used second line to diagnose wet AMD if **optical coherence tomography** does not exclude wet AMD.

Management

Refer suspected cases to an ophthalmologist for assessment and management.

Dry AMD

There is no specific treatment for **dry age related macular degeneration**. Management focuses on lifestyle measure that may slow the progression:
- Avoid smoking
- Control blood pressure
- Vitamin supplementation has some evidence in slowing progression

Wet AMD

Anti-VEGF medications are used to treat **wet age related macular degeneration**. ***Vascular endothelial growth factor*** is involved in the development of new blood vessels in the retina. Medications such as **ranibizumab**, **bevacizumab** and **pegaptanib** block VEGF and slow the development of new vessels. They are injected directly into the **vitreous chamber** of the eye once a month. They slow and even reverse the progression of the disease. They typically need to be started within 3 months to be beneficial.

Diabetic Retinopathy

Diabetic retinopathy is a condition where the blood vessels in the **retina** are damaged by prolonged exposure to **high blood sugar levels** (**hyperglycaemia**), causing a progressive deterioration in the health of the retina.

Pathophysiology

Hyperglycaemia leads to damage to the **retinal small vessels** and **endothelial cells**. Increased **vascular permeability** leads to leakage from the blood vessels, **blot haemorrhages** and the formation of **hard exudates**. Hard exudates are yellow/white deposits of **lipids** in the retina.

Damage to the blood vessel walls leads to **microaneurysms** and **venous beading**. **Microaneurysms** are where weakness in the wall causes small bulges. **Venous beading** is where the walls of the veins are no longer straight and parallel and look more like a string of beads or sausages.

Damage to **nerve fibres** in the retina causes fluffy white patches to form on the retina called **cotton wool spots**.

Intraretinal microvascular abnormalities (**IMRA**) is where there are dilated and tortuous **capillaries** in the retina. These can act as a **shunt** between the arterial and venous vessels in the retina.

Neovascularisation is when growth factors are released in the retina causing the development of new blood vessels.

Classification

Diabetic retinopathy can be split into two broad categories: **non-proliferative** and **proliferative**, depending on whether new blood vessels have developed. Non-proliferative is often called **background** or **pre-proliferative retinopathy** as it can develop to proliferative retinopathy. A condition called **diabetic maculopathy** also exists separate from non-proliferative and proliferative diabetic retinopathy.

These conditions are classified based on the findings on fundus examination.

Non-proliferative diabetic retinopathy
- **Mild**: microaneurysms
- **Moderate**: microaneurysms, blot haemorrhages, hard exudates, cotton wool spots and venous beading
- **Severe**: blot haemorrhages plus microaneurysms in 4 quadrants, venous beating in 2 quadrates, intraretinal microvascular abnormality (IMRA) in any quadrant

Proliferative Diabetic Retinopathy
- Neovascularisation
- Vitreous haemorrhage

Diabetic Maculopathy
- Macular oedema
- Ischaemic maculopathy

Complications of Diabetic Retinopathy

- *Retinal detachment*
- *Vitreous haemorrhage* (bleeding in the vitreous humour)
- *Rebeosis iridis* (new blood vessel formation in the iris)
- *Optic neuropathy*
- *Cataracts*

Management

- *Laser photocoagulation*
- *Anti-VEGF* medications such as *ranibizumab* and *bevacizumab*
- *Vitreoretinal surgery* (keyhole surgery on the eye) may be required in severe disease

Hypertensive Retinopathy

Hypertensive retinopathy describes the damage to the small blood vessels in the retina relating to **systemic hypertension**. This can be the result of years of **chronic hypertension** or can develop quickly in response to **malignant hypertension**. There are a number of signs that occur in the retina in response to hypertension in these vessels.

Silver wiring or *copper wiring* is where the walls of the arterioles become thickened and sclerosed causing increased reflection of light on examination.

Arteriovenous nipping is where the arterioles cause compression of the veins where they cross over. This is again due to sclerosis and hardening of the arterioles.

Cotton wool spots are caused by *ischaemia* and *infarction* in the retina causing damage to nerve fibres.

Hard exudates are caused by damaged vessels leaking *lipids* onto the retina.

Retinal haemorrhages are caused by damaged vessels rupturing and releasing blood into the retina.

Papilloedema is caused by **ischaemia** to the **optic nerve**, resulting in optic nerve swelling (**oedema**) and blurring of the disc margins.

Keith-Wagener Classification

- Stage 1: Mild narrowing of the arterioles
- Stage 2: Focal constriction of blood vessels and AV nicking
- Stage 3: Cotton-wool patches, exudates and haemorrhages
- Stage 4: Papilloedema

Management

Management is focused on controlling the blood pressure and other risk factors such as smoking and blood lipid levels.

Cataracts

Cataracts occur when the **lens** in the eye becomes cloudy and opaque. This reduces **visual acuity** by reducing the light that enters the eye.

The job of the **lens** is to focus light coming in to the eye on to the **retina** at the back of the eye. It is held in place by **suspensory ligaments** attached to the **ciliary body**. The ciliary body contracts and relaxes to focus the lens. When the ciliary body contracts it releases tension on the suspensory ligaments and the lens thickens. When the ciliary body relaxes it increases the tension in the suspensory ligaments and the lens narrows. The lens is nourished by the surrounding fluid and doesn't have a blood supply. It grows and develops throughout life.

Most cataracts develop over years in the presence of risk factors. **Congenital cataracts** occur before birth and are screened for using the **red reflex** during the neonatal examination.

Risk Factors

- Increasing age
- Smoking
- Alcohol
- Diabetes
- Steroids
- Hypocalcaemia

Presentation

Symptoms are usually **asymmetrical**, as both eyes are affected separately. It presents with:
- Very slow reduction in vision
- Progressive blurring of vision
- Change in colour vision with colours becoming more brown or yellow
- **"Starbursts"** can appear around lights, particularly at night time

A key sign for cataracts is the loss of the **red reflex**. The lens can appear grey or white when testing the red reflex. This might show up on photographs taken with a flash.

TOM TIP: It is useful in exams to distinguish the causes of visual problems based on the symptoms. Cataracts cause a generalised reduction in visual acuity with starbursts around lights. Glaucoma causes a peripheral loss of vision with halos around lights. Macular degeneration causes a central loss of vision with a crooked or wavy appearance to straight lines.

Management

If the symptoms are manageable no intervention may be necessary.

Cataract surgery involves drilling and breaking the lens to pieces, removing the pieces and implanting an **artificial lens** into the eye. This is usually done as a day case under local anaesthetic. It generally gives good results.

It is worth noting that cataracts can prevent the detection of other pathology such as macular degeneration or diabetic retinopathy. Once cataract surgery is performed these conditions may be detected. Therefore, the surgery may treat the cataract but they may still have poor visual acuity due to other problems.

Endophthalmitis

Endophthalmitis is a rare but serious complication of cataract surgery. It is **inflammation** of the inner contents of the eye, usually caused by infection. It can be treated with **intravitreal antibiotics**, injected directly into the eye. Endophthalmitis can lead to loss of vision and loss of the eye itself.

Pupil Disorders

The pupil is formed by a hole in the centre of the iris. There are a number of conditions that cause abnormally shaped or sized pupils.

Pupil Constriction
There are **circular muscles** in the **iris** that cause pupil constriction. They are stimulated by the **parasympathetic nervous system** using **acetylcholine** as a **neurotransmitter**. The fibres of the parasympathetic system innervating the eye travel along the **oculomotor** (**third cranial**) nerve.

Pupil Dilation
The **dilator muscles** of the pupil are arranged like spokes on a bicycle wheel, travelling straight from the inside to the outside of the iris. They are stimulated by the **sympathetic nervous** system using **adrenalin** as a **neurotransmitter**.

Abnormal Pupil Shape

Trauma to the sphincter muscles in the iris can cause an irregular pupil. This could be caused by cataract surgery and other eye operations.

Anterior uveitis can cause **adhesions** (scar tissue) in the iris that make the pupils misshapen.

Acute angle closure glaucoma can cause ischaemic damage to the muscles of the iris and an abnormal pupil shape, usually a **vertical oval**.

Rubeosis iridis (neovascularisation in the iris) can distort the shape of the iris and pupil. This is usually associated with poorly controlled diabetes and diabetic retinopathy.

Coloboma is a **congenital malformation** in the eye. This can cause a hole in the iris and an irregular pupil shape.

Tadpole pupil is where there is spasm in a segment of the iris causing a misshapen pupil. This is usually temporary and associated with **migraines**.

Causes of Mydriasis (Dilated Pupil)

- Third nerve palsy
- Holmes-Adie syndrome
- Raised intracranial pressure
- Congenital
- Trauma
- Stimulants such as cocaine
- Anticholinergics

Causes of Miosis (Constricted Pupil)

- Horners syndrome
- Cluster headaches
- Argyll-Robertson pupil (in neurosyphilis)
- Opiates
- Nicotine
- Pilocarpine

Third Nerve Palsy

A third nerve palsy causes:
- **Ptosis** (drooping upper eyelid)
- **Dilated non-reactive** pupil
- **Divergent strabismus** (squint) in the affected eye. It causes a "**down and out**" position of the affected eye.

The third cranial nerve is the **oculomotor nerve**. It supplies all the **extraocular muscles** except the **lateral rectus** and **superior oblique**. Therefore, when these muscles are no longer getting signals from the oculomotor nerve, the eyes moves outward and downward due to the effects of the lateral rectus and superior oblique still functioning without resistance.

It also supplies the **levator palpebrae superioris**, which is responsible for lifting the upper eyelid. Therefore, third nerve palsy causes **ptosis**.

The oculomotor nerve also contains **parasympathetic fibres** that innervate the **sphincter muscle** of the **iris**. Therefore, **third nerve palsy** causes a **dilated fixed pupil**.

The oculomotor nerve travels directly from the brainstem to the eye in a straight line. It travels through the **cavernous sinus** and close to the **posterior communicating artery**. Therefore, **cavernous sinus thrombosis** and a **posterior communicating artery aneurysm** can cause compression on the nerve and third nerve palsy.

Causes of a Third Nerve Palsy

Third nerve palsy can be *idiopathic*, without a clear cause.

A third nerve palsy **with sparing of the pupil** suggests a *microvascular* cause as the *parasympathetic fibres* are spared. This may be due to:
- Diabetes
- Hypertension
- Ischaemia

A **full third nerve palsy** is caused by compression of the nerve, including compression of the *parasympathetic fibres*. This is called a "**surgical third**" due to the structural pathology. It may be due to:
- Idiopathic
- Tumour
- Trauma
- Cavernous sinus thrombosis
- Posterior communicating artery aneurysm
- Raised intracranial pressure

Horner Syndrome

Horner syndrome is a triad of:
- *Ptosis*
- *Miosis*
- *Anhidrosis* (loss of sweating)

They may also have **enopthalmos**, which is a sunken eye. Light and accommodation reflexes are not affected.

Horner syndrome is caused by damage to the **sympathetic nervous system** supplying the face.

The journey of the **sympathetic nerves** to the head is relevant for the causes of Horner syndrome. The sympathetic nerves arise from the **spinal cord** in the chest. These are **pre-ganglionic nerves**. They enter the **sympathetic ganglion** at the base of the neck and exit as **post-ganglionic nerves**. These post-ganglionic nerves travel to the head, running alongside the **internal carotid artery**.

The location of the Horner syndrome can be determined by the **anhidrosis**. Central lesions cause **anhidrosis** of the arm and trunk as well as the face. Pre-ganglionic lesions cause **anhidrosis** of the face. Post-ganglionic lesions do not cause **anhidrosis**.

The causes can be remembered as the 4 Ss, 4 Ts and 4 Cs. S for Sentral, T for Torso (pre-ganglionic) and C for Cervical (post-ganglionic).

Central lesions (4 Ss)
- S - **S**troke
- S - Multiple **S**clerosis
- S - **S**welling (tumours)
- S - **S**yringomyelia (cyst in the spinal cord)

Pre-ganglionic lesions (4 Ts):
- T - **T**umour (Pancoast's tumour)
- T - **T**rauma
- T - **T**hyroidectomy
- T - **T**op rib (a cervical rib growing above the first rib and clavicle)

Post-ganglionic lesions (4 Cs)
- C - **C**arotid aneurysm
- C - **C**arotid artery dissection
- C - **C**avernous sinus thrombosis
- C - **C**luster headache

Congenital Horner syndrome is associated with **heterochromia**, where there is a difference in colour of the iris on the affected side.

Cocaine eye drops can be used to test for Horner syndrome. Cocaine acts on the eye to stop **noradrenalin re-uptake** at the **neuromuscular junction**. This causes a normal eye to dilate because there is more noradrenalin stimulating the dilator muscles of the iris. In Horner syndrome, the nerves are not releasing noradrenalin to start with, so blocking re-uptake does not make a difference and there is no reaction of the pupil.

Alternatively, a low concentration **adrenalin eye drop** (0.1%) won't dilate a normal pupil but will dilate a Horner syndrome pupil.

Holmes Adie Pupil

A Holmes Adie pupil is a unilateral dilated pupil that is sluggish to react to light with slow dilation of the pupil following constriction. Over time the pupil will get smaller. This is caused by damage to the **post-ganglionic parasympathetic fibres**. The exact cause is unknown but may be viral.

Holmes Adie syndrome is where there is a **Holmes Adie pupil** with absent **ankle** and **knee reflexes**.

Argyll-Robertson Pupil

An Argyll-Robertson pupil is a specific finding in **neurosyphilis**. It is a **constricted** pupil that **accommodates** when focusing on a near object but **does not react to light**. They are often irregularly shaped. It is commonly called a "**prostitutes pupil**" due to the relation to neurosyphilis and because "**it accommodates but does not react**".

Eyelid Disorders

Blepharitis

Blepharitis is **inflammation** of the **eyelid margins**. It causes a gritty, itchy, dry sensation in the eyes. It can be associated with dysfunction of the **Meibomian glands**, which are responsible for secreting oil onto the surface of the eye. It can lead to **styes** and **chalazions**.

Management is with hot compresses and gentle cleaning of the eyelid margins to remove debris using cotton wool dipped in sterilised water and baby shampoo.

Lubricating eye drops can be used to relieve symptoms:
- **Hypromellose** drops are the least viscous. The effects last around 10 minutes.
- **Polyvinyl alcohol** drops are the middle viscous choice. It is worth starting with these.
- **Carbomer** drops are the most viscous and lasts 30 to 60 minutes.

Stye

Hordeolum externum is an infection of the **glands of Zeis** or **glands of Moll**. The glands of Moll are sweat glands at the base of the eyelashes. The glands of Zeis are sebaceous glands at the base of the eyelashes. A stye causes a tender red lump along the eyelid that may contain pus.

Hordeolum internum is infection of the **Meibomian glands**. They are deeper, tend to be more painful and may point inwards towards the eyeball underneath the eyelid.

Styes are treated with hot compresses and analgesia. Consider topic antibiotics (i.e. chloramphenicol) if it is associated with conjunctivitis or symptoms are persistent.

Chalazion

A chalazion occurs when a **Meibomian gland** becomes blocked and swells. It is often called a **Meibomian cyst**. It presents with a swelling in the eyelid that is typically not tender, however it can be tender and red.

Treatment is with hot compresses and analgesia. Consider topic antibiotics (i.e. chloramphenicol) if acutely inflamed.

Rarely if conservative management fails surgical drainage may be required.

Entropion

Entropion is where the eyelid turns inwards with the lashes against the eyeball. This causes in pain and can result in **corneal damage** and **ulceration**.

Initial management is by taping the eyelid down to prevent it turning inwards. Definitive management is with surgical intervention. When the eyelid is taped down it is essential to prevent the eye drying out by using regular lubricating eye drops.

A same day referral to ophthalmology is required if there is a risk to sight.

Ectropion

Ectropion is where the eyelid turns outwards with the inner aspect of the eyelid exposed. It usually affects the bottom lid. This can result in **exposure keratopathy** as the eyeball is exposed and not adequately lubricated and protected.

Mild cases may not require treatment. Regular lubricating eye drops are used to protect the surface of the eye. More significant cases may require surgery to correct the defect.

A same day referral to ophthalmology is required if there is a risk to sight.

Trichiasis

Trichiasis is inward growth of the eyelashes. It results in pain and can cause corneal damage and ulceration.

Management by a specialist is to remove the eyelash (**epilation**). Recurrent cases may require electrolysis, cryotherapy or laser treatment to prevent the lash regrowing.

A same day referral to ophthalmology is required if there is a risk to sight.

Periorbital Cellulitis

Periorbital cellulitis (also known as **preorbital cellulitis**) is an eyelid and skin infection in front of the **orbital septum** (in front of the eye). It presents with swelling, redness and hot skin around the eyelids and eye.

It is essential to differentiate it from **orbital cellulitis**, which is a sight and life threatening emergency. CT scan can help distinguish between the two.

Treatment is with **systemic antibiotics** (oral or IV). Preorbital cellulitis can develop into orbital cellulitis, so vulnerable patients (e.g. children) or severe cases may require admission for observation while they are treated.

Orbital Cellulitis

Orbital cellulitis is an infection around the eyeball that involves tissues behind the **orbital septum**.

Key features that differential this from periorbital celluitis is pain on eye movement, reduced eye movements, changes in vision, abnormal pupil reactions and forward movement of the eyeball (proptosis).

This is a medical emergency that requires admission and IV antibiotics. They may require surgical drainage if an abscess forms.

Conjunctivitis

Conjunctivitis is **inflammation** of the **conjunctiva**. The conjunctiva is a thin layer of tissue that covers the inside of the eyelids and the *sclera* of the eye. There are three main types:
- Bacterial
- Viral
- Allergic

Presentation

Conjunctivitis presents with:
- Unilateral or bilateral
- Red eyes
- Bloodshot
- Itchy or gritty sensation
- Discharge from the eye

Conjunctivitis does **not** cause pain, photophobia or reduced visual acuity. Vision may be blurry when the eye is covered with discharge, however when the discharge is cleared the acuity should be normal.

Bacterial conjunctivitis presents with a **purulent discharge** and an inflamed conjunctiva. It is typically worse in the morning when the eyes may be stuck together. It usually starts in one eye and can spread to the other. It is highly contagious.

Viral conjunctivitis is common and usually presents with a clear discharge. It is often associated with other symptoms of a viral infection such as dry cough, sore throat and blocked nose. You may find tender *preauricular* lymph nodes (in front of the ears). It is also contagious.

Differential Diagnosis of Acute Red Eye

A common exam topic and clinical challenge is to differentiate between the causes of an acute red eye. The more serious differentials tend to cause pain and reduced visual acuity.

Painless Red Eye
- Conjunctivitis
- Episcleritis
- Subconjunctival haemorrhage

Painful Red Eye
- Glaucoma
- Anterior uveitis
- Scleritis
- Corneal abrasions or ulceration
- Keratitis
- Foreign body
- Traumatic or chemical injury

Management

Conjunctivitis usually resolves without treatment after 1-2 weeks.

Advise on good hygiene to avoid spreading (e.g. avoid sharing towels or rubbing eyes and regularly washing hands) and avoiding the use of contact lenses. Cleaning the eyes with cooled boiled water and cotton wool can help clear the discharge.

If bacterial conjunctivitis is suspected antibiotic eye drops can be considered, however bear in mind it will often get better without treatment. **Chloramphenicol** and **fusidic acid** eye drops are both options.

Patients under the age of 1 month of age with conjunctivitis need urgent ophthalmology review as **neonatal conjunctivitis** can be associated with **gonococcal infection**. This can cause loss of sight and more severe complications like pneumonia.

Allergic Conjunctivitis

Allergic conjunctivitis is caused by contact with *allergens*. It causes swelling of the *conjunctival sac* and *eye lid* with a significant watery discharge and itch.

Antihistamines (oral or topical) can be used to reduce symptoms.

Topical *mast-cell stabilisers* can be used in patients with chronic seasonal symptoms. They work by preventing mast cells releasing histamine. These require use for several weeks before showing any benefit

Anterior Uveitis

Anterior uveitis is inflammation in the anterior part of the uvea. The **uvea** involves the *iris*, *ciliary body* and *choroid*. The **choroid** is the layer between the *retina* and the *sclera* all the way around the eye. Sometimes *anterior uveitis* is referred to as *iritis*.

It involves *inflammation* and *immune cells* in the *anterior chamber* of the eye. The anterior chamber of the eye becomes infiltrated by *neutrophils*, *lymphocytes* and *macrophages*. This is usually caused by an *autoimmune* process, but can be due to *infection*, *trauma*, *ischaemia* or *malignancy*. Inflammatory cells in the anterior chamber cause *floaters* in the patient's vision.

Anterior uveitis can be *acute* or *chronic*. Chronic anterior uveitis is more *granulomatous* (has more *macrophages*) and has a less severe and longer duration of symptoms, lasting more than 3 months.

Associations

Acute anterior uveitis is associated with *HLA B27* related conditions:
- Ankylosing spondylitis
- Inflammatory bowel disease
- Reactive arthritis

Chronic anterior uveitis is associated with:
- Sarcoidosis
- Syphilis
- Tuberculosis
- Herpes virus

Presentation

Anterior uveitis usually presents with **unilateral** symptoms that start spontaneously without a history of trauma or precipitating events. They may occur with a flare of an associated disease such as **reactive arthritis**. Symptoms include:
- Dull, aching, painful red eye
- **Ciliary flush** (a ring of red spreading from the cornea outwards)
- Reduced visual acuity
- Floaters and flashes
- Sphincter muscle contraction causing **miosis** (constricted pupil)
- **Photophobia** due to ciliary muscle spasm
- Pain on movement
- Excessive tear production (**lacrimation**)
- Abnormally shaped pupil due to **posterior synechiae** (**adhesions**) pulling the iris into abnormal shapes

Management

NICE clinical knowledge summaries on red eye say patients with potentially sight threatening causes of red eye should be referred for same day assessment by an ophthalmologist. They need fully slit lamp assessment of the different structures of the eye and intraocular pressure measurement to establish the diagnosis.

The ophthalmologist will guide treatment choices:
- **Steroids** (oral, topical or intravenous)
- **Cycloplegic-mydriatic** medications such as **cyclopentolate** or **atropine** eye drops. **Cycloplegic** means paralysing the ciliary muscles. **Mydriatic** means dilating the pupils. Cyclopentolate and atropine are **antimuscarinic** medications that block the action of the **iris sphincter muscles** and **ciliary body**. These dilate the pupil and reduce pain associated with ciliary spasm by stopping the action of the ciliary body.
- **Immunosuppressants** such as **DMARDS** and **TNF inhibitors**
- Laser therapy, cryotherapy or surgery (vitrectomy) are also options in severe cases.

Episcleritis

Episcleritis is benign and self limiting **inflammation** of the **episclera**, the outermost layer of the sclera. The episclera is situated just underneath the **conjunctiva**.

It is relatively common in young and middle aged adults and is not usually caused by infection. It is often associated with inflammatory disorders such as **rheumatoid arthritis** and **inflammatory bowel disease**.

Presentation

Episcleritis usually presents with acute onset unilateral symptoms:

- Typically not painful but there can be mild pain
- Segmental redness (rather than diffuse). There is usually a patch of redness in the lateral sclera.
- Foreign body sensation
- Dilated episcleral vessels
- Watering of the eye
- No discharge

Management

If in doubt about the diagnosis, refer to ophthalmology.

Episcleritis is usually self limiting and will recover in 1 to 4 weeks. In mild cases no treatment is necessary. Lubricating eye drops can help symptoms.

Management is with simple **analgesia**, **cold compresses** and **safety net advice**.

More severe cases may benefit from systemic **NSAIDs** (e.g. naproxen) or topical steroid eye drops.

Scleritis

Scleritis involves **inflammation** of the full thickness of the **sclera**. This is more serious than **episcleritis**. It is not usually caused by infection.

The most severe type of scleritis is called **necrotising scleritis**. Most patients with necrotising scleritis have visual impairment but may not have pain. It can lead to **perforation of the sclera**. This is the most significant complication of scleritis.

Associated Systemic Conditions

There is an associated systemic condition in around 50% of patients presenting with scleritis. This may be:
- Rheumatoid arhtritis
- Systemic lupus erythematosus
- Inflammatory bowel disease
- Sarcoidosis
- Granulomatosis with polyangiitis

Presentation

Scleritis usually presents with an acute onset of symptoms. Around 50% of cases are bilateral.
- Severe pain
- Pain with eye movement
- Photophobia
- Eye watering
- Reduced visual acuity
- Abnormal pupil reaction to light
- Tenderness to palpation of the eye

Management

NICE clinical knowledge summaries on red eye say patients with potentially sight threatening causes of red eye should be referred for same day assessment by an ophthalmologist.

Management in secondary care involves:
- Consider an underlying systemic condition
- **NSAIDS** (topical or systemic)
- **Steroids** (topical or systemic)
- **Immunosuppression** appropriate to the underlying systemic condition (e.g. methotrexate in rheumatoid arthritis)

Corneal Abrasions

Corneal abrasions are scratches or damage to the **cornea**. They are a cause of red, painful eye. Common causes are:
- Contact lenses
- Foreign bodies
- Finger nails
- Eyelashes
- Entropion (inward turning eyelid)

If the abrasion is associated with the use of **contact lenses** there may be infection with **pseudomonas**.

An important differential diagnosis to consider is **herpes keratitis**. This will require treatment with antiviral eye drops.

Presentation

- History of contact lenses or foreign body
- Painful red eye
- Foreign body sensation
- Watering eye
- Blurring vision
- Photophobia

Diagnosis

A **fluorescein stain** is applied to the eye to diagnose a corneal abrasion. This is a **yellow-orange** colour. The stain collects in abrasions or ulcers, highlighting them.

Slit lamp examination may be used in more significant abrasions.

Management

NICE clinical knowledge summaries on red eye say patients with potentially sight threatening causes of red eye should be referred for same day assessment by an ophthalmologist. It may be managed in primary care where there are appropriate skills.

Management in secondary care:
- Simple analgesia (e.g. paracetamol)
- Lubricating eye drops can improve symptoms
- Antibiotic eye drops (i.e. chloramphenicol)
- Bring the patient back after 1 week to check it has healed
- Cyclopentolate eye drops dilate the pupil and improve significant symptoms, particularly photophobia. These are not usually necessary.

Uncomplicated corneal abrasions usually heal over 2 to 3 days.

Herpes Keratitis

Keratitis is inflammation of the **cornea**. There are a number of causes of keratitis:
- **Viral** infection with **herpes simplex**
- **Bacterial** infection with **pseudomonas** or **staphylococcus**
- **Fungal** infection with **candida** or **aspergillus**
- **Contact lens acute red eye** (**CLARE**)
- **Exposure keratitis** is caused by inadequate eyelid coverage (e.g. eyelid ectropion)

Herpes simplex infection is the most common cause of keratitis. This is called **herpes simplex keratitis**. It can cause inflammation in any part of the eye, however it most commonly affects the epithelial layer of the cornea. Herpes simplex keratitis can be **primary** or **recurrent**.

Herpes keratitis usually affects only the **epithelial layer** of the cornea. If there is inflammation of the **stroma** (the layer between the **epithelium** and **endothelium**), this is called **stromal keratitis**. This is associated with complications such as **stromal necrosis, vascularisation** and **scarring**, and can lead to **corneal blindness**.

Presentation

- Painful red eye
- Photophobia
- Vesicles around the eye
- Foreign body sensation
- Watering eye
- Reduced visual acuity. This can vary from subtle to significant.

Diagnosis

Staining with **fluorescein** will show a **dendritic corneal ulcer**. **Dendritic** describes the appearance of branching and spreading of the ulcer.

Slit lamp examination is required to find and diagnose keratitis.

Corneal **swabs** or **scrapings** can be used to isolate the virus using a viral culture or PCR.

Management

NICE clinical knowledge summaries on red eye say patients with potentially sight threatening causes of red eye should be referred for same day assessment by an ophthalmologist.

Management options in secondary care:
- Aciclovir (topical or oral)
- Ganciclovir eye gel
- Topical steroids may be used along side antivirals to treat stromal keratitis

Corneal transplant may be required after the infection has resolved to treat corneal scarring caused by stromal keratitis.

Subconjunctival Haemorrhage

Subconjunctival haemorrhages are a relatively common condition where one of the small blood vessels within the **conjunctiva** ruptures and release blood into the space between the **sclera** and the **conjunctiva**. They often appear after episodes of strenuous activity, such as heavy coughing, weight lifting or straining when constipated. It can also be caused by trauma to the eye.

TOM TIP: Most cases are idiopathic and the patient is otherwise healthy, however there are a number of conditions that may have predisposed them to developing a subconjunctival haemorrhage. When a patient turns up with a subconjunctival haemorrhage use it as a clue to think about other conditions that may have contributed:
- *Hypertension*
- *Bleeding disorders (e.g thrombocytopenia)*
- *Whooping cough*
- *Medications (warfarin, NOACs and antiplatelets)*
- *Non-accidental injury*

Presentation

A subconjunctival haemorrhage appears as a patch of **bright red** blood underneath the conjunctiva and in front of the sclera. It covers the white of the eye. It is painless and does not affect vision.

There may be a precipitating event such as a coughing fit or heavy lifting.

They can be confidently diagnosed based on a simple history and examination.

Management

Subconjunctival haemorrhages are harmless and will resolve spontaneously without any treatment. This usually takes around 2 weeks.

Think about the possible causes such as hypertension and bleeding disorders. These may need investigating further.

If there is a foreign body sensation **lubricating eye drops** can help relieve symptoms.

Posterior Vitreous Detachment

The **vitreous body** is the gel inside the eye that maintains the structure of the eyeball and keeps the **retina** pressed on the **choroid**. The vitreous body is made up of **collagen** and **water**. With age it becomes less firm and less able to maintain its shape. **Posterior vitreous detachment** is a condition where the vitreous body comes away from the retina. It is very common, particularly in older patients.

Presentation

Posterior vitreous detachment is a painless condition. It may be completely asymptomatic or there may be:
- Spots of vision loss
- Floaters
- Flashing lights

Management

No treatment is necessary. Over time the symptoms will improve as the brain adjusts.

Posterior vitreous detachment can predispose patients to develop retinal tears and retinal detachment. These conditions can present in a very similar way. It is essential to exclude and assess the risk of a **retinal tear** or **detachment** with a thorough assessment of the **retina**. This is usually done by an optometrist or ophthalmologist.

Retinal Detachment

Retinal detachment is where the the **retina** separates from the **choroid** underneath. This is usually due to a **retinal tear** that allows **vitreous fluid** to get under the retina and fill the space between the retina and the choroid. The outer retina relies on the blood vessels of the choroid for its blood supply. This makes retinal detachment a **sight threatening** emergency that needs to be quickly recognised and treated.

Risk Factors

- Posterior vitreous detachment
- Diabetic retinopathy
- Trauma to the eye
- Retinal malignancy
- Older age
- Family history

Presentation

Retinal detachment is a painless condition that can present with:
- Peripheral vision loss. This is often sudden and described as a shadow coming across the vision.
- Blurred or distorted vision
- **Flashes** and **floaters**

Management

Patients presenting with painless flashes and floaters should have a detailed assessment of the retina by someone with the appropriate skillset to detect **retinal tears** and **retinal detachment**. Any suspicion of retinal detachment requires immediate referral to ophthalmology for assessment and management.

Management of **retinal tears** aims to create adhesions between the retina and the choroid to prevent detachment. This can be done using:
- Laser therapy
- Cryotherapy

Management of **retinal detachment** aims to reattach the retina and reduce any traction or pressure that may cause it to detach again. This needs to be followed by treating any retinal tears. Reattaching the retina can be done using one of three options:
- **Vitrectomy** involves removing the relevant parts of the vitreous body and replacing it with oil or gas.
- **Scleral buckling** involves using a silicone "buckle" to put pressure on the outside of the eye (the sclera) so that the outer eye indents to bring the choroid inwards and in contact with the detached retina.
- **Pneumatic retinopexy** involves injecting a gas bubble into the vitreous body and positioning the patient so the gas bubble creates pressure that flattens the retina against the choroid and close the detachment.

Retinal Vein Occlusion

Central retinal vein occlusion occurs when a blood clot (**thrombus**) forms in the **retinal veins** and blocks the drainage of blood from the retina. The **central retinal vein** runs through the **optic nerve** and is responsible for draining blood from the retina.

There are four branched veins that come together to form the central retinal vein. Blockage of one of the branch veins causes problems in the area drained by that branch, whereas blockage in the central vein causes problems with the whole retina.

Blockage of a retinal vein causes pooling of blood in the retina. This results in leakage of fluid and blood causing **macular oedema** and **retinal haemorrhages**. This results in damage to the tissue in the retina and loss of vision. It also leads to the release of **VEGF**, which stimulates the development of new blood vessels (**neovascularisation**).

Presentation

Blockage of one of these retinal veins causes **sudden painless loss of vision**.

Risk Factors

- Hypertension
- High cholesterol
- Diabetes
- Smoking
- Glaucoma
- Systemic inflammatory conditions such as **systemic lupus erythematosus**

Fundoscopy

Fundoscopy examination is diagnostic of retinal vein occlusion. It give characteristic findings:
- Flame and blot haemorrhages
- Optic disc oedema
- Macula oedema

Other Tests

The **Royal College of Ophthalmologists** guidelines from 2015 suggest checking for possible associated conditions in patients presenting with retinal vein occlusion:
- *Full medical history*
- *FBC* for leukaemia
- *ESR* for inflammatory disorders
- *Blood pressure* for hypertension
- *Serum glucose* for diabetes

Management

Patients with suspected retinal vein occlusion should be referred immediately to an ophthalmologist for assessment and management.

Management in secondary care aims to treat **macular oedema** and prevent complications such as **neovascularisation** of the retina and the iris and glaucoma. The options for this are:
- Laser photocoagulation
- Intravitreal steroids (e.g. a dexamethasone intravitreal implant)
- Anti-VEGF therapies (e.g. ranibizumab, aflibercept or bevacizumab)

Central Retinal Artery Occlusion

Central retinal artery occlusion occurs when something blocks the flow of blood through the **central retinal artery**. The **central retinal artery** supplies the blood to the retina. It is a branch of the **ophthalmic artery**, which is a branch of the **internal carotid artery**.

The most common cause of occlusion of the retinal artery is **atherosclerosis**. It can also be caused by **giant cell arteritis**, where **vasculitis** affecting the **ophthalmic** or **central retinal artery** causes reduced blood flow.

Risk Factors

Risk factors for retinal artery occlusion by atherosclerosis are the same as for other cardiovascular disease:
- Older age
- Family history
- Smoking
- Alcohol consumption
- Hypertension
- Diabetes
- Poor diet
- Inactivity
- Obesity

Those at higher risk for retinal artery occlusion secondary to *giant cell arteritis* are white patients over 50 years of age, particularly females and those already affected by *giant cell arteritis* or *polymyalgia rheumatica*.

Presentation

Blockage of the central retinal artery causes *sudden painless loss of vision*.

There will be a *relative afferent pupillary defect*. This is where the pupil in the affected eye constricts more when light is shone in the other eye compared to when it is shone in the affected eye. This occurs because the input is not being sensed by the ischaemic retina when testing the direct light reflex but is being sensed by the normal retina during the consensual light reflex.

Fundoscopy will show a *pale retinal* with a *cherry red spot*. The retina is pale due to a lack of perfusion with blood. The cherry red spot is the macula, which has a thinner surface that shows the red coloured choroid below, which contrasts with the pale retina.

Management

Patients with suspected central retinal artery occlusion should be referred immediately to an ophthalmologist for assessment and management.

Giant cell arteritis is an important potentially reversible cause. Therefore older patients are tested and treated for this if suspected. Testing involves an *ESR* and *temporal artery biopsy* and treatment is with high dose systemic *steroids*.

Immediate Management
If the patient presents shortly after symptoms develop there are certain things that can be tried to attempt to dislodge the thrombus. None of these have a strong evidence base. Some examples are:
- Ocular massage
- Removing fluid from the anterior chamber to reduce intraocular pressure.
- Inhaling *carbogen* (a mixture of 5% carbon dioxide and 95% oxygen) to dilate the artery
- Sublingual *isosorbide dinitrate* to dilate the artery

Long Term Management
Long term management involves treating reversible risk factors and secondary prevention of cardiovascular disease.

Retinitis Pigmentosa

Retinitis pigmentosa is a *congenital inherited condition* where there is *degeneration* of the *rods* and *cones* in the retina. There are many different genetic causes. Some causes involve *isolated* retinitis pigmentosa whereas others result in *systemic diseases* associated with the condition. They vary in age at presentation and prognosis.

In most genetic causes the *rods* degenerate more than *cones*, leading to *night blindness*. They get decreased *central* and *peripheral* vision.

Presentation

The presentation can vary depending on underlying causes. Family history is very important. In most causes the symptoms start in childhood.
- **Night blindness** is often the first symptom
- **Peripheral vision** is lost before the **central vision**

Fundoscopy

Fundoscopy will show **pigmentation**. This is described as "**bone-spicule**" pigmentation. **Spicule** refers to sharp, pointed objects. **Bone-spicule** is used to refer to the similarity to the networking appearance of **bone matrix**.

The pigmentation is most concentrated around the **mid-peripheral** area of the retina.

There can be associated narrowing of the arterioles and a waxy or pale appearance to the optic disc.

Associated Systemic Diseases

There are several genetic systemic diseases that involve retinitis pigmentosa. It is not worth learning the names and details but it is worth being aware they exist. Some examples are:
- **Usher's syndrome** causes hearing loss plus retinitis pigmentosa
- **Bassen-Kornzweig syndrome** is a disorder of fat absorption and metabolism causing progressive neurological symptoms and retinitis pigmentosa
- **Refsum's disease** is a metabolic disorder of **phytanic acid** causing neurological, hearing and skin symptoms and retinitis pigmentosa

Management

General management involves:
- Referral to an ophthalmologist for assessment and diagnosis
- Genetic counselling
- Vision aids
- Sunglasses to protect the retina from accelerated damage
- Driving limitations and informing the DVLA
- Regular follow up to assess vision and check for other potentially reversible conditions that may worsen the vision such as cataracts

There isn't a huge amount of evidence supporting options to slow the disease process. Some options that may be considered by a specialist in certain scenarios include:
- Vitamin and antioxidant supplements
- Oral acetazolamide
- Topical dorzolamide
- Steroid injections
- Anti-VEGF injections

Gene therapy is a potential future treatment that could alter the disease process and lead to better outcomes.

INDEX

ABCD2 score 269
Absence seizures 284
Acoustic neuroma 291
Acromegaly 61
Acute angle closure glaucoma 310
Acute asthma 116
Acute chest syndrome 185
Acute coronary syndrome 10
Acute interstitial nephritis 258
Acute kidney injury 247
Acute left ventricular failure 14
Acute lymphoblastic leukaemia 187
Acute myeloid leukaemia 188
Acute tubular necrosis 259
Addisonian crisis 56
Adrenal insufficiency 44
Age related macular degeneration 311
AIDS 164
Alcohol dependence 71
Alcohol withdrawal 73
Alcoholic liver disease 71
Alloimmune haemolytic anaemia 180
Alpha 1 antitrypsin deficiency 87
Alpha-thalassaemia 182
Anaemia 173
Anaemia of chronic kidney disease 251
Analgesic headache 303
Ankylosing spondylitis 217
Ann Arbor staging system 190
Anterior uveitis 323
Antibiotic coverage 140
Antibiotics 138
Anticoagulation (AF) 29
Antiphospholipid syndrome 230
Aortic regurgitation 25
Aortic stenosis 24
Aplastic crisis 185
Argyll-Robertson pupil 319
Arrhythmias 31
Arterial blood gas 120
Arteriovenous fistula 254
Asbestosis 123
Ascites 78
Asthma 113
Atherosclerosis 6
Atlantoaxial subluxation 209
Atrial fibrillation 26
Atrial flutter 32
Atypical pneumonia 110
Autoimmune haemolytic anaemia 179

Autoimmune hepatitis 84
B-type natriuretic peptide (BNP) 15
Bacillus cereus 155
Bacteria 136
Barretts oesophagus 96
BCG vaccine 161
Behçet's disease 236
Benign essential tremor 282
Beta-thalassaemia 182
BiPAP 121
Blepharitis 320
Blood 171
Blood film 172
Bone marrow biopsy 187
Bone mineral density 241
Bradycardia 36
Brain tumours 289
Budd-Chiari syndrome 205
Campylobacter 155
Carbimazole 49
Cardiac arrest rhythms 32
Cardiovascular disease 6
Cataracts 315
Cellulitis 147
Centor criteria 149
Central pontine myelinolysis 66
Central retinal artery occlusion 331
Cerebellopontine angle tumours 291
Cervical spondylosis 303
CHADS-VASc score 31
Chalazion 320
Charcot-Marie-Tooth 296
Chest drain 126
Chest infections 144
Child-Pugh score 76
Cholangiocarcinoma 91
Chondrocalcinosis 239
Chronic heart failure 17
Chronic kidney disease 249
Chronic lymphocytic leukaemia 188
Chronic myeloid leukaemia 188
Chronic obstructive pulmonary disease 117
Chronic tubulointerstitial nephritis 259
Churg-Strauss syndrome 234
CLO test 95
Cluster headaches 306
Coeliac disease 103
Complex regional pain syndrome 287
Conjunctivitis 322
Conn's Syndrome 63

Cor pulmonale 19
Corneal abrasions 326
Coronary arteries 10
Coronary artery bypass graft (CABG) 9
CPAP 122
Crohn's disease 99
Cryptogenic organising pneumonia 123
CT pulmonary angiogram (CTPA) 128
Cushing's syndrome 42
Cystitis 145
Deep vein thrombosis 202
Delirium tremens 73
Dermatomyositis 229
DEXA scan 241
Dexamethasone suppression test 43
Diabetes insipidus 66
Diabetic nephropathy 258
Diabetic retinopathy 313
Dialysis 252
Diffuse cutaneous systemic sclerosis 223
Discoid lupus erythematosus 221
DMARDS 212
Dressler's syndrome 13
Echocardiography (echo) 16
Ectropion 321
Empyema 125
Endopthalmitis 316
Endoscopic retrograde cholangio-pancreatography 91
Enhanced liver fibrosis (ELF) test 81
Entropion 320
Eosinophilic granulomatosis with polyangiitis 234
Epilepsy 283
Episcleritis 324
ERCP 91
Eron classification of cellulitis 148
ESBL bacteria 138
Essential thrombocythaemia 196
Extended spectrum beta lactamase bacteria 138
Extradural haemorrhage 272
Extrinsic allergic alveoli's 123
Eyelid disorders 320
Facial nerve palsy 287
FAST tool 269
FEV1 112
FibroScan 75
Flu 152

Focal nodular hyperplasia (of the liver) 93
FRAX tool 241
FVC 112
G6PD deficiency 179
Gastro-oesophageal reflux disease 94
Gastroenteritis 154
Giant cell arteritis 227
Giardiasis 156
Glaucoma 308
Gliomas 291
Glomerulonephritis 256
Goodpasture syndrome 258
Gout 238
Granulomatosis with polyangiitis 234
Growth hormone 41
Guillain-Barré syndrome 297
Haemochromatosis 85
Haemolytic anaemia 178
Haemolytic disease of the newborn 180
Haemolytic transfusion reactions 180
Haemolytic uraemic syndrome 261
Haemophilia 201
HAS-BLED score 31
Headaches 301
Heart block 36
Heart sounds 22
Helicobacter pylori 95
Hemiplegic migraine 304
Henoch-Schonlein purpura 234
Heparin induced thrombocytopenia 200
Hepatic encephalopathy 79
Hepatitis 81
Hepatocellular carcinoma 91
Hepatorenal syndrome 79
Hereditary elliptocytosis 179
Hereditary spherocytosis 178
Herpes keratitis 327
HIV 164
Hodgkin's lymphoma 189
Holmes Adie pupil 319
Hormonal headache 303
Horner syndrome 318
Huntington's chorea 292
Hyperaldosteronism 63
Hyperkalaemia 264
Hyperparathyroidism 62
Hypersensitivity pneumonitis 123
Hypertension 19
Hypertensive retinopathy 314
Hyperthyroidism 48
Hypothalamus 40
Hypothyroidism 50
Idiopathic pulmonary fibrosis 122
IgA nephropathy 257

Immune thrombocytopenic purpura 199
Incretins 59
Inflammatory bowel disease 99
Influenza 152
Inotropes 16
Insulin 60
Interferon-gamma release assays 162
Internuclear ophthalmoplegia 275
Interstitial lung disease 122
Intra-abdominal infections 150
Intracerebral haemorrhage 272
Intracranial haemorrhage 270
Iron deficiency anaemia 175
Irritable bowel syndrome 101
Kawasaki disease 235
Korsakoffs syndrome 74
Lambert-Eaton myasthenic syndrome 296
Leukaemia 185
Libmann-Sacks endocarditis 231
Limbic encephalitis 108
Limited cutaneous systemic sclerosis 222
Liver cancer 91
Liver cirrhosis 74
Liver transplant 93
Lumbar puncture 158
Lung cancer 106
Lung function tests 111
Lymphangioleimyomatosis 301
Lymphoma 189
Malaria 166
Mantoux test 162
MELD score 76
Membranous glomerulonephritis 257
Meningiomas 291
Meningitis 157
Mesothelioma 108
Methicillin-resistant staphylococcus aureus 137
Microangiopathic haemolytic anaemia 180
Microscopic polyangiitis 234
Migraines 304
Mitral regurgitation 24
Mitral stenosis 24
Monoclonal gammopathy of undetermined significance 191
Motor neurone disease 278
Mouth ulcers 236
MRSA 137
Multiple myeloma 191
Multiple sclerosis 274
Murmurs 22
Myasthenia gravis 293
Myasthenic crisis 295
Myelodysplastic syndrome 197

Myelofibrosis 196
Myeloma 191
Myeloproliferative disorders 195
NAFLD 80
Nailfold capillaroscopy 224
Neurofibromatosis 298
Neuropathic pain 286
Neutropenic sepsis 143
Non alcoholic fatty liver disease 80
Non-Hodgkin lymphoma 191
Non-invasive ventilation 121
Novel anticoagulants (NOACS) 30
NSTEMI 10
Obstructive sleep apnoea 134
Open angle glaucoma 308
Optic neuritis 277
Orbital cellulitis 321
Orthopnoea 17
Osmotic demyelination syndrome 66
Osteoarthritis 207
Osteomalacia 243
Osteoporosis 240
Osteosarcoma 245
Otitis media 149
Pacemakers 37
Paget's disease of the bone 244
Palindromic rheumatism 209
Paraneoplastic syndromes 107
Parathyroid axis 41
Parkinson's disease 279
Parkinson's-plus syndromes 281
Paroxysmal nocturnal dyspnoea 17
Paroxysmal nocturnal haemoglobinuria 180
PCP pneumonia 110
Peak flow 112
Peptic ulcers 96
Percutaneous coronary intervention (PCI) 9 & 12
Periorbital cellulitis 321
Peripheral neuropathy 297
Peritoneal dialysis 253
Pernicious anaemia 177
Phaeochromocytoma 68
Phrenic nerve palsy 107
Pituitary 40
Pleural effusion 124
Pneumocystis jiroveci 110
Pneumonia 108
Pneumothorax 125
Polyarteritis nodosa 235
Polycystic kidney disease 265
Polycythaemia vera 196
Polymyalgia rheumatica 225
Polymyositis 229
Portal hypertension 77
Posterior vitreous detachment 329
Primary biliary cirrhosis 88
Primary sclerosis cholangitis 89

Prosthetic valve replacement 25
Pseudogout 239
Psoriatic arthritis 214
Pulmonary embolism 126
Pulmonary fibrosis 122
Pulmonary hypertension 129
Pulmonary oedema 14
Pupil disorders 316
Pyelonephritis 145
Radioactive iodine 49
Radiofrequency ablation 34
Rapid urease test 95
Reactive arthritis 216
Recurrent laryngeal nerve palsy 107
Reflux 94
Renal artery stenosis 63
Renal bone disease 251
Renal dialysis 252
Renal transplant 255
Renin-angiotensin system 41
Retinal detachment 329
Retinal vein occlusion 330
Retinitis pigmentosa 332
Rhabdomyolysis 262
Rheumatoid arthritis 208
ROSIER tool 269
Salmonella 155
Sarcoidosis 131
Schirmer test 232
Schober's test 218
Scleritis 325
Sengstaken-Blakemore tube 78
Sepsis 141
Sepsis six 143
Septic arthritis 151
Septic shock 141
Severe sepsis 141
Shigella 155
Short synacthen test 45
SIADH 64
Sickle cell anaemia 183
Sinusitis 149
Sjogren's syndrome 231
Skin infection 147
Small cell lung cancer 106
Soft tissue infection 147
Spirometry 111
Stable angina 8
Statins 7-8
Status epilepticus 285
STEMI 10
Stroke 268
Stye 320
Subarachnoid haemorrhage 273
Subconjunctival haemorrhage 328
Subdural haemorrhage 271
Supraventricular tachycardias (SVT) 33

Syndrome of inappropriate anti-diuretic hormone 64
Systemic lupus erythematosus 219
Systemic sclerosis 222
Tachycardia 32
Takayasu's arteritis 235
Temporal arteritis 227
Tension headaches 302
Tension pneumothorax 126
Thalassaemia 181
Third nerve palsy 317
Thrombocytopenia 198
Thrombolysis 129
Thrombophilia 203
Thrombotic thrombocytopenic purpura 199
Thyroid axis 40
Thyroid function tests 46
Thyroid storm 49
Tonsillitis 148
Torsades de pointes 34
Transcatheter aortic valve implantation (TAVI) 26
Transjugular intra-hepatic portosystemic shunt 77
Trichiasis 321
Trigeminal neuralgia 303
Triptans 305
Troponins 11
Tuberculosis 160
Tuberous sclerosis 300
Type 1 diabetes 52
Type 2 diabetes 56
Ulcerative colitis 99
Urinary tract infections 145
Urine dipstick 145
Varices 77
Vasculitis 232
Venous thromboembolism 202
Ventilation-perfusion (VQ) scan 128
Ventricular ectopics 35
Viral meningitis 158
Vitamin B12 deficiency 177
Von Willebrand disease 200
Warfarin 30
Water deprivation test 67
Wegener's granulomatosis 234
Wernicke's encephalopathy 74
Wilson disease 86
Wolff-Parkinson-White syndrome 34
Yersinia enterocolitica 156

Printed in Great Britain
by Amazon